People with Multiple Sclerosis

People with Multiple Sclerosis

Condition, Challenges and Care

Paul J. Bull
Independent Researcher, UK

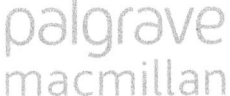

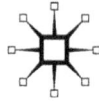 © Paul J. Bull 2015

All rights reserved. No reproduction, copy or transmission of this publication may be made without written permission.

No portion of this publication may be reproduced, copied or transmitted save with written permission or in accordance with the provisions of the Copyright, Designs and Patents Act 1988, or under the terms of any licence permitting limited copying issued by the Copyright Licensing Agency, Saffron House, 6–10 Kirby Street, London EC1N 8TS.

Any person who does any unauthorized act in relation to this publication may be liable to criminal prosecution and civil claims for damages.

The author has asserted his right to be identified as the author of this work in accordance with the Copyright, Designs and Patents Act 1988.

First published 2015 by
PALGRAVE MACMILLAN

Palgrave Macmillan in the UK is an imprint of Macmillan Publishers Limited, registered in England, company number 785998, of Houndmills, Basingstoke, Hampshire RG21 6XS.

Palgrave Macmillan in the US is a division of St Martin's Press LLC, 175 Fifth Avenue, New York, NY 10010.

Palgrave Macmillan is the global academic imprint of the above companies and has companies and representatives throughout the world.

Palgrave® and Macmillan® are registered trademarks in the United States, the United Kingdom, Europe and other countries.

ISBN: 978–1–137–45705–9

This book is printed on paper suitable for recycling and made from fully managed and sustained forest sources. Logging, pulping and manufacturing processes are expected to conform to the environmental regulations of the country of origin.

A catalogue record for this book is available from the British Library.

A catalog record for this book is available from the Library of Congress.

For Christine

Contents

List of Figures		viii
List of Tables		ix
Acknowledgements		xi
List of Abbreviations		xiii
1	Introduction	1
2	Multiple Sclerosis: A Brief Overview of the Illness	19
3	Research on People with MS: Definitions, Data Sources and Methodologies	41
4	What Type of Person Suffers from MS?	83
5	How Many People Have MS? A Case Study of the UK	110
6	The Impact of MS	159
7	The Care of People with MS	213
8	Conclusion	260
Notes		273
References		276
Index		301

List of Figures

5.1	Worldwide prevalence of MS by nation state	112
5.2	UK regional MS prevalence rates	117
5.3	MS admissions to NHS hospitals in Scotland 1997–2009 by Health Board Area	129
5.4	MS admissions to NHS hospitals in England 1998–2005 by Strategic Health Authority Area	140
6.1	Hypothetical impact of MS on a person's life	166

List of Tables

1.1	Selected neurological conditions in the UK	12
2.1	Type of MS by selected regional and national survey	28
3.1	The number of PwMS diagnosed using the A&M and poser criteria for selected regional populations in the UK	47
3.2	The definition of MS used in recent UK regional studies	55
3.3	The most important source for recent regional surveys of PwMS	57
4.1	Surveys of PwMS	84
4.2	Female to male ratios in regional MS studies since 1985	86
4.3	The ages of PwMS: summary statistics from regional research	94
4.4	The distribution of PwMS and the population of the countries of the UK by age group	96
4.5	Distribution of PwMS by age group and female/male ratios for selected regions	97
5.1	Estimates of the number of PwMS in the four countries of the UK in 2010	115
5.2	The principal regional MS prevalence studies published since 1985	120
5.3	UK regional MS prevalence rates by year of study	123
5.4	UK regional MS prevalence studies ranked by prevalence rate	124
5.5	Population of Northern Ireland and the north of Northern Ireland MS study area: selected characteristics in 2001	131
5.6	Regional MS annual incidence rates in the UK	143
5.7	Prevalence of PwMS/100,000 in 1981 by region in Australia and place of birth	154
6.1	Kurtzke's Expanded Disability Status Scale	168
6.2	Factors aiding successful and unsuccessful adjustment to MS	178
6.3	Domains of care for people with MS as identified by Gruenewald et al. (2004)	181
6.4	The MS Impact Scale (MSIS-29)	183
6.5	Original areas of importance identified by the LMSQoLS	184
6.6	LMSQoL scores by disease state and ambulation status	186

6.7 Average group scores for the physical and psychological
    components of the MSIS-29   188
6.8 The ten subject-event combinations producing most and
    least subjective happiness   201
6.9 Mean annual costs per PwMS by category (£s in 2006/7)   202

Acknowledgements

Trying to write a book that covers a vast amount of research within a strict word limit presents the author with the awkward task of deciding what to include and what to exclude. In this case this issue was solved in a pragmatic way by concentrating on the research I knew best, the research undertaken mainly on people with multiple sclerosis in the United Kingdom. This was not out of any arrogance that believed British research to be best because I know it is not, but more out of my own limited cerebral capacity that could cope with little more. I must therefore apologise for any excellent research on people with MS I have omitted.

The early reading and ideas sorting for this book became possible through a small research grant from the MS Society and an Honorary Research Fellowship at the University of Sheffield. I would like to thank both organisations for their support and especially their library staffs for sourcing many obscure references. I would also like to thank the library staff of my local branch library in Prettygate Colchester for undertaking a similar task. Without their dedicated bibliographic skills, this book would never have been produced.

The skills of Ed Oliver, cartographer at the School of Geography, Queen Mary University of London, in producing the maps in Chapter 5 and the figure in Chapter 6 must also get a special mention.

Throughout the writing of this book many people offered advice, provided information and commented on various chapters. I would like to thank them all for their assistance. They include Reece Andrew, Wendy Baird, Verity Brack, Sarah Briggs, Doug Brown, Chris Bull, Andrew Church, Lee Dunster, Isabel Dyck, Gill Green, Beth Greenhough, Siobhan Hart, Barbara Harvey, Ed Holloway, Isla Mackenzie, Stuart Nixon and Steve Royle.

Two further scholars, Iain Chalmers and Tony Gatrell, deserve particular thanks because without their wise invaluable counsel and warm encouragement at strategic moments this book may never have been completed.

Thanks must also go to the editorial and production teams at Palgrave Macmillan for making this book a reality. It is also important to acknowledge a number of copyright permissions including the MS Society for the front cover picture, the map in Figure 5.1 based on information from the Atlas of MS, published by the Multiple Sclerosis International Federation and Eiona Roberts for her poem in Chapter 1.

Finally, I must thank my wife Christine, for allowing me the time and space to write this book and, when the work was going badly, for putting up with my bad moods with such grace and understanding. I owe her far more than these feeble words can say.

List of Abbreviations

A&M	Allison and Millar
ABI	acquired brain injury
ARMS	Action into Research for Multiple Sclerosis (former MS charity in UK)
BMS	benign MS
CCSVI	chronic cerebrospinal venous insufficiency
CIS	clinically isolated syndrome
CNS	central nervous system
CSF	cerebrospinal fluid
DMD	disease modifying drugs
EBV	Epstein-Barr virus
EDSS	Expanded Disability Status Scale
GHS	General Household Survey
GP	general practitioner
GPRD	general practice research database
IM	infectious mononucleosis
MND	motor neurone disease
MRI	magnetic resonance imaging
MS	multiple sclerosis
MSIF	MS International Federation
MwMS	members of the MS Society with MS
NARCOMS	North American Research Committee on MS
NHS	National Health Service (UK)
NHNN	National Hospital for Neurology and Neurosurgery
NICE	National Institute for Health and Care Excellence
NSF	National Service Framework
PCT	primary care trust
PRISMS	Prevention of Relapses and Disability by Interferon beta-1a Subcutaneously in Multiple Sclerosis
PPMS	primary progressive MS
PwMS	people with multiple sclerosis
RCP	Royal College of Practitioners
RRMS	relapsing remitting MS
SPMS	secondary progressive MS
SRD	sustained reduction in disability

SWIMS	South West Impact of MS Project
UK	United Kingdom
US	United States
VEP	visual evoked potential
WHO	World Health Organization

1
Introduction

1.1 Setting the scene

In March 2008, the *London Times* newspaper included a 12-page supplement on multiple sclerosis (MS) that painted a thoroughly depressing picture of living with the illness. It said that 'people with MS are more likely to get divorced, lose their job, to end up in poverty, take their own lives, and to die on average five to ten years earlier than the general population. Living with a chronic long-term condition like MS without care or support is a recipe for becoming isolated, dependent on state benefits and – in the worse cases – written off by life' (p.2). This publication coincided with the MS Society of Great Britain and Northern Ireland's biennial MS Life conference that also included a stern reminder from the Cambridge neurologist Alasdair Coles of some of the less palatable aspects of having MS, especially lower life expectancy and lower income than expected accompanied by the almost inevitability of disability progression, in a presentation on MS 'risks, placebos and myth busting'.[1] Was the prognosis of having MS really that dreadful? Could the information sources on which such dire assertions were based be believed?

The Times supplement went on to state (again on p.2) that there were 'many hundreds of thousands of people across the United Kingdom (UK) living with MS.' The strong implication of this phrase must be that many hundreds of thousands of people in the UK actually had MS. But, that was definitely wrong because the admittedly apocryphal and increasingly moribund official estimate of the number of people with the disease in the UK at that time was only 85,000, to be revised upwards to 100,000 in 2009. And, while there is a very good case to be made to suggest that even this latest total was too frugal, as shown in Chapter 5, it would not be underestimated by many hundreds of thousands. What may be true, however, was that there may be many hundreds of thousands of people in the UK closely related to the illness as relatives and friends of those with MS and as health professionals caring for people with MS (PwMS). Such a spectacular exaggeration for the apparent sake of hyperbole probably does not help the MS cause in any way but what it surely demonstrates is that the printed word may not always tell the truth about this condition. It may therefore always pay to be sceptical and cautious about what is said in print about MS. The published record had definitely been wrong once about the PwMS in the UK so perhaps it could have been wrong on other occasions too especially about some of the worst implications of having the illness. This book is an attempt to find out.

Two years later, in August 2010, the doom and gloom rhetoric about MS in the press continued with, for example, another supplement on MS in the *Independent* newspaper this time offering the thoughts of the Chief Executive of the MS Trust, one of the UK's main MS charities, stating that 'the sad facts are that a diagnosis of MS can impact on many life plans. 50 per cent of people with MS will be out of work within 5 years of diagnosis; 75 per cent of married people with MS get divorced and many people put off having a family for fear of not being able to cope.' Now, it may be justifiable to give such grim statistics in the context of trying to raise awareness, sympathy and thereby charitable funds for the MS cause, but to present them as if they were the immutable consequences of the natural history of the disease was going too far. Whether a person with MS loses their job or lives in poverty is not just a function of their neurological disease but, probably more importantly, is also a function of the way in which their society treats them. For example, a disabled person need not necessarily be unemployed if their society offers them the appropriate support and encouragement in the work place. And, the same argument applies to poverty, physical isolation and many other elements of people's lives too, all of which can be encompassed within the well-known 'social model of disability' (Oliver 1996), that a society through the creation of systematic barriers and negative attitudes can be held responsible for the limits to activity (disability) experienced by its impaired citizens. In other words, people are disabled just as much by the society in which they live as by their own bodies. What is more, societies in different parts of the world differ hugely in their attitudes and behaviours and to assume otherwise is naïve. Thus, it may possibly be true that in the recent past in say North America (Glantz et al. 2009, Julian et al. 2008) or Denmark (Pfleger et al.

2010a and 2010b), where significant research has been undertaken in this area, PwMS had a higher rate of unemployment, divorce or even suicide than their national averages, it does not necessarily imply that they should also be true for the UK. To demonstrate that reliable British evidence would need to be presented.

In her writing for the *Independent,* the Chief Executive of the MS Trust went on to advise that PwMS should 'Be wary and don't believe everything you hear or read about MS – you may end up frightening yourself or find people dealing in false hope.' It would appear that such sagely comment should be applied to what she had just reported too. Indeed, as Rose et al. (2000, 22) counsel in their 'MS at your Fingertips', PwMS should be careful not to be misled by newspaper and TV reports. More importantly though, these observations help to raise the more general question: what do we really know about PwMS in, for example, their numbers, demographic characteristics, geography, state of health, access to health care, quality of life and what level of certainty can be placed on what is published about them; what can be trusted? This book is an attempt to answer these questions with particular emphasis on PwMS in the UK. Unfortunately, because of space limitations it is not possible to treat the other major MS nations of the world in as much detail as the UK. However, what will be possible is to place the UK evidence in the context of broader international trends in the MS world; a comparative analysis to improve our understanding of the UK case that may provide a template for similar analyses in other nations.

1.2 Sources of evidence

The evidence used in this book comes primarily from a range of different published sources, books, magazines and mainly academic journal articles, but also from the Internet. It is important to note that the quality assurances that can be given for these different sources vary enormously. For the latter, the Internet, no assurance can be given what-so-ever on the veracity of the material available (Cooke 2001). Any individual or organisation can set up an attractive, authoritatively looking website on this medium and make virtually any claims they wish with little chance of sanction. Any material gleaned from this source must therefore be treated with extreme caution, subject to the most vigorous scrutiny and only accepted as valid if other corroboration is available.

The most reliable evidence in theory used in this analysis should come from peer-reviewed academic journal articles. Here the editorial process should help guarantee a publication's worth because it will include experts in the field judging the work's quality, competence and suitability for publication. Such a process is expected to eliminate clear errors of method, bias and interpretation. As the epidemiologist Bhopal (2002, 281) noted, 'There is a widespread view that only work that has passed the scrutiny of peers is reliable and trustworthy.' In addition, where the research has needed the collection of personal evidence including medical records the work will initially have had to have received the sanction of a local research ethics committee and then include a statement of the authors' conflicts of interest; both helpful indicators of research competence and integrity.

Although peer review may be the best way of achieving reliable worthy publishing so far developed, it is far from infallible. Indeed, as shown in this volume, much of the published research on the lives of PwMS in the UK suffers from problems of method, available data options and interpretation that limit its value. Thus, it would not be true to say that all errors are avoided in the academic publishing process. Nor would it be true to say that all defensible research work is accepted for publication. There are many reasons why unreasonable judgements can be made. Some degree of bias on the part of reviewers and editors is unavoidable, but this is probably a relatively benign influence. It is also possible for genuine mistakes to be made even in the best organised system of review when very busy people are working to tight deadlines. More pernicious reasons exist, however, to include the deliberate suppression by powerful individuals and organisations of material that challenges their views and practices. This may be less of an issue in the social sciences than in medical science where, for commercial reasons, a pharmaceutical company may refuse to release results or deliberately delay their release, as has certainly occurred relating to research on drugs for MS.[2]

In terms of all published work, be it formal research journals, specialist magazines, trade journals or books, it is not just the editorial function that is crucial for its credibility, it is also important to ask why a particular publication exists and whose interests it serves. It can be argued that a research journal, for example, exists to further the advancement of knowledge and understanding in a particular area of inquiry. In such a situation it would be the quality of the original research and the thoroughness of the editorial process that determines information quality and integrity. However, even here such apparent benign altruism is superficial. Most academic journals are profitable commercial operations for their publishers and if they were not they would not exist. Furthermore, a journal's economic success can be best achieved by securing a high impact factor or citation index in its field that in turn is secured by getting the best research and researchers to publish in that journal. At the same time the researchers themselves need to publish in academic journals to advance their careers and the higher the journal is ranked the better it will be for them. Nevertheless, for relatively inexperienced academic researchers, there can often be a trade-off between the chances of getting published and the impact rating of the journal with a lower ranked journal sometimes being chosen to improve their chances of publication. Thus, it is not always the case that the most important, original and ground-breaking work is published in the 'top' ranked journals.

It is important to realise at this point that research is not just a simple iterative process in which finding X leads on to finding Y within a community of cooperative scientists, even if that may be the long-term logic behind it. Research is a social process too involving personal relationships with all the usual personality clashes, egos and petty rivalries imaginable. Such obstacles to the smooth progress of knowledge are rarely aired in print except perhaps in the memoirs and diaries of retired luminaries. It was therefore both unexpected and revealing to note in a review paper on MS incidence and prevalence the following observation by Zivadinov and colleagues (2003, 71) after managing to secure original data from only approximately 20 per cent of the authors of more than 90 studies: 'There were various reasons, such as no response, no availability of the original data, or no collaboration if not included in the authorship.' The latter bares testament to the pressure to publish in today's academic world along with the time pressures many researchers experience, and while the former may represent simple bad manners collectively they symbolise the often fragmented, isolated dysfunctional professional and social worlds of much of today's research community.

In a similar way books serve two clear interests, a commercial one and the ambitions and goals of their authors. They must be read cautiously with the latter in mind that should have been made clear at the beginning of the volume. Nevertheless, to get on a library shelf a book will normally have passed through a number of different quality assessments: the authors themselves, an editor or editorial board, a publisher and their reviewers and then the librarian or library committee. At each stage, different quality and suitability criteria will need to be met before a book will be accepted. By contrast, trade journals and some magazines may serve only a commercial interest that could make their evidence and opinions of questionable worth.

The charity sector forms another important element of the publishing world involved in providing material both for and on the MS community in the UK. It involves three main charities with a national reach: The MS Society of Great Britain and Northern Ireland (now the MS Society), The MS Trust and the smaller MS Resource Centre (now MS-UK). In addition, Northern Ireland has its own Action MS regional charity, the Federation of MS Therapy Centres offers material on its particular interventions and many MS Society branches produce their own local newsletters. The three main charities produce two very different forms of publication. First, they publish a large range of factsheets on many aspects of the MS condition and specific therapies for use by PwMS, the people who care for them and related health professionals. These often can be downloaded online or ordered in hard copy and have usually been compiled by recognised experts. The high quality of such material provided by both the MS Society and the MS Trust has been recognised by the award of The Information Standard. This means that they have persuaded the independent operators of this scheme, Capita, that the processes and systems used to produce their information publications are accurate, impartial, balanced, evidence-based, accessible and well-written (The Information Standard website).

The MS Society, the MS Trust and MS-UK also publish magazines. The former publishes *MS Matters* six times a year and *MS Research Matters* twice a year for which both an editor and editorial boards exist that at least for *MS Matters* is clearly stated on page 2 along with the standard disclaimer: 'Articles signed by the authors represent their views rather than those of the MS Society'. For the MS Trust's quarterly *Open Door* magazine no such statement exists, and it therefore remains formally unclear how and who makes decisions on the inclusion of written material. For MS-UK the *New Pathways* Magazine is produced every other month.

For MS professionals and researchers, the MS Society produces an *MS Network* Newsletter three times a year, guided by an 11-strong editorial board of MS professionals, along with online and hard copy library access facilities. Similarly the MS Trust publishes a quarterly *Way Ahead* Newsletter and a regular Information Update listing important yet difficult to access journal articles. The *MS Network* and *Way Ahead* newsletters usually include short research-based articles but in the latter it is not clear how they are judged for inclusion. And, because no peer-review function may have taken place, they must be treated with appropriate prudence.

The MS-UK's *New Pathways* is different from the magazines of the other two charities. It begins inauspiciously with the statement: 'New Pathways and its publishers do not guarantee the accuracy of statements made by contributors or advertisers or accept responsibility for any statement which they express in this publication.' This means that anything published in this magazine cannot be directly accepted as true; it must first be corroborated by other evidence. The enthusiast for this publication would probably defend its disclaimer by suggesting that it simply does not have the resources thoroughly to scrutinise everything it might publish and, such a position is a price worth paying for the magazine's varied exposure of different forms of therapies and experiences that the MS public would otherwise never encounter. Indeed, they would probably go further to praise *New Pathways*' editors for their candour. Their critics, however, would argue that such a disclaimer gives *New Pathways* carte blanche for irresponsible publishing, stressing that it is wrong to raise false hopes among the MS community for new therapies that may ultimately prove impotent. After all, it is worth remembering that the history of MS has been regularly punctuated by the trumpeting of new 'wonder' therapies that have not worked (Murray 2005). In general, therefore, the concern with *New Pathways* would be that it relies too much on anecdote and personal testament and that such a standard of evidence is not rigorous enough to lead to safe therapeutic practice. Instead they would argue that the only way it is possible to know if anything truly makes a difference to disease progression or symptom relief is through scientific scrutiny and experiment, usually necessitating some form of clinical trial. To suggest otherwise is both odious and irresponsible; the peddling of false hope as psychologically destructive as the prescribing of ineffective drugs.

There will be no attempt here to resolve this debate other than to suggest that it raises a fundamental conundrum of MS set firmly in the context of a therapeutic vacuum. On the one hand there are elements of the MS media including *New Pathways* that present tempting accounts of therapies that appear to have helped alleviate the symptoms of some PwMS that have no formal medical approval. Should PwMS try such therapies especially when formally licensed drugs are either ineffectual or non-existent? On the other hand, the medical establishment will advise PwMS for their own safety only to use properly tested and licensed therapeutic regimens. But, can PwMS, and especially those having a difficult time with their illness, be expected to wait years, if not decades, for the treatments they need to be developed and tested? In many cases the risks of getting some relief from their suffering now by trying an informal therapy may appear worth taking.

In one sense at least the gulf between the two stereotypical positions presented above may be narrowing a little. Since 2003 neurologists in the UK have had formal approval from the National Institute for Clinical Excellence (now the National Institute for Health and Care Excellence or NICE) in their Guidelines on MS care (NICE 2003, 28–9) to explore the use of some complementary therapies. However, the reasons for the lack of general encouragement of non-conventional therapies by neurologists are clear. Either they have been shown not to alter the disease course as in the case of the Cari Loder therapy or as yet there is not enough reliable evidence to support them. In such a situation neurologists cannot recommend their use; to do so would be unethical, irresponsible and almost certainly lead to legal action if matters went wrong. So until a new therapy has progressed positively through the formal testing and licensing channels neurologists cannot recommend its use (Prasad and Bell 2008).

1.3 MS research: treatments to patients

The much more practically relevant question to ask at this point is why some seemingly promising therapies and interventions in MS that have built up anecdotal and even modest scientific community support have not been developed to the point where they may be available in the clinic? First of all there have been some, of which perhaps the cannabis-based Sativex manufactured by GW Pharmaceuticals trialled for neuropathic pain and spasticity, is the most recent and high-profile example. The second crucially important point to make though is just how difficult it is to bring a possible therapy, especially a chemical compound, from showing theoretical and then anecdotal promise to clinical application. For example, Matthews (2008, 23) points out that the cost of the successful development of a drug from molecule discovery to therapeutic application including its marketing costs could be as high as $1 billion and could take between 12 and 20 years, or up to half the working life of a research scientist. In addition, fewer than 1 in 10 possible drugs actually make it through the 3 phases of clinical trials to the clinic. As Archibald and colleagues (2011) suggested in an open letter to the British Prime Minister on the safety of medicines, more than 90 per cent of potential new drugs fail in clinical trials and that recouping the costs of these failures is the major reason for the high and rising costs of new medicines. Indeed, drugs can fail at all stages of their development process with, for example, research on the drug Dirucotide for Secondary Progressive MS (SPMS) being abandoned by Eli Lilly and BioMS late in its development process after it failed to prevent the disease worsening in a major phase III study of 612 people with SPMS.

The huge sums of money involved in such activity can be gleaned from the fact that the original deal between these two companies was to give Lilly the drug's worldwide rights in exchange for an upfront payment of $87 million, plus milestone payments of up to $410 million along with escalating royalties as the drug won increasing international approval (MS Trust website on news items).

Thus, two of the main reasons for the slow pace of drug development in MS, as in many other conditions, are the costs involved, linked to the chances of their manufacturers making a profit, and the long time it takes to assess their usefulness and safety to secure regulatory approval. This book though is more concerned with research in the social sciences about PwMS than research on the production of MS therapies although the two are closely related in an analysis of the provision of care. In this case, although the funding required is at least two orders of magnitude less with fewer commercial complications because it would have been carried out mainly in the higher education sector, judged by the quantity and quality of publications so far there has only been modest interest shown in carrying out academic research on PwMS in the UK. Two important points directly follow from this. First, it makes the detailed analysis of such work a manageable exercise for one major essay. Second, it has meant that a great deal of material on the PwMS in the UK has had to be obtained from non-social science publications. Indeed, most has had to come from research undertaken by neurologists and other health-care professionals. This is unfortunate because research on PwMS offers major opportunities for developing real understanding not only of their lives directly, but also to set such research within a number of wider contexts that could include disability studies, coping with chronic illness, the costs of medical care, quality of life assessment, the use of formal and alternative therapies and the adequacy of state care provision. It is one of the intentions of this book to demonstrate that the MS community is a fertile ground for future research in the social sciences and in many ways to offer a provisional sifting of the relevant information. It therefore in one sense offers a preface for such work.

As shown in this analysis, even with peer-review assessment errors still sometimes appear; a point that emphasises a fundamental theme of this book, that it is not good enough to accept the findings even in the most respected outlets uncritically; they must always be thoroughly scrutinised. Furthermore, such a position also necessitates that review article observations based on such material cannot be accepted at face value either; wherever possible the original research publications must be sought for close examination. Thus, this book is an attempt at a critical examination of the existing research evidence on a particular group of people in the UK defined by their proximity to a specific illness, MS, to include those actually with the condition and, where possible, those ensnared in its web through the bonds of kinship, friendship and care. It is possible that the result of such an endeavour will be to show that much of the material in the public domain on PwMS is of a highly speculative, tentative and sometimes even implausible nature that would be better to ignore than use as the basis for any policy prescription or personal care plan. Some may view this exercise as unnecessarily destructive and negative, fearing a form of Pyrrhic denouement in which nothing worth keeping is left. Such a view should be resisted. It is only through the constant challenging of existing research in every logical way possible that its integrity and value can be established. The ideas and descriptions that survive such exercises are worth keeping, plausible and reliable. Those that do not survive must be improved and replaced or abandoned altogether. In a similar vein Bhopal (2002, 285) goes much further remarking that 'critical appraisal is important because much of what we know as the truth is wrong, sometimes dangerously so.'

It is well known that in the past serious errors of judgement have been made by well-meaning medical scientists and clinicians leading to patient deaths and disabilities for which Skrabanek and McCormick (1992) detailed some of the most notorious in their 'Follies and Fallacies in Medicine'. It is also well known that similar tragic mistakes with seemingly plausible (at the time) efforts have been made to ameliorate the effect of MS as ably reviewed by Murray (2005, 391–503). And, it is likely similar dreadful mistakes are being made today with unregulated stem cell implantation, the Liberation treatment and even in the use of some disease modifying drugs (DMDs). What is certainly less well understood is that patient lives and wellbeing have regularly been put in jeopardy in the past, and for which Chalmers (2007) uses the adjective 'lethal', by the deliberate under-reporting and suppression of research findings by many different elements of the medical research community when less than satisfactory findings ensued. In order for scientists to make accurate decisions about their future projects and for patients and their doctors to make the right decisions about their care, it is vital that they all have access to all relevant research evidence. This has led directly to Chalmers and colleagues (Chalmers 2007, Chalmers and Glasziou 2009) advocating the speedier and more complete publication of research findings (positive or negative), greater ease of access to all forms of research publications and for more systematic research reviews of clinical evidence so researchers have a sound base of existing knowledge from which their work can progress without the need for much duplication of effort. Now, the equivalent position may not be so dramatic or critical in the social science of medical conditions' research such as MS, but the need for regular incisive audits still exists. It is the intention of this book to provide such a review for MS considering in particular research on the 100,000 or so people in the UK who have to live with the illness and to a lesser extent on those who try to assuage its consequences, both carers and health-care professionals.

1.4 MS in a wider disease context

There can be no doubt MS is a serious medical condition that for many represents an understandably fearful diagnosis because of a number of the disease's principal characteristics. First, it is a chronic or long-lasting, illness. And, given MS is incurable then for the sufferer it is a disease for life, an indefinite sentence. Second, it is a neurological disorder, involving the way the brain and nervous system work. There will therefore be worries that personal control of bodily and cognitive functions could be lost. Neurological illnesses such as MS are not like heart disease or renal failure because they have the almost unique ability to 'dehumanize' in how they affect a patient's ability to function. There is therefore with MS not only the very real prospect of clear overt symptoms that are impossible to hide from the populace of physical disability and the need to use a stick or wheelchair, but also the perhaps more frightening hidden symptoms of cognitive impairment, pain and fatigue. Finally, MS is regarded as an autoimmune disease, in which a person's own body is trying to destroy parts of itself, so in a very real physical sense, and in a potentially psychologically damaging sense too, it is the person's own fault they are ill. Nevertheless, no matter how unpalatably depressing such thoughts may be to anyone with a chronic autoimmune neurological condition, it may be perversely reassuring to know that they are not alone. They are in fact part of a huge community of chronically ill people with neurological, autoimmune and disabling conditions. For example, according to the 2000–1 General Household Survey, 32 per cent of the British population had a long-standing health problem, with 19 per cent having a condition that limited their activities in some way. Remarkably similar figures for the latter were also available from the 2001 Census of Population, in which 18.2 per cent of the population claimed they had a long-term illness, health problem or disability that limited their activities, and the 2001 Labour Force Survey in which 19 per cent of the working-age population was classified as long-term disabled (Ackroyd

2003, 33–4). Clearly PwMS in the UK are part of the third of the entire British population with a long-term illness, but the number of PwMS who have their activities limited by their condition is not yet clear. That is investigated in Chapter 6 along with the proportion who are unfortunate enough to be so physically disabled they are part of the wheelchair community, for which the best estimate for England at the start of the twenty-first century was 1.2 million (Sapey et al. 2005, 504).

More specifically in terms of neurological diseases it is possible that 10 million people in the UK have such a condition that imposes a significant long-term effect on their lives. Their afflictions range from sudden onset ones such as acquired brain injury (ABI) and stroke, intermittent ones such as epilepsy, progressives such as MS, Motor Neurone Disease (MND) and Parkinson's through to more stable conditions such as Cerebral Palsy. They make up 19 per cent of UK's National Health Service (NHS) hospital admissions (Royal College of Physicians et al. 2008, 2) and lead to 350,000 people in the UK needing help with most of their activities of daily living (NHS National Workforce Projects 2008, 3). The numbers of people experiencing the major neurological conditions in the UK at the beginning of the twenty-first century are listed in Table 1.1 from which it can be seen that MS is neither one of the principal afflictions such as migraine, epilepsy and Alzheimer's, nor one of the less common ones such as Huntingdon's and MND. These

Table 1.1 Selected neurological conditions in the UK

Condition	Incidence. Numbers per 100,000 population	Prevalence. Numbers per 100,000 population	Number.	Year of the source of the original evidence
Alzheimer's	25,000 in more than 65 year-olds.	1,000	700,000	1996
Brain Injury (moderate and severe)	15	228	135,000	2000
Cerebral Palsy		156	110,000	Soc*
Epilepsy	80	500	300,000	2000
Migraine	400	15,000	8,000,000	1999
Huntington's		13.5	6,000	Soc*
Motor Neurone Disease	2	7	4,000	Soc*
Multiple Sclerosis	4	144	100,000	Soc*
Parkinson's	17	200	120,000	Soc*
Stroke	240	500	300,000	1996

Source: Neurological Alliance (2003), 8–11.

Soc* – Best estimate available from the disease support charity at time of publication.

results are supported by the comparative evidence on neurological disorders given by the NHS National Workforce Projects (2008, 34–5). Here the prevalence (per 100,000 population) for traumatic brain injury with long-term problems was 1,200, Epilepsy was 763, Parkinson's 200, Cerebral Palsy 186, MS 120, early onset dementia 67, Huntington's 14 and MND 7.

A different route to estimating neurological disease prevalence from the patients attending the National Hospital for Neurology and Neurosurgery (NHNN) in London between 1 January 1995 and 1 July 1996 presents a slightly different view. In this case, in what Robertson (2000, 663) referred to as a 'rare and detailed insight into the burden of neurological disease' of the 625 neurological disorders observed, lifetime disease prevalences were able to be calculated from a set of 27,658 patients. Of these, stroke at 9/1,000 population, was at the top of the list with active epilepsy in a mid-range at 5/1,000 whereas MS was on a par with Parkinson's disease at 2 per 1,000 (MacDonald et al. 2000, 670). Finally, and probably most depressingly, according to the *Lancet Neurology* (2010, 9 (1), 1) in a Leading Edge comment the global burden of MS during the next decade along with other neurological conditions such as stroke, epilepsy, dementia and Parkinson's disease, 'all look set to increase.'

Autoimmune diseases are those in which the immune system attacks other cells in its own body causing inflammation and pain. Such illnesses include many common present day conditions such as Rheumatoid Arthritis, Lupus, thyroid disorders, Celiac Disease, Type 1 Diabetes and MS. Obtaining figures on the prevalence of these conditions in the UK is difficult, but it is believed that 4.26 per cent of the UK population have Diabetes, 1 in 100 people suffer from Rheumatoid Arthritis, of which the majority are women, and 1 in 200 men and 1 in 500 women have Ankylosing Spondylitis in which the bones of the spine begin to fuse together (taken from the respective disease support charity websites). The other diseases of this nature, including MS, may be less common but collectively they form a major challenge for the UK care and health services. However, with these conditions comes the concern that if a person has one of these diseases, then he/she may be more susceptible than the general population of getting another; a general genetic susceptible to autoimmune disorders. According to Somers et al. (2006) from a review of published research papers from around the world, while some autoimmune diseases displayed some comorbidity this was not a general phenomenon. For MS specifically the evidence was far from equivocal, although on balance not good. For example, Canadian evidence from

5,031 MS patients demonstrated no excess risk in common autoimmune diseases in PwMS or in their immediate families compared with spousal controls (Ramagopalan et al. 2007). However, the comparator here was a very limited one. Unfortunately, in a much wider ranging inquiry in Denmark looking at 42 different autoimmune diseases, the prognosis was not so positive (Nielson et al. 2008). In a comparison of 12,403 patients on the Danish MS Register and 20,174 of their first degree relatives with the general population, MS patients were at an increased risk of generating Ulcerated Colitis and Pemphigoid but at a reduced risk of Rheumatoid and Temporal Arthritis. Their first degree relatives were at an increased risk of Crohn's disease, Addison's disease and Polyarteritis Nodosa. For the British case Somers et al. (2009) also discovered using evidence from the UK General Practice Research Database between 1990 and 1999 that there was a strong negative association between MS and Rheumatoid Arthritis, a modest positive association with Thyroiditis for women and no link with Type 1 Diabetes. More recently, however, the latter's relationship with MS has attracted growing interest because of their apparent genetic and environmental aetiological similarities (Handel et al. 2009a).

1.5　The range of perspectives into life with MS

Many of the diseases in these categories present major challenges for bio-medical scientists not only in trying to understand the basic mechanisms of their origins and development but also in designing remedial and curative therapies. Certainly in the case of MS, there are important discoveries still to be made from the laboratory to the consulting room and, while this may make this area of research exciting for the neuroscientist as the many aetiological theories of MS are debated and refined, it makes it all the more perplexing for the person with MS trying to comprehend what may be going on inside their heads to make their nervous system fail. In an attempt to distil some of the main elements of the MS condition therefore the next chapter presents a broad overview of the illness. However, it is important to emphasise that this is not a book about the MS disease; it is about the people who have this illness and the people who help them to cope with it. In this context, there are huge opportunities for meaningful insights to be made too in healthcare provision, resource allocation, human behaviour and the indomitable spirit of PwMS to overcome whatever life may throw at them. Indeed, the fact that MS can be so socially intrusive, life-changing and emotional has proved a rich vein of experience for writers of TV and film fiction. Recent TV appearances of PwMS on British TV would include the Bill, Waterloo Road, Hollyoaks, Doctors, West Wing and Neighbours (Miller 2008, Gray 2011) while internationally between 1941 and 2006, 33 films have had an MS theme that have progressed from 'disaster' stories and heroic coping to more modern ones of adapting to changing family and friendship relationships (Karenberg 2008). Perhaps the most famous though have been the two movies about the talented cellist Jacqueline du Pre who died of MS in 1987 aged 42, 'Duet for One' and 'Hilary and Jackie'. One of the most recent films of this genre is the thought-provoking 'Lourdes' with the intriguing strap-line 'There's no justice in miracles!' about Christine, a non-believer, who is apparently cured of her MS on a visit to the sanctuary. But is it a real cure, or has she just snapped into remission?

PwMS too have tried to capture what it is like to live with their illness through a range of different art media including painting, sculpture, poetry and prose. Such work has served two complementary purposes; to inform, to try to let the rest of society have some idea of what it is like to live with MS, and therapeutically, even cathartically, to help themselves cope with their affliction. Good examples of representations in paintings and sculpture of the way in which MS may distort the senses and the world in which PwMS live can be found on the MS Society's website. Collections of their creative writings are available, for example, in the two 'MS Talent' edited volumes by Lake and Evans (2007 and 2009), with a good example of the best of this work being the movingly rhythmical poem 'Where do you go?' by Eiona Roberts (Lake and Evans 2007, 94–5) that captures beautifully much of the emotional turmoil and frustration of living with MS.

> Where do you go
> When your body deserts you,
> When your mind is as active as ever it was?
> To whom do you turn
> When life overwhelms you,
> But the cogs keep on turning
> When they should be on pause?
>
> Who bears the brunt
> Of frustration and tears?
> When your brain cells say 'Yes',
> But your body says 'No!'?
> To whom can you turn when you're trapped in the prison

> Of a body that's failing,
> But your mind just won't go?
>
> Who picks up the pieces
> Strewn all around you
> When your bits fall apart
> Or no longer comply?
> Who pays the price
> For the anger and sorrow
> For questions you throw out
> Knowing there's no real reply?

In his discussion of the patient's view Honigsbaum (2009, 194) suggests that 'direct unmediated accounts of illnesses are rare, and accounts that vividly capture the subjective experience rarer still.' This is not the case with MS. Autographical accounts of variable quality and perception on 'how I lived with my MS' are only too common. They range from the work of PwMS who have obtained celebrity or notoriety within and outside the MS world through writings by health-care professionals with MS who can relate their experiences to their medical knowledge, to the more mundane descriptions of the daily grind of living with a disabling condition.

The former includes Car Loder's (1996) *Standing in the sunshine* about the discovery of her ill-fated 'cure', the American Marlo Donato Parmelee's (2009) *Akward bitch: my life with MS* on working in London with MS in high fashion at Donna Karan and *Higgy: matches, microphones and MS* by the former sportsman Alistair Hignell (2011). The works by health-care workers include the doctors Burnfield (1985) *Multiple sclerosis: a personal exploration*, Forsyth (1988) *Multiple sclerosis: exploring sickness and health* and more recently Cuthbert (2010) *Keeping balance: a psychologist's experience of chronic illness and disability* all of which include elements of touching personal interest and humour. For example, Burnfield admits that he continued to take a daily supplement of Evening Primrose Oil not really because he thought it was doing him any good but irrationally just in case he might get worse if he stopped. The more mundane accounts include Roberts (2007) *Stumbling along: a journey with the master of surprises* and Timpson (2010) *MS: the gloves are off.* In this style of writing, the authors often appear to derive amusement and solace from using the letters MS as the initials for the way in which they relate to their illness. For example, Roberts rather modestly refers to her MS as a 'Master of Surprises' and has the temerity to call her illness 'just an inconvenience' (2007, 67) while struggling with a walking stick, vertigo, an uncooperative bladder and heat intolerance on a Pembrokeshire coastal path! Similarly, the irrepressible Meg Kingston (2010, 14) refers to her MS as a 'MonSter', 'a separate, malevolent presence that has more control over my body than I do.' By contrast, Val Evans in *MS Matters* 84, 2009 believes her disease signifies a 'Missing Self' and much more prosaically Sue Le Blond (2008), who wrote the novel 'Down to a Sunless Sea' about the relationships between the women in the lives of the friends William Wordsworth and Samuel Taylor Coleridge, suggested her MS was responsible for creating a Miserable Sod (MS Matters 85, 2009, 5). However, according to his daughter Rayne in an address to the MS Life conference in 2006 all of these are eclipsed by the direct approach of the late black American comedian Richard Pryor to his MS: 'more shit!'

Honigsbaum (2009, 195) goes on to argue that the importance of patient-centric accounts is that 'they remind us that to attempt, as the neurosciences have been doing in recent years, to reduce illnesses and the mental states associated with illness to biology and mere brain processes, is to lose sight of what it means to be human....in capturing the essence of their suffering they create a bridge from their time to our own.' This may well be true. But, although personal testimony, or the 'patient's voice', will form some of the supporting material in the following argument, introduced to add a contrasting texture to the analysis, it is not the principal focus. General verifiable evidence on the MS community is the main objective. Thus, when individually authored material is encountered it will be treated with appropriate caution because it is susceptible to problems of accurate recall and serious 'point of view' bias. Indeed, it could be insensitively suggested that such a position is doubly relevant in the case of testimony from PwMS because a large minority will most likely have some sort of cognitive deficit as a direct consequence of their illness. But, given the main objective of this text certain types of evidence will be more valuable than others. For example, the findings of research using representative sampling techniques will be more useful than case studies. However, as will become clear, this sort of material is rarely available in an unambiguous form and usually not available at all. In such cases the reasons for the inadequacy of the evidence will be made clear. Nevertheless, it is important also to make clear that this is not to denigrate more individualistic qualitative study evidence, merely to note it is not the most appropriate material for the task this book seeks to undertake.

This book therefore is about trying to establish the basic evidence about PwMS especially in the UK, that some may wish to call the facts. In so doing this book seeks answers to the following questions:

What sorts of people get MS? Do some particular groups of people suffer more than others? [Chapter 4]

How many people in the UK have MS and where do they live? [Chapter 5]

How does MS affect people's lives; the impact of MS? [Chapter 6]

What sort of care do PwMS need? And, do they receive it? [Chapter 7]

Before these substantive issues are considered a brief description of the illness known as MS is given in the next chapter and an overview of some of the major problems of trying to carry out research on the MS community is presented in Chapter 3.

2
Multiple Sclerosis: A Brief Overview of the Illness

2.1 Disease overview

Multiple Sclerosis (MS) is a disease of the human central nervous system (CNS), of the brain, spinal cord and optic nerves, in which nerve tissue is damaged and destroyed. Conventionally the principal element of this destruction is the erosion of the myelin sheath surrounding nerve fibres or axons, by immune cells that have crossed the blood-brain barrier to enter the CNS. Here these cells mistakenly identify myelin as alien tissue and attack it causing lesions of acute inflammation. These lesions leave behind hardened scars or plaques, areas of sclerosis that from their nineteenth-century pathological analysis became the eponymous characteristic of this disease. In these lesions the mass of immune cells squeezed into a small space and the damaged myelin interfere with signals trying to travel along the underlying nerve fibres. Such messages may be partially blocked, slowed down, diverted into other nerve fibres or in the most severe cases stopped altogether. Thus, the control by the brain of the bodily parts to which the affected nerves are connected can be impaired to a lesser or greater degree. This is the familiar, common understanding of the proximate cause of MS symptoms by most commentators. It is 'a demyelinating disorder'. The very essence of the disease therefore is to do with the integrity of myelin surrounding nerve fibres (Rose et al. 2000, 2; Wade and Green 2001, 6; MS Society 2010a, 3). It also directly follows that certain targets for therapeutic intervention are suggested such as damping down an over-active immune system, preventing immune cells crossing the blood-brain barrier into the CNS and enhancing the body's own myelin repair capability. Indeed, it will be shown in what follows that research to achieve these goals has progressed apace over the recent past with some notable successes in the former in terms of what became known as Disease Modifying Drugs (DMDs). Unfortunately, recent research has also rediscovered what was in fact pointed out by Charcot in his original descriptions of the disease in the 1860s (Murray 2005), that the MS disease process is much more complicated than simply myelin destruction because it involves damage and destruction of their underlying axons too. Such a finding is particularly depressing because as currently understood axonal tissue cannot be replaced or repaired. Thus, anyone who believed the answers to the whole MS disease conundrum were close to being revealed is mistaken. They are not and almost certainly still many years away. People with MS (PwMS) are not going to be 'cured' soon. The destructive nature of their illness may be slowed substantially by a number of different drugs but for the majority symptom control will be the fundamentally important part of their on-going care.

There is some encouraging research news from recent neurological work. It may well be that the brain has the remarkable ability of both functional and structural plasticity to help compensate for any damage it may sustain. In the former other parts of the brain may take over from damaged areas whereas in the latter active rerouting of signals may occur (Doidge 2008, Tomassini 2008). When this is added to the body's innate, if imperfect, myelin repair mechanisms not all MS lesions need necessarily result in overt or long-lasting clinical symptoms or even permanent impairment. A number of important points follow from these observations. The first must be that the body, at least in the early stages of MS, can take positive action to try to overcome any damage it may sustain. The brain and spinal cord therefore become a battle ground between the MS forces of nerve tissue destruction and the body's counterattacks of remyelination and cerebral reorganisation. Second, it suggests that not all demyelination lesions need cause overt clinical symptoms either in the short or longer term; it will depend on where in the brain they take place. Indeed, in some studies of early MS, only one in ten active CNS lesions produced clear clinical events (Zajicek et al. 2007, 38). This must also suggest that MS may be causing damage to parts of the brain without the individual actually knowing about it. In fact pre-clinical MS has now been identified by research in France in which patients showed demyelinating lesions and cerebrospinal fluid abnormalities up to 2.25 years before any overt clinical signs of MS (Lebrun et al. 2008). What this might imply for their longer-term neurological health, however, is unknown. But, most importantly it indicates that MS may have a prodromal phase that may be used to identify individuals at risk of developing the condition (Ramagopalan et al. 2010). Third, it results in some parts of the brain being more 'eloquent' at producing clinical signs when demyelinated than others. Again, according to Zajicek et al. (2007, 78) it will be the optic nerves, spinal cord and brain stem with exceptional high densities of nerve pathways and relatively thin myelin sheaths that will produce clinical symptoms from relatively small areas of inflammation. The fourth important implication must be that when patients present with their first symptom of demyelination that will ultimately lead to definitive MS, they could be at many different stages of neurological damage that in turn might demand different treatment regimes. The final important point to note is that at the start of the 2010s the observable brain damage and lesion load is dependent on what Magnetic Resonance Imaging (MRI) can resolve. It is always possible and, indeed almost certain, that additional tissue damage will be taking place too at a scale this technology cannot yet 'see', that may or may not generate clinical symptoms.

The first overt clinical symptom suggestive of MS is referred to as a Clinically Isolated Syndrome (CIS). It can be hugely variable in character, with some of the most common CIS presentations that have proved to be a prelude to definitive MS being double vision, blurred vision, poor balance and co-ordination, muscle weakness (often in legs), stiffness or spasticity in muscles, altered sensation (e.g., numbness, tingling or a burning feeling in any part of the body), slurred speech, fatigue inappropriate to activity, bladder and bowel problems, impotence, forgetfulness and poor concentration (Burgess 2002, 21), with one of the most unusual being 'erotomanic' delusions in a female patient in the American military (Smith 2009). It is also important to emphasise that for reasons already described the CIS event is unlikely to reflect the first MS lesion in the CNS although it may be the first indication of anything amiss to the sufferer and their physicians. There may be many more 'silent' areas of demyelination in the CNS that have failed to elicit any clear clinical symptoms. However, many such lesions can today be observed with the aid of MRI (Bakshi et al. 2008) although, as we have already intimated, not all. Nevertheless, in some cases this has helped to lead to a relatively quick diagnosis of MS after the CIS. In the past a second definitive neurological event consistent with additional demyelination, or relapse, had to occur before a diagnosis of MS could be given. This is no longer the case and may be a potentially crucial development because many neurologists believe early intervention with DMDs will slow MS disease activity and delay the onset of permanent disability. However, it must be stressed that such a view is a recent phenomenon. In 2002 for example Dalton et al. (2002, 52) were arguing for a three year follow-up time after the CIS to confirm a definitive diagnosis of MS. They announced bluntly that there was 'currently no evidence that the long term prognosis is more favourably modified by therapeutic intervention at a first presentation with a clinically isolated syndrome.' Even then only 38 per cent of their cohort of 50 patients with a first demyelinating event could be confirmed as definite MS at 3 years.

No matter how the initial signs of MS may be treated, it will not stop PwMS worrying about the damage taking place in their CNS, if and when the next relapse will take place and of which part of their anatomy they may begin to lose control. The start of a relapse is often clear and distinct in both time and functionality. For example, the vision in an eye may suddenly become blurred or the control of part of a limb abruptly lost. In the early stages of the disease such events may be relatively transient with only modest if any residual disability afterwards. Furthermore, where a relapse has an initially serious and distressing effect, a course of corticosteroids may be administered to reduce the underlying inflammation and hasten the relapse's demise. However, for a number of less tangible and palpable MS symptoms such as fatigue, numbness, light headedness, pins and needles and possibly even pain the start and finish of a relapse may be far from clear cut. Therefore, the formal definition of a relapse as 'an episode of neurological dysfunction attributable to a lesion within the CNS lasting at least 24 hours, not attributable to fever, against a stable clinical background of at least a month' (Zajicek et al. 2007, 18), must be regarded as a construct for the precision of scientific inquiry only, to allow comparisons between different studies undertaken at different times and places, rather than of any practical use to the sufferer whose experiential reality will be much more uncertain and fuzzy. Nevertheless, using this formal definition of a relapse, that may miss some of the most unpleasant symptoms of the illness, PwMS tend initially to experience one relapse every one to two years (MS Society 2010a, 5; Zajicek et al. 2007, 10). Furthermore, for their first relapse after CIS some PwMS may wait many years. For example, the mean time to first relapse for patients with relapsing remitting MS (RRMS) in North Cambridgeshire in 1993 was 3.4 years with 95 per cent having a first relapse within 10 years (Robertson et al. 1995, 74). That, of course, meant 5 per cent waited more than 10 years for this relapse. Similarly, for people with RRMS in Rochdale in 1989, the mean time to the first relapse was 4.6 years with a maximum for 1 patient of 26 years (Shepherd and Summers 1996, 416).

The period between relapses is known as a remission and leads to this most common of presenting forms of MS being called RRMS.

Approximately 85 per cent of all cases of MS in the United Kingdom (UK) present initially with this form of the disease.

The rate of relapse is hugely variable. Some PwMS experience only very mild attacks separated by relatively long periods of remission of many years. Such a mild form of RRMS is sometimes referred to as Benign MS (BMS). Nevertheless, at some time in the future their situation may change. For example, in a follow up study of 379 patients with definite or probable MS in South Wales in 1985, only 19 per cent of those with benign disease in 1985 remained so 20 years later (Hirst et al. 2008a). For the 10 per cent or so of the UK MS population who experience this form of the illness, it is important to note that at the moment it is only possible to give such a definition retrospectively; there are no early indicators of such a course at the CIS presentation. However, this may soon change because recent research has suggested genetic differences between people with severe and benign forms of the illness (Deluca et al. 2007). Furthermore, it has also been observed that, while locomotor disability may be absent or minimal in BMS, cognitive impairment occurs in many cases (Rovaris et al. 2008). It is also worth noting that this form of MS may also be problematic emotionally because it can take such a long time to diagnose with transient non-specific symptoms; difficult for the clinician to formalise and difficult for the patient to articulate other than knowing something is wrong.

At the other extreme some unfortunate PwMS experience many relapses in quick succession with barely time to recover from the first before another begins. These individuals during the second decade of twenty-first century qualify for the most potent of DMDs such as Tysabri and Fingolimod (Gilenya) to try to dampen their disease activity that also carry the greatest risk of serious side effects. They represent one extreme of a usually unspoken 'relapse rule of thumb' of MS prognosis, the more frequently relapses take place the more likely they are to occur in the future along with its corollary, the less frequently relapses occur the less frequent they will take place in the future, although usually expressed less brutally (Degenhardt et al. 2009). Between these two cases, however, there is a great deal of uncertainty. But, in general this suggests that the timing of lesion formation and their related relapses may not be random temporal processes.

In many cases the site of nerve damage in the CNS directly results in clinical symptoms such that, for example, damage to the optic nerve can lead to impaired vision; lesions in the spinal cord to spasticity, leg weakness, bladder and bowel problems; brainstem damage to double vision and nystagmus; attacks in the cerebellum to balance difficulties and tremor (MS Trust 2004, 15). However, why certain locations in the CNS are 'chosen' for assault is not known. Perhaps detailed analysis of demyelinating syndromes with definitive brain lesion geographies such as Devic's disease (Neuromyelitis Optica, NMO) in which the optic nerves and spinal cord are targeted may help unravel an otherwise seemingly random process. However, research from America suggests that once a first demyelinating event has taken place in the CNS there would appear to be an increased chance of the next and second assaults occurring in exactly the same sites at least relating to the spinal cord and optic nerves (Mowry et al. 2009a). Thus, it may be that patients with early RRMS have relatively localised recurrent clinical relapses; weakened sites appearing to be chosen for further attacks. But, what may determine the location of the attack in the first place is unknown. This American research has gone on to show that the severity and recovery success from a first or second demyelinating event are good predictors of the severity and recovery success of the second and third relapses (Mowry et al. 2009b). Thus, the depressing conclusion must be that those with aggressive attacks and poor recovery will continue in this fashion in the early stages of their illness without therapeutic intervention. But what triggers a relapse? There have been many suggestions such as stress, trauma, infections and vaccinations but none so far has been shown to be generally true although it is possible some may be potential triggers for some people (MS Society 2010a). However, there is one profoundly important deduction to be drawn from the available evidence on the relapsing remitting form of MS: its relentless presence for those afflicted and that another attack at some time in the future is an odds-on certainty!

Two important challenges for future MS research to help PwMS plan their lives with more confidence directly follow. First, attempts must be made to try to stop the progress of the disease by limiting the scale of myelin damage, axonal loss and the number of relapses. The second challenge is to be able to predict the future course of the condition from early presentation characteristics. While there has been little progress on the latter, and some successes in the former with for example DMDs, these two concerns will feature regularly throughout this discussion.

There comes a point in some MS lesions, especially where multiple attacks have taken place at the same site at different points in time, when the damage is too serious to be repaired by the body's own resources and the rerouting of signals impossible. At such points the nerve functioning will be seriously disrupted. Worse, the axon itself may be transected stopping the movement of signals along its length permanently because mammals have no natural ability of nerve fibre regeneration and repair (Zajicek et al. 2007, 8). Thus, any resulting disability will be permanent. In other words, if persistent demyelination becomes a significant precursor to the loss of axons in MS, then this will be associated with MS disease progression and disability. Over time, therefore, as more axons are broken and disappear completely from the CNS, disability will appear to be progressive. At such a point a critical milestone in the MS disease process has been reached, a point at which a PwMS will experience a slow and unremitting worsening of their ability to function and, if this continued deterioration lasts for at least six months, an individual will be classified as having Secondary Progressive MS (SPMS) that Zajicek et al. (2007, 18) call 'a more insidious progressive course'. It is worth being reminded at this point what the ominous word 'insidious' means: sinister, dangerous, menacing, treacherous, proceeding secretly and subtly. The progressive forms of MS are certainly all these and more. In approximately 50 per cent of all cases of RRMS, signs of such permanent loss of function will commence by 10 years after CIS presentation according to the MS Trust (2004, 27). The MS Society's document (2010a) 'What is MS?' goes further to say that 65 per cent of RRMS cases will become SPMS within 15 years of diagnosis. And, in a recent study in British Columbia of more than 5,000 PwMS with an RRMS onset, the median time to SPMS for those who had had no DMD treatment was 21.4 years after diagnosis (Koch et al. 2011), perhaps rather longer than one might have expected from the British evidence. But, this could simply be explained by rather earlier ages at diagnosis. Thus, for people in the UK who are usually diagnosed with MS around the age of 30 to 35, most will have reached their SPMS phase by their early 50s. For children with MS the time to reaching the secondary progressive phase varies hugely but the majority will be much earlier than the average person with SPMS beginning at the depressingly early age of 30 years according to Banwell et al. (2007).

One of the principal questions in the shift to SPMS for which there is as yet no definitive answer is whether the use of DMDs will postpone the time of SPMS. Certainly one of the reasons for arguing for the earliest start possible to this form of therapy is to prevent persistent myelin damage that in turn should limit axonal harm and the production of permanent disability. Unfortunately, as Young (2008, 15) makes clear, the evidence that DMDs 'can postpone or block the change to secondary progressive MS is unconvincing.' And, even if they could postpone the start of SPMS, it is unlikely that they will stop it happening completely because so far it would seem that the switch from RRMS to

SPMS is one of the few predictable qualities of the affliction. Or, as Coles (2008, 19) ominously put it, there is a 'near inevitability that RRMS will become SPMS if you wait long enough.'

Are there any factors directly related to the risk of secondary progression development for RRMS patients? For the UK there is no convincing material on this issue, but for other countries there are suggestions that male gender, motor onset symptoms and higher age at onset are directly related to the speed with which SPMS emerges from RRMS (Confavreux and Vukusic 2008, Koch et al. 2008a and 2011, Tremlett et al. 2008a). The latter relationship interestingly suggests that the older the time of disease onset the shorter the time to the beginning of SPMS. It is almost as if there is a small age range in which SPMS begins irrespective of when the disease commences.

It is important to realise that when SPMS begins it does not mean the demyelination process ceases although new inflammatory activity may calm down. It is possible for the degenerative and demyelination processes to be taking place at the same time in different parts of the CNS. Indeed, some experts when categorising the various types of MS include a progressive type with superimposed relapses as a distinct form. It would also be true to say that axonal loss measured by the shrinking of the volume of the CNS, or atrophy, has been observed from the earliest moments of MS and is now used as a marker of the disease's progression, with the atrophy of different parts of the brain being associated with different clinical outcomes.

The cause or causes of axonal damage and worse of axon loss (axonopathy) in MS are yet other elements of the condition that remain uncertain. Inflammation during relapses may cause some axonal damage, so may the change in the axonal environment after demyelination. However, it is also possible that axonopathy may be the result of a completely independent neurodegenerative process (Wilkins and Scolding 2008). In other words, the process responsible for creating permanent disability in MS, the most serious consequence of the condition for most sufferers, is unknown. This is truly a scary and invidious observation. As a result, finding the causes of axon damage and loss and then creating 'neuro-protection' therapies to stop them taking place must now become a major focus for bio-medical research in MS.

For some individuals the MS disease course appears to be progressive from the very start with few if any relapses and little sign of any remission. Thus, any resulting disability becomes permanent, increasing through time at varying rates both between individuals and for any particular person. This form of MS is known as Primary Progressive MS (PPMS). It appears to be associated with lesions being much more concentrated in the spinal cord than elsewhere in the CNS and with an older age at diagnosis (Miller and Leary 2007, MS Society 2008). But, why this form of MS should be so resoundingly different from RRMS is unknown. Some have suggested it may be less associated with nerve cell damage through inflammatory demyelination and much more dependent directly on the death of nerve cells (Zajicek et al. 2007, 166), that reinforces the need to rework some of Charcot's nineteenth-century observations on the illness. Could apoptosis (programmed cell death) play an important part in this form of MS and to a much greater extent than in other forms of the illness (Zajicek et al. 2007, 10)? It is certainly believed that nerve cell death by whatever route is the almost certain proximate cause of acquired permanent disability. Could it be that processes of axonal loss are only obliquely related to demyelination? There must be an aching worry therefore that the focus of so much research effort on myelin damage and repair has missed the most destructive aspect of the MS disease completely. Now that would be invidious! For people with PPMS, therefore, there is very little reliable knowledge and few if any available therapies (MS Society 2008). The UK MS Society has in place an on-going project to identify and test potential neuro-protection agents, but the pessimists might argue that the understanding of the disease processes at play in this form of MS may be many years away for one fundamentally important reason, their complexity. It is much easier to understand any bio-medical process when the number of potential variables at play is at a minimum which usually means as early as possible in any disease. Unfortunately, PPMS does not tend to reveal itself until a person is more than half their way through their expected life span that adds a number of age-related complications to an already complex situation. This makes progress in comprehending what is happening in this form of MS extremely difficult that in turn must be regarded as another invidious state of affairs.

From the descriptive work on the different forms MS may initially take, two main types have been identified, RRMS that is the main starting form for most people with the illness and PPMS. Some regional studies in the UK have been able to distinguish between the individuals with these types of onset. For example, in North Cambridgeshire in 1993, 78 per cent of the 373 cases began as RRMS with the remaining 22 per cent experiencing a progressive course from onset (Robertson et al. 1995, 74). Similar proportions were also discovered in PwMS in Rochdale in 1988 where 190 cases (74.8 per cent) had initially RRMS, 50 cases (19.7 per cent) an initially progressive course with 6 uncertain cases and 8 with a single demyelinating episode (Shepherd and Summers 1996, 416). For South Glamorgan in 2005 a much smaller proportion of progressive MS from onset occurred. Here only 44 individuals, 7.7 per cent, had PPMS, with the RRMS percentage being commensurately higher at 92.3 (529 cases) (Hirst et al. 2009, 389). Thus, in the broadest of terms between 10 and 20 per cent of the newly diagnosed with MS in the UK towards the end of the twentieth century appear to have begun with a progressive form of the condition and at least 80 per cent beginning with a relapsing remitting form.

The relative distribution of the five types of MS noted above for three selected regions of the UK and two national surveys of MS charity members are portrayed in Table 2.1. These distributions represent three different forms of information collection. The three regional surveys were attempts at complete enumeration of all PwMS in their areas with assessment of disease type by consultant neurologists. Thus, in terms of disease type they should be regarded as highly accurate. In this context perhaps the 13 per cent of cases that could not be allocated to a specific type in the Plymouth survey should be a cause for concern. However, it is also possible that this could be a more honest reflection of how fuzzy the boundaries really are between the categories of this typology. As a result, this form of information must be regarded as giving only the broadest possible indication of the types of MS experienced by people in the UK for it is not known the extent to which these regions may be representative of the UK as a whole. This is especially so when it is understood that MS type descriptions in the two GB-wide surveys were based on the assessments of each PwMS who responded and not on

Table 2.1 Type of MS by selected regional and national survey

Type of MS	North N. Ireland 1996	Leeds 1999	Plymouth 2001	MS Society members in GB, 2003	MS Trust mailing list GB
RRMS (%)	35.0	26	46	33.6	35.5
Benign (%)	12.9	12		9.0	
SPMS (%)	39.6	40	30	28.0	37.2
RPMS (%)		7			
PPMS (%)	12.5	15	12	17.9	27.3
CIS (%)			9		
Unknown (%)			13	11.6	
Total cases	280	481	402	912	

Sources: McDonnell and Hawkins (1998, 425–26), Ford et al. (2002, 263), Fox et al. (2004, 57), Green et al. (2007, 529) and Orme et al. (2007, 57).

expert testimony. The MS Society evidence does, however, come from a random survey of its members which suggests it has greater representativeness and therefore credibility than the MS Trust information that came in response to a self-selecting mail survey. In the broadest of terms, this evidence suggests than BMS accounts for approximately 10 per cent of all cases of MS in the UK, and if this category can be subsumed within RRMS, then this form of the condition accounts for a minimum of 35 per cent of all cases up to a maximum of approximately 45 per cent. Indeed, if the 10 per cent of the relapsing progressive PwMS in Leeds can be added to the RRMS category, then 45 per cent may be nearer the true picture. Thus, given the best estimate for the number of PwMS in the UK at the start of the twenty-first century was 100,000 (see Chapter 5) this would indicate that between 35,000 and 45,000 people had a relapsing form of MS. There was rather more unanimity among the surveys in Table 2.1 on the proportion of people with primary progressive disease. In this case approximately 15 per cent of the MS population (or 15,000 people) would appear appropriate excepting the survey of MS Trust members that is 10 per cent higher. This possibly aberrant result may be accounted for in two ways. First of all because the membership of the MS Trust may be on average older than the mean age for all PwMS leading relatively to more progressive cases in their ranks. The second reason may be due to the self-selecting nature of this quality of life survey in which those with most to grumble about and those most able to grumble responded proportionately more. Finally, these results indicate that SPMS accounted for between 30 and 40 per cent of all cases of MS in the UK, or between 30,000 and 40,000 individuals.

In their 2008 review of MS in the *Lancet*, Compston and Coles referred to this MS-type classification as 'clinical empiricism' pointing out that it helped little with the understanding of the processes at work in MS, the area where they argued any new typology should focus. This may well be so, but to make such an observation demonstrated how superficial and provisional their (two of the world's leading experts) understanding of the MS disease processes must be. That really is invidious!

But, what causes the MS disease processes to begin in the first place and why does it appear to progress indefinitely? In considering the recent evidence on MS causality and making particular use of some excellent review articles, two common themes emerge, complexity and uncertainty; the former in the large number of possible individual and interacting influences implicated and the latter in simply the lack of knowledge of whether all possible causes have been at least listed and knowing how they might causally inter-react with one another. As

Ascherio and Munger (2007, 504) pointed out with profound understatement 'the true determinants of MS have been hard to pin down.' Meanwhile Giovannoni and Ebers (2007) refer to MS as a complex autoimmune disease, not attributable to a single gene or environmental factor. Therefore numerous possible causes are likely and for the individual with MS it will almost certainly mean that the cause of their own particular MS will never be discovered. What is more, this raises the possibility, if not certainty, that the initial triggers for the illness may be very different from those that promote its progress. As Goodin (2009) suggested in his causal model of MS, different environmental factors may act on the genetically susceptible at the time of their birth, in early childhood and in early adulthood to produce a chronic MS response. Thus, demonstrating causality becomes extremely difficult because of a long and complex natural history. One of the additional factors to take into account in the last 20 or so years is the effect of the therapeutic action by DMDs in changing the course of the disease. Indeed, given the seriousness of MS once these drugs became available to administer it would have been unethical to withhold them. But, what this means for those interested in researching MS aetiology and epidemiology is the increasing impossibility of finding someone with the disease in which the 'true' natural history has been allowed to unfold without interruption.

In an attempt to understand how MS may come about it is important to consider the three components of time, person (their genetic make-up) and place (the varying environments in which they lived). In MS the first component, time, is crucial because the illness is a chronic one that evolves usually for the worse over a long period of time. As such its progress, as has already been intimated, may be influenced by many different elements along the way, including therapeutic action. But, because the disease shows some time or age-related traits such as when it becomes clinically apparent and when certain symptomatic milestones are reached hints at its aetiology have been suggested.

Within any given environment, people vary in their susceptibility to developing MS because of their genetic make-up. For example, at the broadest level it is known that MS susceptibility varies between the sexes, ethnicities and age groups (see Chapter 4). It is also known that MS occurs more often in close family members than in the general population and that family clusters do occur suggesting some form of genetic inheritance pattern (Compston 2011, 18). For example, five different regional enquiries into MS in the UK reported on their patients' family histories of the disease. Robertson et al. (1995, 74) observed that

17 per cent of their MS patients in North Cambridgeshire in 1993 had an additional family member with the condition but the closeness of the kinship bonds were not reported. This was also not noted in the research in Rochdale in 1989 and Jersey / Guernsey in 1991 where 10.8 per cent (Shepherd and Summers 1996, 417) and 13 per cent (Sharpe et al. 1995, 24) respectively reported familial MS. Ford et al. (2002, 262) in Leeds progressed the family links one step further by observing that 9 per cent of the 176 incident cases of MS between 1996 and 1999 reported either a first- or a second-degree relative with the condition. Extending the familial linkage even more to third-degree relatives produced the much higher rate of 22.6 per cent for the prevalent cases in north Northern Ireland in 1996 (McDonnell and Hawkins 1998, 426).

Nevertheless, the inherited MS risk appears to be a small one. For example, Burgess (2002, 12) noted from work by Robertson et al. (1996a) in Cambridgeshire the age-adjusted risk of developing MS for relatives of an individual already diagnosed. For a parent the risk was 2.0 per cent, for a sibling 3.8 per cent, a child 1.8 per cent, a nephew/niece 1.6 per cent, an aunt/uncle 0.9 per cent and a first cousin 0.9 per cent. However, it is not known how representative this study may be of the UK generally or how stable such proportions of at risk relatives may be through time.[1] MS inheritance though is not of a directly predictable fashion as in Cystic Fibrosis or Huntingdon's disease. It is an inherited risk that must also be stimulated by exposure to environmental triggers. Good evidence for this assertion comes from the observation that among genetically identical twins most do not develop the illness when their sibling has MS (Compston 2011, 18). Indeed, the importance of the environment may be seen to grow when it is realised that MS concordance between identical twins appears to vary between countries: 25 per cent in the UK, 15 per cent in Italy and 35 per cent in Canada (Amor and van Noort 2012, 38).

The search for the genes associated with MS susceptibility and development have expanded at great speed in the recent past. For example, in 2008 Sawcer reported that while only four genes related to MS susceptibility had been identified by that time he anticipated probably as many as 100 would be at work. By 2011, after a major international effort involving almost 250 researchers worldwide studying the DNA of 9,772 PwMS and 17,376 unrelated healthy controls supported by major improvements in computing power and data handling techniques, the situation was very different. By then 23 known genetic associations were confirmed, 29 new genetic variants identified and an additional five had been strongly implicated with MS susceptibility

(The International Genetics Consortium and the Wellcome Trust Case Control Consortium 2011). Thus, MS is not the result of a single aberrant gene, and some form of simple gene therapy would therefore not be appropriate as a 'cure'. Nor would it be possible, if the background ethics could be ignored, to eradicate the illness by 'encouraging' those with MS not to have any progeny. What is more, it is known that many of these genes are involved in the workings of the immune system adding support to the view that MS is a complex autoimmune disorder. However, what this form of research has not yet been able to discern are the genes involved in nerve tissue injury and repair and why MS develops differently in different people. What this means is that the pool of knowledge about MS is not at a point where the people who will develop MS can be predicted, along with the course a person's MS may take and who will benefit most with fewest side effects from available DMD therapies. More recently though it has been suggested that, although there may be many different genes implicated in the inherited risk of MS, one gene dominates, the major histocompatibility complex, that is crucial for the body to mount immune responses (Amor and van Noort 2012, 37).

There are two further complications to an understanding of the relationship between a person's genes and their susceptibility to MS. The first concern stems from Ebers' observation on the 2009 MS Life Conference CD that genes may change their function under different environmental circumstances to trigger an MS immune response; in other words environmental factors may switch a gene on to produce damaging immune cells, and thereby influence the risk of developing MS. Such 'epigenetic' effects, however, make the whole search for the genetic background to MS causality and progression much more complex. The second complication refers to the view that genetic make-up is just part of the answer to MS susceptibility, the others being the environments in which people live and the way they behave within them that may furnish the triggers to an MS immune response and the speed of its progression. As Bhopal (2002, 294) claimed, 'Genetic factors provide the stage in the great drama of disease causation, but the environment is the leading player.' This does not mean that genetic make-up is a bit-part player. Far from it, if the view of Goodin (2009) is to be taken seriously that because of their genetic make-up more than 99 per cent of individuals seem incapable of developing MS regardless of the environmental exposures they may experience. But, given according to Giovannoni and Ebers (2007) no evidence exists of non-genetic transmission of MS within families, for those who have the relevant MS genes it must be environmental impacts that account for MS susceptibility differences between places and individuals.

Many different types of environmental agent, risk factor or trigger have been implicated in the aetiology of MS and in the rate of its progress (Ebers 2008). These have included microbes of many kinds that people may catch, many aspects of the area in which people live to aspects of personal behaviour, lifestyle, consumption and experience from food, drink and drugs to trauma and stress. None, however, have been shown to be the sole causal agent in the genetically susceptible (Ascherio and Munger 2007, Giovannoni and Ebers 2007). Thus, it must be accepted that the disease may genuinely have a number of different possible causes that may act alone or in conjunction with one another, either at the same time, or more probably sequentially through a person's life, to produce an MS response. It is also possible that they could act serially to accelerate the disease's impact. Furthermore, the possibility must exist for someone to experience more than one MS trigger during their lives.

Giovannoni and Ebers (2007, 266) point out that, even if there were overwhelming circumstantial evidence for a positive link between an environmental factor and MS prevalence, proving such a link is causal '...is complicated and may take years or even decades to achieve.' For some this may appear as difficult and as futile as searching for Lewis Carol's elusive 'Snark'; a point emphasised by Compston's (2009, 1145) observation that the search for 'an environmental cause of multiple sclerosis remained stubbornly unproductive.' But, this should not stop researchers trying because many possible causes may prove to be things that can be avoided or at least reduced to a minimum by changes in behaviour or by inexpensive ameliorative action. There may even be the prospect of MS being preventable. So the search for the causes of MS and its progression must continue.

One of the most persistent and compelling observations about the geographical distribution of MS suggestive of causation is its latitudinal variation with the highest regional prevalence rates typically furthest from the equator (see Chapter 5). Though latitude may be correlated with many physical, chemical, biological and social factors, the possibility that sunlight intensity may be a causal factor naturally emerged. Could it be that people subjected to relatively high levels of ultraviolet (UV) radiation would have the lowest relative levels of MS? Certainly Kurtzke (1967) observed in Switzerland an inverse correlation between altitude (a proxy for sunlight intensity) and MS prevalence. Could this mean that where sunlight intensity is very high MS propensity will be low unless people lived in the shade much of the time? Evidence from Middle East countries and especially for their women who in traditional households spend much of their lives indoors and when out of doors are fully covered would be useful in this regard, but no reliable evidence exists (Al-Hashel et al. 2008). There is some weak evidence from mortality rates of PwMS in both the United States (US) and the UK of a protective effect of sunlight. For example, in the UK skin cancer mortality in PwMS was found to be 50 per cent less than would have been expected by Goldacre et al. (2004). Similarly, in the US MS mortality rates appeared to be higher in low sunlight areas and for indoor activities, especially in high sunlight areas, where deaths from skin cancers increased (Freeman et al. 2000). However, in this case there was the potential for reverse causation confounding the explanation such that PwMS spent more time indoors because their MS, including heat intolerance, made them incapable of outdoor work. These sorts of results raise the question as to when in a person's life could a latitude or UV affect operate? Could it be a causative factor with a particular time within a person's life to be effective or was it both causative and relevant to a person's whole MS history? Migration studies, reviewed in Chapter 5, indicated that whatever the impact of location, or environmental risk factor may be, it appeared to operate before early adolescence because those who moved their place of residence before that time tended to follow the MS prevalence trend of their destination area and, those who migrated after that time followed the MS trend of their area of origin. Further research has tended to suggest that the important trigger events may be earlier in a person's life and could even be before they are born. For example, work on the season of birth of PwMS from both Canada, the UK and Denmark has indicated that significantly more PwMS were born in May and less in November than would otherwise be expected (Koch et al. 2008b). In other words, mothers to be who tended to experience the least amount of direct sunshine during their pregnancies had the greatest chance of giving birth to someone who would eventually develop MS. Furthermore, for Newfoundland and Labrador, Sloka and colleagues (2008) found trends in MS incidence better correlated with UV levels of the first year of life than the latitude or the locale of their first MS episode. In addition, Tremlett et al. (2008b) found relapse rates inversely related to vitamin D levels and positively related to Upper Respiratory Tract infections in a prospective study of PwMS in Tasmania. Could such evidence be suggestive that vitamin D plays a protective part in MS aetiology both in the mother during pregnancy, a very long time before diagnosis, and then throughout a person's life?

Vitamin D is obtained primarily from the exposure of the skin to UV radiation and the farther from the equator a person lives the lower the chances of producing enough of this vital vitamin. Vitamin D can also be obtained from a limited range of foodstuffs such as fish, and there is some limited evidence that where fish eating is high, that is a high vitamin D dietary intake, such as in Japan, among the Inuit people in the high Arctic or even in coastal Norway, MS prevalence is low (Brustad et al. 2004). Unfortunately, carrying out accurate research on eating habits is notoriously difficult not least because of the problems of recall over the long period required for a chronic illness, but also because of the many other factors involved. Furthermore, such studies have become even more problematic for the modern era because a person's diet is no longer confined to what their local area can seasonally produce because of efficient preserving technologies and the ease of transporting food of any kind around the planet. Nevertheless, if an association between the development and progression of MS and vitamin D deficiency can be established, it leads directly to an effective preventative public health strategy of vitamin D as a dietary supplement. Indeed, Ascherio and Munger (2007) were so convinced by the evidence on the association between MS prevalence, progression and vitamin D, they called for a randomised controlled trial to discover its preventative properties saying, 'increasing vitamin D levels among adolescents and young adults could reduce MS risk' (Ascherio and Munger 2007, 508). And, 'protection could be achieved with doses of vitamin D supplements regarded as safe...there appears to be no reason to wait' (Ascherio and Munger 2007, 510). Meanwhile Gillie argued for vitamin D supplementation in Scotland where he claimed in the *Times* (Monday, 15 September 2008) its MS incidence was high in part due to low levels of vitamin D from that country's low levels of sunlight, its population's poor diet and their tendency to live in tenements. However, such public health schemes may be thought to offer little for the individual because most would not have developed the condition anyway. Furthermore, they may offer little politically because there may be few grateful voters when success means nothing happens.

To be expected a counter argument by Albert et al. (2009) soon emerged suggesting low levels of vitamin D in PwMS and other autoimmune diseases may be the result and not the cause of their morbidity. They suggested that autoimmune diseases were caused by persistent pathogens, probably unidentified very slow growing bacteria and, while vitamin D supplementation was being advised universally, global autoimmunity continued to rise. In such circumstances, vitamin D supplementation would make things worse not better.

The relationship between vitamin D and MS represents potentially two different modifiable aspects of a person's life, where they live and what they consume. In terms of the latter many people have believed that what they eat and drink has had a direct influence on their chance of developing MS and will continue to have an effect on their disease's progression and relapses to the point that a range of specialised therapeutic diets have been advocated such as the Best Bet Diet (Graham 2010, 39–49) although, according to the dietician Payne (2012, 7), there is no credible research evidence to support their use. However, according to Ascherio and Munger (2007, 509–10) although 'moderate effects cannot be excluded', there is no strong or persuasive evidence to link MS incidence or progression with vitamin C, E, beta-carotene or fruit and vegetable consumption more generally, or to antibiotics, antihistamines and the tetanus vaccination. Furthermore, Giovannoni and Ebers (2007) could find no clear link with alcohol consumption, recreational drugs or the contraceptive pill. This latter view, however, may need some revision because cannabis is now accepted as having a symptom-relief impact forming the basis of the anti-spasticity drug Sativex (see Chapter 7) and, while neither taking the contraceptive pill nor age of first birth is related to an increased risk of MS (Ascherio and Munger 2007, 509), the sex hormone oestrogen is beginning to attract increased research interest because of its possible impact on disease activity during pregnancy. In this case it is believed to be responsible for a non-inflammatory immune response that settles down MS-disease activity during pregnancy. However, this benefit is temporary because the disease often rebounds afterwards.

On one aspect of consumption there appears to be complete unanimity; smoking is bad for PwMS! Smoking appears to increase the risk of getting MS, especially among women (Sundstrom et al. 2008), increases the rate of progression, brain shrinkage and relapse rates (Zivadinov et al. 2009), accelerates transition from RRMS to SPMS (Hernan et al. 2005) and even increases the risk of children developing MS who are subjected to passive smoking (Tardieu and Mikaeloff 2008). What is more, the earlier a person starts smoking the greater the risk of starting with MS, the faster the rate of progression and the greater the severity of the disease. Finally, all these effects seem to be dose dependent such that the more a person smokes the worse the likely MS impacts (Handel et al. 2011). But, from Swedish research this unremitting gloom does not seem to extend to an increased risk of getting MS among children whose mothers smoked during pregnancy (Montgomery et al. 2008). Handel and colleagues (2011) interestingly raise the intriguing prospect that it might not be nicotine directly that is having the negative MS impacts but other elements of the pollutants smoking generates that in turn would help to account for its passive smoking effects. It is also possible that smoking could increase the risk of a person developing upper respiratory tract infections that are regarded as MS risk factors too. Could tobacco smoking, therefore, either directly or indirectly, through the pollutants released be implicated in the growth of MS in women or the changing geography of MS in the UK, or anywhere else in the world? Or more generally, could it be that changing smoking patterns is one of the important dimensions of a broader cultural view that MS is the product of a multifaceted 'Westernization' of the world that has been employed to try to explain the growing rates of MS in Japan and eastern Asia (Osoegawa et al. 2009). What is certainly clear is that in order to understand the causes and development of MS anywhere in the world an understanding of changing behavioural and consumption patterns of its people is vitally important.

The search for a transmissible agent such as a bacterium or virus that may act as a trigger for MS either in the first instance or for subsequent relapses, has been a continuous one for many years and many possible microbes have been implicated such as measles, rubella, canine distemper, human herpes virus-6 and chlamydia pneumonia bacterium. As Compston (2009, 1144–45) exclaimed, 'Rarely in the history of research in multiple sclerosis is there not a current microbial favourite for the cause of the disease.' Indeed, after cataloguing the number of PwMS in Greater London between 1960 and 1972 paying particular attention to the disease among immigrant groups and the age at which MS might strike, Dean and colleagues (1976, 864) argued that MS was the product of a viral infection the immunity to which was usually acquired during childhood, concluding, 'The key to the mystery of multiple sclerosis appears to be within our grasp.' Unfortunately, nothing could have been further from the truth, because no infectious causal agent for MS has resisted determined scrutiny so far with perhaps the current hot favourite the Epstein-Barr Virus (EBV). EBV is a particular successful virus infecting the vast majority of people on the planet and persisting in the body indefinitely. Infection typically occurs in early childhood and is either asymptomatic or indistinguishable from other childhood infections. In western societies, however, the initial infection is often delayed until adolescence or early adulthood, possibly due to better hygiene, when it causes Glandular Fever or Infectious Mononucleosis (IM) in 35 to 50 per cent of cases (Goodin 2009). What has now been established with some certainty is that the risk of developing MS after IM appears to be relatively high. For example, Giovannoni and Ebers (2007, 265) reported that in a large Danish study of 25,000 patients the risk of developing MS after IM was more than twice what should have been expected and that this heightened risk persisted for more than 30 years and was uniformly distributed across all investigated strata of sex and age. Similarly, in a major study in Canada using a longitudinal database with 14,362 MS cases plus 7,671 spousal controls that inquired about their history of Measles, Mumps, Rubella, Varicella and IM and vaccinations for Measles, Mumps, Rubella, Hepatitis B and Influenza, found only IM to be associated with an increased risk of MS later in life. Finally, the meta-analysis by Handel and colleagues (2010) from 18 articles that included 19,390 MS patients and 16,007 controls firmly established an increased risk of MS following IM with no significant evidence to suggest this relationship varied with either latitude or sex ratio. But, the material used in this case was heavily dominated by Caucasian samples; the importance of the IM-MS relationship still needs to be explored for other ethnic groups. Furthermore, it is not yet understood why MS risk should be associated so strongly with IM and not with asymptomatic EBV infection. Nevertheless, late-onset IM and its increased risk of MS may be part of the explanation of why MS is often associated with professional occupations and higher levels of educational achievement (see Chapter 4). It is in institutions of higher education in particular that the sexual activity of adolescent students will permit the rapid spread of the EBV and its associated infections.

Two further areas of possible trigger factors for MS, or at least for relapses, include the micro-environment in which people live over which they have some control and events in their lives over which they probably have very little control. In terms of the latter, there is persistent anecdotal evidence that stressful and traumatic events in people's lives such as bereavement and serious accidents can cause relapses in MS and even trigger the disease de novo. While there would appear to be little material on these issues generally in terms of trauma, there is substantial evidence from Denmark that it is not a causal factor. For example, in an examination of 150,868 subjects from the Danish Patient Registry admitted to hospital for cerebral concussion, contusion or skull fracture between 1977 and 1992 aged less than 55 years and then linked to the Danish MS Registry up to the end of 1999 for the subsequent development of MS, there was no indication that head injury of any severity affected the risk of acquiring MS later in life for either the group as a whole or the male and female subgroups separately (Pfleger et al. 2009).

According to Fleming and Cook (2006), the character of the microenvironment in which people live may be a contributory factor in the development of their MS through the so-called 'hygiene hypothesis'. This postulates that the early immune system needs to be challenged to develop properly to allow it to beat threats later in life and that the increasingly sterile conditions in which people tend to live with their antibiotics, vaccines, cleaning products and quarantine behaviours prevents this from happening properly. If infection availability could be measured by the presence of older siblings, then both Canadian and Danish research provided no support for the hygiene hypothesis (Giovannoni and Ebers 2007). Interestingly, it may be worth pondering where MS prevalence is at its lowest, in countries closest to the equator, that are probably the unhealthiest places in the world as far as the presence of microbial life is concerned. Could these places represent an example of the hygiene hypothesis 'writ large'? Or, could it be that the populations in these areas are benefitting from their immune systems being moderated by gut parasites such as hookworms; a technique being actively tested by Constantinescu at the Nottingham University Hospital NHS Trust (MS Society website).

On MS, Handel and colleagues (2010, 2) argue, 'It is becoming increasingly clear that a multitude of genetic and environmental factors interact at different times during the course of an individual's life to determine disease susceptibility'. And, Goodin (2009) has proposed an MS causal model to represent this complexity in which three sequential environmental risk factors are implicated for the genetically susceptible. The first risk factor acts near birth, the second during childhood and the third long after, and while vitamin D deficiency and EBV may be the first two factors no suggestion is offered for the third; an observation symptomatic of the lack of understanding of MS aetiology. Indeed, this limited clarity on the cause or causes of MS continues to lead to many different and new suggestions. For example, Corthals (2011) has claimed that MS is caused by faulty lipid metabolism, Berer and Krishnamoorthy (2012) implicate gut microbiopta and Zamboni et al. (2009) argue for a vascular cause of MS. The latter in particular, discussed more thoroughly in Chapter 7, has caused a great deal of interest recently especially among patient groups. In this view it is argued that MS is the result of chronic cerebrospinal venous insufficiency (CCSVI), a constriction in the veins from the brain to the heart that causes a backflow of blood into the brain. This in turn leads to iron deposition that results in immune cells entering the CNS to cause the damage seen in MS. What is so appealing about his view is that it leads to a clear relieving therapy, vein widening or angioplasty that is not, however, without risk.

This brief overview of the MS condition indicates that in order to comprehend fully how people develop the illness in the first place and then how it progresses within them three vital elements are needed. First, an understanding of the genes that make people susceptible to MS is required. These genes are now being identified at an increasing pace. But, it is also now accepted that there may be an important genetic component in controlling the rate at which MS progresses too and that genes may interact with the environment to respond differently in different situations. Thus, the genetic component of MS pathogenesis is becoming increasingly complicated. The second required element is an understanding of the biological processes that lead to both MS inflammatory and degenerative responses in the CNS. By contrast, the third required element involves the social and economic processes that enable people to acquire the MS susceptibility genes in the first place and then locates them in the wrong place at the wrong time, or undertake a particular form of behaviour that triggers an MS-related response.[2] Thus, as Churchill exclaimed about Russian decision making at the start of the Second World War, so might the MS condition be thought of as 'a riddle wrapped in a mystery inside an enigma' (W. Churchill 10/01/1939).

3
Research on People with MS: Definitions, Data Sources and Methodologies

3.1 Introduction

This chapter considers the principal challenges facing research on people with Multiple Sclerosis (PwMS) and in so doing details some of the inadequacies of the research that has already been carried out. Most of these issues stem from three main sources: the nature of the disease itself including its definition and diagnosis, the available information sources and the ways in which they have been used to answer research questions, that is their methodologies. It then proceeds to consider the four main approaches to research adopted so far to provide the descriptive evidence and insight into the lives of PwMS employed in this book: regional counts of PwMS, the growth of registers of PwMS, mass surveying of PwMS and detailed small group qualitative analyses.

MS is a multifaceted complex disease with many evolving difficulties for the unwary researcher, not least its fertile and elastic nosology. For example, there were at least three different sets of diagnostic criteria for MS used in the world at the start of the twenty-first century (WHO and MSIF 2008), by Schumacher, Poser and McDonald, with an earlier scheme by Allison and Millar (A&M) regularly used in the United Kingdom (UK) and the Americas before that time. Such variability and change is perhaps to be expected in a rapidly developing area of medical science, that is the expected outcome of an iterative scientific method in which new discoveries and technologies change the way MS is perceived, measured and treated. What is more, for similar reasons one should expect such a process to continue. Nevertheless, from a research interpretation perspective it might raise the question as to whether the disease called MS in the 1980s is the same disease as that called MS at the start of the twenty-first century?

Two further aspects of the disease that cause all MS researchers concern are first its huge variability in presenting symptoms and second its chronic nature. The first of these issues not only raises the problem of being able to muster a large enough size of sample to give most variations a chance to be represented properly, it also challenges the ingenuity of researchers to design generalised effect measures in which many different dimensions can be included. While the second issue, that MS for a sufferer is much more of a life sentence than a death sentence means that its full effect needs to be traced over whole life times, not truncated ones, life times that may not be very different from the general populace. Thus, for most PwMS their lives from Clinically Isolated Syndrome (CIS) or diagnosis to death will be much longer than the working life of any MS research worker; it is simply not possible for them to follow the entirety of the changing behaviour of a person with MS as their disease unfolds. One possible way around this problem is to take a cross-sectional approach by looking at PwMS at different ages and stages of the disease at one particular point in time. This, however, must always be in the knowledge that the life of someone with MS of 60 years of age at the start of the twenty-first century may be very different from an equivalent person in 1960 or probably from one in 2060 in terms of the society in which they live, the medical support they can expect to receive and the environment to which they are exposed. Another way to overcome this longevity problem is through the keeping of disease registers, data bases of PwMS for specific places that are maintained for many years. Indeed, they are vital if the impacts of various disease milestones such as diagnosis, relapses, conversion to secondary progressive MS (SPMS), and the taking of disease modifying drugs (DMDs) on the health and behaviour of PwMS are to be explored thoroughly. Similarly, they would be necessary if the effect of preventative medical interventions were to be researched. The development of such register-based material is considered in detail later in this chapter.

A further area to bedevil social research on PwMS concerns interpretative difficulties stemming from poor methodological and data source decisions. These have either been inappropriate for the questions posed or too weak to support the research conclusions. In particular, poor sample definition has often seriously compromised research conclusions. This has been particularly irksome because in a number of important cases it has led to promising research with the possibility of delivering meaningful insights into the behaviour and lives of PwMS producing less than secure results.

3.2 The definition and diagnosis of MS

There is no single test or single clinical feature sufficient for the diagnosis of MS. There are now a number of useful tests, using visual evoked potential (VEP) techniques, MRI or the analysis of the cerebrospinal fluid (CSF) obtained by lumbar puncture, that can produce results suggestive of MS. But, none is sufficient on its own or even together definitively to diagnose MS. Therefore, its diagnosis remains primarily a clinical one dependent on the skill and experience of the neurologist to interpret the presenting symptoms, signs, test results and medical histories of their patients. To aid this process a number of diagnostic criteria have been suggested. In the UK, the relatively liberal classification of A&M in 1954 was usually employed until the 1980s when the more precise and restrictive Poser criteria (Poser et al. 1983) became the norm. Meanwhile, in the United States (US) the Schumacher criteria,[1] that are still in use in many parts of the world today (WHO and MSIF 2008, Evans et al. 2013), became the accepted standard and according to Murray (2005, 321) after three years of wrangling. It too was superseded by the Poser criteria in the mid-1980s, that in turn has been replaced by the McDonald criteria in 2001 (McDonald et al. 2001) and its update in 2005 (Polman et al. 2005). However, these systems are still under debate, under constant review and far from universally understood as often disgruntled neurologists try to apply them (Hawkes and Giovannoni 2010). Thus, in some respects this book is about a disease that has no adequate mode of identification or definition; it is about a fuzzy and unstable concept. Some researchers may find such a situation alarming and wholly unsatisfactory while others may view it as an exciting challenge.

For the development of the MS diagnostic criteria, three powerful motivations seem to have been in play, not all of which were necessarily pulling in the same direction. First, there has been the introduction of new laboratory and technological developments to aid the diagnostic process. The second motivation seems to have been the closely related desire to make the diagnosis of MS more precise, to limit as far as possible the chances of getting the diagnosis wrong, so that scientists around the world could be sure they were all referring to exactly the same disease. As Poser et al. (1983, 227) stated, 'there is a need for more exact criteria than existed earlier in order to conduct therapeutic trials in multicenter programs, to compare epidemiological surveys, to evaluate new diagnostic procedures and to estimate the activity of the disease process in MS.' In essence, therefore, they were designed specifically 'to restrict therapeutic trials and other research protocols to patients with definite MS' (Poser et al. 1983, 230). In this scheme the use of laboratory evidence from CSF was introduced. However, such a scheme could easily produce a large set of individuals whose diagnosis of MS could not yet be given but who almost certainly had the disease. These individuals may be particularly problematic for the physician especially if they had undergone a series of potentially uncomfortable tests such as lumbar punctures that were not yet positive for MS.

By 2001 McDonald et al. (2001, 121) had changed tack somewhat, the third motivation, saying they had set out to 'create diagnostic criteria that could be used by the practicing physician and that could be adopted, as necessary, for clinical trials', what Polman et al. (2005, 840) said was to provide a 'better and more reliably diagnosis of MS, balancing early diagnosis with the need to avoid false positive diagnosis.' In these McDonald criteria Magnetic Resonance Imaging (MRI) scans were introduced along with a definition of primary progressive MS (PPMS), but of equal importance seemed to have been the desire to help the practicing clinician make a diagnosis with all the uncertainties of real life subjects rather than just concentrating on an increasingly accurate definition of the disease that excluded more and more potential subjects. It could be argued, therefore, that indirectly there was a sense in which they were trying to help the patient secure a speedy diagnosis.

There were four guiding principles that permeated all these criteria to come to a decision about an MS diagnosis. First, there must be the separation, or a dissemination, in time and space (distinctly different parts of the human central nervous system [CNS]), of at least two attacks of neurological dysfunction, that is more than one CNS lesion. What McHugh et al. (2008, 84) called 'an unswerving principle in the diagnosis of MS in general neurology practice.' Second, no other possible explanation or diagnosis could be used to account for the signs and symptoms displayed. Third, historical accounts of symptoms, while possibly suggestive of MS, were not enough; objective clinical evidence of lesions was necessary. Fourth, the diagnosis must be undertaken by a consultant neurologist or at least someone experienced in clinical neurology.

The A&M diagnostic criteria for MS (Forbes et al. 1999, 1034) were based on the signs and symptoms of patients neurological histories in which three possible states were identified:

1. Early MS in which there existed a recent history of relapsing remitting symptoms and little physical disability.

2. Probable MS when some physical disability was present set within a relapsing remitting history that could only be explained by multiple lesions in the CNS.
3. Possible MS concerned mainly with a progressive disease course but with insufficient evidence to demonstrate scattered CNS lesions although no other cause could be found.

The Poser et al. (1983) criteria for a diagnosis of MS were far more specific and detailed. They began with a set of five definitions:

1. Only individuals with an age of onset between 10 and 59 years should be included. The upper limit though is more than often ignored in UK regional work (see e.g., Rice-Oxley et al. 1995, Fox et al. 2004).
2. An attack or exacerbation (relapse): the occurrence of a symptom or symptoms of more than 24 hours constitutes an attack.
3. Remission: a definite improvement of signs or symptoms that has been present for at least 24 hours. A remission must last at least one month (30 days) to be considered significant.
4. 'Laboratory support' is used only to indicate the examination of CSF for oligoclonal bands (OB) and increased production of immunoglobulin G (IgG).
5. Paraclinical evidence: The demonstration by means of various tests and procedures of the existence of a lesion of the CNS. For example, using VEP to measure the time for a flashing image to pass along the optic nerves is one such procedure as were the nascent brain imaging technologies at that time.

Before delving any further into Poser's precise definitions, however, it was clear that much of what might legitimately be regarded as being part of the MS experience was being purposefully ignored, regarded as unworthy of inclusion, illegitimate. There was no space for short-duration symptoms, for example, such as heat intolerance, Lhermitte's Sign and temporary vertigo no matter how typical they may be of the condition. Indeed, Poser et al. (1983, 228) admit that Lhermitte's sign is really a symptom of MS. Nor was there room for the often longer lasting symptoms of uncertain duration with fuzzy beginnings and endings such as numbness, low mood, cognitive difficulties and fatigue; all sacrificed on the alter of scientific precision, despite often being regarded as classic initial presentations (Burgess 2002, 21). These exclusions may very well be for perfectly laudable scientific reasons but did they need to be so exclusive for the giving of a diagnosis to a concerned patient?

The Poser system included two main groups, definite MS and probable MS, each with two subgroups, clinical and laboratory supported:

A. Clinically definite MS (CDMS);
   1. Two attacks and clinical evidence of two separate lesions.
   2. Two attacks, clinical evidence of one lesion and paraclinical evidence of another, separate lesion.
B. Laboratory supported definite MS (LSDMS)
   1. Two attacks; either clinical or paraclinical evidence of one lesion and CSF OB/IgG.
   2. One attack; clinical evidence of two separate lesions and CSF OB/IgG.
   3. One attack; clinical evidence of one lesion and paraclincal evidence of another, separate lesion, and CSF OB/IgG.

For the inclusion of PPMS, steady progression for at least 6 months must take place.

C. Clinically probable MS (CPMS)
   1. Two attacks and clinical evidence of one lesion.
   2. One attack and clinical evidence of two separate lesions.
   3. One attack; clinical evidence of one lesion and paraclinical evidence of another, separate lesion.
D. Laboratory-supported probable MS (LSPMS)
   1. Two attacks and CSF OB/IgG.

The inclusion of the 'probable' MS category may have appeared unusual. Indeed, the authors suggested that it 'may matter very little' (p.230) to the physician. It was designed to present a second cohort of PwMS to the research community whose diagnosis was not quite as certain as the definite group. For the patient, however, it was no solution because above all else they needed certainty, a confirmation of their condition. A probable MS diagnosis just prolonged their agony of waiting.

The Poser system was certainly in stark contrast to its much more liberal predecessor by A&M. For example, when diagnostic criteria were compared in a study of MS prevalence in Tayside in Scotland in 1996, of the 880 cases subsumed by the A&M regime 153 were excluded by the definite and probable categories of the Poser classification, a 17 per cent reduction (Forbes et al. 1999). Similar large proportions for this 'suspected' MS group were also found in studies in Sussex (Rice-Oxley et al. 1995) at 18 per cent, north Northern Ireland (McDonnell and Hawkins 1998) and Leeds at 13 per cent (Ford et al. 1998, 607) and 14 per cent (Ford et al. 2002) but, much smaller for Rochdale (Shepherd and Summers 1996) at 9 per cent and only 4 per cent in Southampton (Roberts et al. 1991). In essence, what this meant was the A&M category of 'possible MS' had been removed temporarily from the diagnostic lexicon. As Poser et al. (1983, 229) stated, 'the traditional possible group is not included because patients so labelled would not be acceptable for research studies.' Perhaps, unfortunately, the term reappeared with the McDonald diagnostic criteria in 2001.

The number of cases of MS classified by both the A&M and the Poser (definite and probable) diagnostic schemes in recent regional epidemiological work in the UK are given in Table 3.1 in which it can clearly be

Table 3.1 The number of PwMS diagnosed using the A&M and poser criteria for selected regional populations in the UK

Area	Year of survey	No. of cases using A&M criteria	No. of cases using Poser criteria		
			definite and probable	suspected	unclassified
Sutton (south London)	1985	195			
South Glamorgan	1985	441	360	60	21
South Hampshire	1987	411	379	16	16
South Glamorgan	1988		379	74	
Rochdale	1989	254	232	22	
South and east Cambridgeshire	1990	374	318	52	4
Guernsey and Jersey	1991	148	129		19
Brighton and mid-Downs	1991		665	105	
South and east Cambridgeshire	1993	441	374	61	6
North Cambridgeshire	1993	449	388	48	13
Lothian / Borders	1995		310	160#;	11
Leeds	1996		526	95	91
North Northern Ireland	1996	288	254	34	
Tayside	1996	880	727	153	
Leeds	1999		625	112	55
Plymouth	2001		387	44	15
Tayside	2002		918*		
North Northern Ireland	2004		370		
South Glamorgan	2005		612		8

Sources: Williams and McKernan (1986), Swingler and Compston (1988), Hennessy et al. (1989), Roberts et al. (1991), Mumford et al. (1992), Sharpe et al. (1995), Rice-Oxley et al. (1995), Shepherd and Summers (1996), Robertson et al. (1995), Robertson et al. (1996b), Rothwell and Charlton (1998), Ford et al. (1998), McDonnell and Hawkins (1998), Forbes et al. (1999), Ford et al. (2002), Fox et al. (2004), Donnan et al. (2005), Gray et al. (2008), Hirst et al. (2009).

* calculated from a prevalence of 236/100,000 and a population in 2001 of 389,012.
\# called 'possible' MS by Rothwell and Carlton (1998, 732), presumably in the A&M sense.

seen that the former are much larger than the latter. However, in addition the Poser criteria not only provided a 'suspected' category of individuals but also resulted in a set of individuals who could not be given a precise 'Poser' classification at all, but who were, nevertheless, thought, and one cannot say suspected, to have MS.

Did this change in the way MS was diagnosed mean that earlier studies of the illness, especially in Scotland and Northern Ireland, significantly overestimated the frequency of the illness? Some researchers have suggested that it did (Forbes et al. 1999, Fox et al. 2004) arguing the most reliable and robust indicator would be the Poser definite and probable MS categories. This would especially be the case if this 'suspected' group of patients did not go on to develop MS. The limited evidence on this issue from the UK came from two studies. The first was on the changing disability of PwMS in SE Wales from 1985 to 2005 (Hirst et al. 2008a). In this case, of the 380 people diagnosed with MS in 1985 by Swingler and Compston (1988), 61 were classified as 'suspected MS', 13.6 per cent of the total (the original table on p.1522 actually reports 60 people). Of these 8 were diagnosed with something else, 18 never had a second inflammatory event, 26 could not be accurately determined and only 9 (15%) eventually fulfilling the Poser criteria for definite or probable MS. Indeed, 3 had already reached clinically definite MS by 1988 (Hennessy et al. 1989, 1086). Thus, MS was initially misdiagnosed in only 3 per cent of cases in this instance. The second set of evidence on the 'suspected' category came from the two studies of MS in the Cambridgeshire Health District in 1990 (Mumford et al. 1992) and 1993 (Robertson et al. 1996b). In the latter it was pointed out that, of the 52 patients with suspected MS in 1990, 11 (21%) had converted to definite or probable MS by 1993, a much faster rate than in the Welsh study, while 69 per cent remained in the 'suspected' category (Robertson et al. 1996b, 276). Thus, the 'suspected' category was as Robertson et al. suggested (1995, 75) 'now accepted as referring to those suspected of having demyelinating disease but without signs or paraclinical evidence of more than one lesion.' It was therefore a device for coping with the transition in diagnostic criteria from A&M to Poser. What is more, as the demarcation between what could be contemplated as MS and what could not became clearer, with experience of applying the Poser criteria and the introduction of McDonald's criteria, this suspected category disappeared.

A relatively high proportion of cases of 'suspected MS' may not have mattered that much when the illness, and those with which it could be easily confused, were incurable and largely untreatable. Indeed, it may have been thought that giving a positive diagnosis of something could be psychologically beneficial for the patient, taking them out of a stressful 'limbo land' of worrying about what dreadful illness they actually had. However, when treatments started to arrive that could actually change the course of the illness, then assured diagnoses became absolutely vital, with those for whom an MS diagnosis was not so certain, no matter how strongly suspected, needing to be excluded. This was especially so when the new medications were awkward to administer, uncomfortable for the patient and even potentially life threatening as well as expensive. Only those definitely with the condition could be contemplated. It is understandable, therefore, that the diagnostic criteria became more restrictive, more certain they included only those definitely with MS.

Certainly these figures indicate at the very least the difficulty of applying consistently MS diagnostic standards by different neurologists in different locations; a point emphasised by Ford and colleagues (1996) regarding the Poser criteria. Here the problem was not with the interpretation of clinical evidence but with historical records in patients' notes in deciding whether earlier relapses had actually occurred. All this material was also strongly suggestive of the difficulty of diagnosing MS at all. From a patient's perspective, however, they indicated that there were many people in the world worrying about their diagnosis that did not quite make it to the elevated heights of definite MS, confined to its definitional penumbra indefinitely until something more positive diagnostically turned up, or they suffered a more overt neurological disturbance. This was not a positive state of affairs.

The McDonald criteria (McDonald et al. 2001) in general followed what has been suggested above but with some crucial developments, most notably the inclusion of strict criteria for the use of MRI evidence to demonstrate dissemination of lesions in time and space. Specifically using the McDonald diagnostic schema a diagnosis of MS may be given if one of the following five sets of criteria were met:

1. Two or more attacks with objective clinical evidence from MRI of two or more lesions
2. Two or more attacks with objective clinical evidence of one lesion plus:
    i. dissemination in space demonstrated by MRI or
    ii. two or more MRI-detected lesions consistent with MS plus positive CSF or
    iii. a further clinical attack implicating a different site.

3. One attack with objective clinical evidence of two more lesions plus:
   i. dissemination in time demonstrated by MRI or
   ii. a second clinical attack
4. One attack with objective clinical evidence of one lesion (CIS) plus:
   i. dissemination in space demonstrated by MRI or
   ii. two or more MRI-detected lesions consistent with MS plus positive CSF and dissemination in time demonstrated by MRI or
   iii. a second clinical attack.
5. Insidious neurological progression suggestive of MS (PPMS) plus:
   i. Positive CSF and dissemination in space demonstrated by MRI or
   ii. Abnormal VEP plus specified brain lesions on MRI and dissemination in time demonstrated by MRI or
   iii. Continuous progression for 1 year.

In addition, these criteria clarified how to identify separate attacks or relapses by proposing the arbitrary time of 30 days between the onset of a first attack from the beginning of a second attack, noting that in adopting such a rule of thumb there was no need to be able to estimate when the first attack actually ended. The McDonald panel also conceded that some patients with an appropriate clinical presentation for a diagnosis of MS may, nevertheless, fail to satisfy some of the criteria for a formal diagnosis of the disease and that these individuals may be considered to have 'possible MS' (McDonald et al. 2001, 122).

What is important to notice here is that these MS diagnostic criteria were essentially for the standard presentations of MS in western European and North American populations where sophisticated technologies are available. Indeed, they have been adopted by 66 per cent of the countries contributing to the WHO/MSIF (2008) Atlas of MS. Nevertheless, in the MS prevalence work of Visser et al. (2012, 721) in north east Scotland, that must be regarded as part of the 'western' world, the lack of available MRI evidence restricted the giving of an MS diagnosis according to the McDonald criteria in 7 per cent of cases. In many poorer parts of the world, however, where MRI technologies may be scarce they may not be so easily applied. For example, with evidence again from the afore-mentioned Atlas of MS (WHO/MSIF 2008, 20), it was noted that in Africa only 0.004 MRI machines existed per 100,000 people compared with 0.31 in Europe. What this material also suggests is that even in the 'west' until all large neurology departments have access to MRI technology those living nearest to these sites have a definite advantage. They will most likely be diagnosed faster than those living further away (Dalton et al. 2002, 47), have the progress of their disease more easily monitored and perhaps as a consequence stand a much better chance of taking part in the clinical trials of new drugs.

The McDonald criteria, however, were not welcomed universally. After comparing them with the Poser criteria and having difficulty allocating four individuals to any of the new categories, surprisingly therefore excluding even more people from a potential diagnosis of MS, Fox et al. (2004, 58) lament, 'it is difficult to see how they are superior to the current Poser criteria.' In fact, in this study of MS in Plymouth in 2001, 446 PwMS were defined using the Poser criteria, of which 44 had suspected MS, whereas using the McDonald criteria 4 were reclassified as 'not MS' (Fox et al. 2004, 58), with no use of the McDonald 'possible' category. And, as a result, the prevalence for definite and probable MS for Plymouth was reduced from 118 per 100,000 inhabitants to 117. Admittedly this is only a very small change, but it is yet another downward pressure on the frequency of people with the illness, in the number of people who can receive a positive diagnosis. Interestingly another UK study to apply both the Poser and McDonald criteria, in north Northern Ireland in 2004 (Gray et al. 2008), made no comment on their relative merits or difficulty of interpretation. By contrast, a third study in South East Wales in 2005 (Hirst et al. 2009) observed that both systems produced the same number of PwMS with the McDonald criteria leading to a greater proportion of definite disease, thereby 'elevating patients to a more secure diagnostic classification' (Hirst et al. 2009, 390).

What some may find difficult to accept in this schema is the number of times waiting for another relapse or episode of demyelination is suggested before a formal diagnosis of MS can be given, for two very different reasons. First, on ethical grounds, that despite in many occasions a second episode is to be expected and a doctor's duty is to relieve suffering nothing is to be done. Second, if the initiation of DMDs as soon as possible is believed to limit future neurological damage, then possible beneficial therapy is not being offered when it should be. There is a third difficult issue too that complicates these ethical matters even further, the knowledge that a small number of patients presenting with a first demyelination episode will not have a second one and go on to lead apparently normal lives with clinically silent MS. Offering uncomfortable and expensive therapy to them when there was no need must be avoided. Unfortunately, at the moment there is no way of identifying such fortunate individuals.

The revision of these criteria by Polman et al. (2005) made a number of technical changes to the ways in which MRI information should be interpreted for a positive diagnosis of MS, including the inclusion of spinal cord damage, and changed the recommendations for the diagnosis of PPMS such that in certain circumstances a CSF analysis may not be necessary. Avoiding the need for a lumbar puncture wherever possible must be viewed as a very positive development because it can have most uncomfortable after effects. They also made one important observation that may signal a change in diagnostic policy for the future. While reaffirming the importance of the dissemination of lesions in time and space in the CNS, they added that 'in a hierarchical fashion, rigorous demonstration of dissemination in time might be more important than dissemination in space' (p.842). This seems a very positive suggestion since it is the confirmation of the processes of inflammation, demyelination and axonal loss in the CNS that are important, not necessarily where in the CNS they are taking place. Furthermore, it is the demonstration of such processes that will impact on what therapeutic interventions may be appropriate. Indeed, one episode of demyelination may be enough to demonstrate that the processes typical of MS are taking place. Of course, experience has shown that in such circumstances there are likely to be a number of silent, sub-clinical, lesions as well that may show up on MRI. But, it may not always be the case. It is possible that only one episode will take place, with the processes either being naturally turned off or operating so slowly that another one simply does not happen; that is a very benign form with no apparent dissemination in time. Similarly, there could easily be no dissemination in space within the CNS; all episodes taking place in one region. For example, in the regional study of MS in Leeds in 1996, 1 per cent of cases, 8 individuals, had recurrent episodes in only one region of the CNS with neither clinical signs nor symptoms of the involvement of another (Ford et al. 1998, 608). The dilemma for the clinician in such situations is to decide whether to start such patients on DMDs knowing the risks, discomfort and costs involved, or to wait for more definite evidence of MS continuance. It would seem the latter is powering these most recent MS definitions not knowledge of the underlying processes. It may also be a worry that these definitional schemes have become rather more concerned with fitting a disease to a name, it must be multiple, than fitting a name to a disease process such as demyelination and axonal loss.

 The use of the McDonald principles for MS diagnosis and especially the increased employment of MRI are expected to speed up the diagnostic process (Polman et al. 2005, 842) and as a direct consequence, therefore, over the following decade or so an increase in MS incidence and prevalence may well be detectable purely because ascertainment practices have improved. No such trend, however, was observable in the MS incidence increase in South East Wales between 1985 and 2005 investigated by Hirst and colleagues (2009, 289). Nevertheless, this must be regarded as a potentially enduring problem of MS epidemiological research. Indeed, a study of the diffusion of MRI techniques through time across the UK, Europe and perhaps prospectively across the second and third worlds with its expected increase in MS diagnoses may be a useful future research project to consider.

However, the earlier diagnosis of MS through time generates major problems for the comparison of different cohorts of PwMS of different dates. For example, it will almost certainly mean that the newly diagnosed with relapsing remitting MS (RRMS) today and in the future will be younger than those of the past and, therefore, may lead to longer time periods from diagnosis to major relapses, serious disability and the onset of progression. This could give the erroneous suggestion to the unwary that early drug treatments, for example, were working in slowing the disease down when in fact nothing of the kind had taken place. Measuring disease mile stones from the CIS may therefore be an advisable development.

Notwithstanding the careful consideration that has been lavished on theses definitional criteria, the formal diagnosis of someone with MS is still a difficult undertaking in which errors even by the most experienced neurologists can be made, not least because there are many different conditions for which MS can be mistaken as Miller et al. (2008) make clear. An indication that such outcomes are possible can be elicited from the study of Gray et al. (2008) on MS in Northern Ireland where it was discovered that of those deemed to have definite MS in 2004 who had undergone appropriate supportive diagnostic tests, 12.2 per cent had normal CSF, 18.6 per cent normal VEP and 4.8 per cent a normal MRI. A further example of the complicated and involved outcomes from MS diagnoses came from the work of Hirst et al. (2008a) in a study of the changing disability of PwMS in South East Wales over a 20-year period from 1985. In that year 380 individuals with either a definite or probable diagnosis of MS using the Poser criteria were identified. By 2005, 10 were considered not to have MS at all because either a consultant neurologist had reviewed the case to decide an alternative diagnosis was more likely or a post mortem had found no pathological evidence of the disease. In other words, the problems of MS diagnosis can be profound.

The issue of speedy diagnosis is an important one for many reasons. There is the view already noted that the earlier the better so as to begin with DMDs although this is not a unanimous view; some are of the belief that a wait for up to three years for confirmed RRMS through relapses will have no deleterious impact on therapeutic impacts (Dalton et al. 2002). While the medical case may be ambiguous, the social case is far less so. First, there is confirming to a worried patient exactly what illness they may have; some find this reassuring. More importantly is the social context in which such a diagnosis is likely to be given, during the late 20s and early 30s of someone's life. This is a crucial time for many people, a time that establishes long-term structures in their lives, potentially for the rest of their lives and most likely expected to be so: jobs, relationships and marriage, major financial commitments such as mortgages for a house, the starting of a family. It is shown in this book that MS affects peoples' lives in very direct ways, but how does the diagnosis itself impact on peoples' decisions at this crucial time? Could it make PwMS question their involvement in long-term relationships for fear of burdening their potential partner with becoming their carer as disability increases, or not being able to support them financially or emotionally? Could it stop an employer offering a permanent job to someone with MS because they do want to take the risk of allowing them time off work for relapses or invest in their training when they may have to retire early due to ill health? Similarly, would a mortgage provider be willing to offer a long-term loan to someone with MS whose long-term earning prospects may be questionable? And, could it also make someone question their lives more fundamentally to decide what they want to do before they die and set about completing them immediately before disability might set in? But, more generally, would a diagnosis of MS speed someone's life up to achieve as much as they can as quickly as they can, slow it down to take as few chances as possible at exacerbating their symptoms, or create completely different behaviours altogether? This is a wholly unexplored avenue for future social MS research.

In what follows much of the empirical evidence on PwMS, especially of a regional nature will come from a transitional period in which the liberal definition of MS of A&M is steadily replaced by the more discriminatory Poser definition which in turn starts to be substituted by the more technically demanding McDonald criteria. This can be seen in Table 3.2 for the regional prevalence research undertaken in the UK between 1985 and 2009. It may also be worth remembering that around the definitions of MS offered by the Poser and McDonald schemas lies a potentially large diagnostic penumbra of individuals who may or may not have the disease and probably worry far too pessimistically about what they actually do have.

Table 3.2 The definition of MS used in recent UK regional studies

Area	Year of survey	MS definition used
Sutton (south London)	1985	A&M
South Glamorgan	1985	A&M, Poser
South Hampshire	1987	A&M, Poser
South Glamorgan	1988	Poser
5 GP Practices in rural Suffolk	1988	A&M
Rochdale	1989	A&M, Poser
South and east Cambridgeshire	1990	A&M, Poser
Guernsey and Jersey	1991	A&M, Poser
Brighton and mid-Downs	1991	Poser
South and east Cambridgeshire	1993	A&M, Poser
North Cambridgeshire	1993	A&M, Poser
Lothian / Borders	1995	Poser
Leeds	1996	Poser
North Northern Ireland	1996	A&M, Poser
Tayside	1996	A&M, Poser
Fife	1996	Not given: based on GP records and judgement
Leeds	1999	Poser
Central Glasgow	2000	Pragmatic – documented evidence of an MS diagnosis by a neurologist
Plymouth	2001	Poser and McDonald
Tayside	2002	Poser
North Northern Ireland	2004	Poser and McDonald
South Glamorgan	2005	Poser and McDonald
Aberdeen city, Orkney and Shetland combined	2009	Poser and McDonald

Sources: Williams and McKernan (1986), Swingler and Compston (1988), Hennessy et al. (1989), Roberts et al. (1991), Lockyer (1991), Mumford et al. (1992), Sharpe et al. (1995), Rice-Oxley et al. (1995), Shepherd and Summers (1996), Robertson et al. (1995), Robertson et al. (1996b), Rothwell and Charlton (1998), Ford et al. (1998), Grant et al. (1998), McDonnell and Hawkins (1998), Forbes et al. (1999), Ford et al. (2002), Murray et al. (2004), Fox et al. (2004), Donnan et al. (2005), Gray et al. (2008), Hirst et al. (2009), Visser et al. (2012).

3.3 Approaches to research on PwMS

In general terms four different styles of approach to research on PwMS can be identified. First, attempts at counting the number of PwMS in a defined area using various modes of ascertainment for prevalence and incidence estimates. Second, the progression of some of these regional information sets into defined data bases or registers to permit the tracking of clinical and demographic evidence through time. Third, the surveying of large numbers of PwMS, using either random or self-selecting techniques contacted either through the afore-mentioned data bases or via patient association membership lists. Finally, the last approach relates to the use of small groups of PwMS for detailed interview to be analysed using qualitative techniques.

3.3.1 Regional counts

Prevalence and incidence research, that has often provided basic demographic evidence on PwMS as well as their frequencies, has depended in the first instance on the identification of lists of PwMS for a specified area. Because, in many parts of the world including the UK no nationally functioning morbidity data base exists for all its citizens, a number of other sources of information, individually and collectively, have had to be used for this task. These have included all the sources of medical and social support as well as patient and disease specific charities. For example, to construct a provisional list of PwMS for the Southampton and South West Hampshire Health Authority area in 1987, eight sources of ascertainment were employed: GPs; hospital activity analyses; local branch of the MS Society; ARMS (Action into Research for Multiple Sclerosis); daily admission books of the regional neurological unit; three local consultant neurologists; local Dependent Disabled Register; Young Disabled Unit (Roberts et al. 1991, 55). Much later in 2001, Fox et al. (2004, 56) also employed eight different sources to compile their provisional list of PwMS in the Plymouth region. These included pre-existing hospital databases and discharge letters; hospital episode statistics; MS Specialist nurse case files; VEP data; MS support groups; community therapy services; letters, phone calls and visits to GPs; nursing homes of which 40 out of 45 responded. Similar multiple sources of information were also required in the construction of regional prevalence and incidence estimates in regional epidemiological research in North America too including hospitals/clinics, physicians, nursing homes and patient associations (Evans et al. 2013) and in the pan-Australia research by Hammond et al. (1988).

When a provisional population of PwMS for an area has been established each entry then needs to have their diagnosis confirmed either through hospital and GP notes or by direct neurological assessment. In these exercises the records of either hospital neurology departments or GPs have invariably been the most profitable sources in correctly identifying prevalent cases of MS as can be seen in Table 3.3 where the most important sources in 23 recent UK regional surveys are given. In this context the evidence from neurology departments was especially

Table 3.3 The most important source for recent regional surveys of PwMS

Area	Year of survey	Data source	Percentage cover of prevalent cases (%)
Sutton (south London)	1985	Hospital records	55 of provisional list.
South Glamorgan	1985	Neuro' Dept	95
South Hampshire	1987	GPs	73
South Glamorgan	1988	Neuro' Dept*	Not given
5 GP Practices in rural Suffolk	1988	GPs	84
Rochdale	1989	Neuro' Dept	79
South and east Cambridgeshire	1990	Neuro' Dept	78
Guernsey and Jersey	1991	GPs	Not given
Brighton and mid-Downs	1991	Insufficient details given	
South and east Cambridgeshire	1993	Neuro' Dept	83
North Cambridgeshire	1993	GPs	67
Lothian / Borders	1995	Neuro' Dept	62
Leeds	1996	Neuro' Dept	59
North Northern Ireland	1996	GPs	80
Tayside	1996	GPs	68
Fife	1996	GPs	95
Leeds	1999	Neuro' Dept*	90*
Central Glasgow	2000	GPs	89
Plymouth	2001	Hospital records	79
Tayside	2002	Neuro' Dept*	Not given
North Northern Ireland	2004	GPs	83
South Glamorgan	2005	GPs	73
Aberdeen city, Orkney and Shetland combined	2009	GPs	93.6

Sources: Williams and McKernan (1986), Swingler and Compston (1988), Hennessy et al. (1989), Roberts et al. (1991), Lockyer (1991), Mumford et al. (1992), Sharpe et al. (1995), Rice-Oxley et al. (1995), Shepherd and Summers (1996), Robertson et al. (1995), Robertson et al. (1996b), Rothwell and Charlton (1998), Ford et al. (1998), Grant et al. (1998), McDonnell and Hawkins (1998), Forbes et al. (1999), Ford et al. (2002), Murray et al. (2004), Fox et al. (2004), Donnan et al. (2005), Gray et al. (2008), Hirst et al. (2009), Visser et al. (2012).

* PwMS carried over from the previous study.

significant because it was the neurologists in these departments who were needed to confirm the MS diagnoses. The lowest proportion accounted for by such a source in this set of studies was in Leeds in 1996 with only 59 per cent of prevalent cases and the highest in South Glamorgan in 1985 at 95 per cent. By contrast, in Sutton in 1985 and for Plymouth in 2004 more general hospital records identified the most PwMS for their areas. Swingler and Compston (1988, 1522) confirm the importance of their collective hospital information by pointing out that the use of their two main hospital sources, discharge notices from the neurology department and hospital activity returns, would have identified 98.9 per cent of all their confirmed cases of MS. However, in the more recent regional epidemiological work evidence of PwMS from GPs has become of much greater importance. For example, they furnished 73 per cent of cases in South Glamorgan in 2005 (Hirst et al. 2009, 387), 89 per cent in central Glasgow in 2000 (Murray et al. 2004, 102), 80 per cent in the most northerly parts of Northern Ireland in both 1996 and 2004 (McDonnell and Hawkins 1998, 425) and 83 per cent (Gray et al. 2008, 882) respectively and in Aberdeen city, Orkney and Shetland combined 94 per cent (Visser et al. 2012). Finally, it is important to note from Table 3.3 that in no case did the membership lists of the national MS charities provide the most confirmed regional cases of MS. The best coverage they ever provided was 42 per cent in South Hampshire in 1987 (Roberts et al. 1991), 39 per cent in south and east Cambridgeshire in 1990 (Mumford et al. 1992) and 31.5 per cent in north Northern Ireland in 2004 (Gray et al. 2008). However, it must be remembered that in these comparisons of regional ascertainment sources not every source was accessible in every region.

What is also important to note is that as medical records became increasingly computerised, the memories of the doctors concerned became less important. Hirst and colleagues (2009, 389) pointed out that such memories were often remarkably accurate because only 8 patients with MS (1.8% of the total) were identified in the GP computerised data bases in 2005 that should have been included in an earlier survey of their region of South Glamorgan in 1985 that relied more on GP memories. Further evidence for the high regard in which GP evidence was held by some researchers may come from the work of Phadke and Downie (1987) in 1980 who bundled all the cases of PwMS they had collected from five other sources into their GP groups who were then asked to remove those no longer on their lists and add any new ones. That is, GPs became the final arbiter of who was included and who was not in their study. A similar approach was adopted in Rochdale in 1989 (Shepherd and Summers 1996) and in Fife in 1996 (Grant et al. 1998). In essence, therefore, very little may have changed from the first attempted regional survey of MS, or disseminated sclerosis as it was called then, by Allison in 1929 for North Wales. He argued that GPs were the ideal source of case ascertainment because MS was a memorable disease due to its rarity and serious symptoms that would lead quickly to the seeking of hospital help. He therefore concluded, 'In this way, the cases in his district, if any, will be known to him' (Allison 1931, 395), if the anachronistic language can be forgiven. Sadly recent evidence no longer supports this view. For example, in Leeds in 1996 the GPs had no records on 44 per cent of the PwMS, and in Plymouth in 2001 the equivalent figure was 26 per cent. It is depressing indeed that for such a potentially devastating disease the doctors responsible for the delivery of primary care appeared to know so few of their MS patients.

In some cases doctors may not release information on some or all their patients with MS for a number of very good reasons. First, there will be those patients with only minor signs of the illness who the doctor is reluctant to tell of their diagnosis who stand little chance to be on any MS list (Robertson et al. 1996b, 277). Second, there may be some doctors who will not supply information on their patients with MS for confidentiality reasons. This occurred in two cases in the 1993 Cambridgeshire investigation by Robertson et al. (1996b, 275). There may be many other reasons too such as pressure of work, but perhaps contemporary information technology may be making this task less onerous and tending to improve GP responses. For example, in South Glamorgan in 1985 only 69 per cent of GPs responded to a request for details of the PwMS on their lists (Swingler and Compston 1988, 1520). But, 20 years later a similar inquiry produced the much better 89 per cent response (Hirst et al. 2009, 387). It is also worth pointing out at this juncture that even when administrative systems are in place the accuracy of GP information can be questioned. Not only may this be in terms of diagnostic accuracy but more especially in updating their records when patient transfers between practices and deaths are concerned. Indeed, Murray et al. (2004) have suggested this could produce a 5 per cent inflation of totals.

3.3.2 Data bases and registers

Some of the most problematic research issues to undertake on PwMS of both a medical and a social nature concern change over time simply because the illness is for life and the lives of PwMS are of almost normal duration. Few researchers, therefore, will be able to follow a person with MS from diagnosis to death and probably fewer funding agencies will have the patience to wait for many years for usable research outputs. Yet such longitudinal evidence is increasingly in demand as new drug, symptomatic-relief therapies, care pathways and preventative regimens are being introduced and trialled, but also as PwMS themselves demand better treatment and a better quality of life. Thus, health organisations and MS-patient support organisations need reliable evidence on the changing lives of PwMS along with their changing needs for support and different forms of care. Unfortunately, very few research organisations seemed to have taken steps to accrue the data to tackle such issues and therefore little evidence of this longitudinal nature is available anywhere in the world and even fewer analyses of such material. There have been a small number of regional studies of change in health-related variables between just two or three points in time in the UK such as in Cambridgeshire (Robertson et al. 1996b), Leeds (Ford et al. 2002), north Northern Ireland (Gray et al. 2008), Tayside (Donnan et al. 2005) and especially in South Glamorgan where some individuals with MS have been tracked since 1985 (Hirst et al. 2008b). But, in none of these examples was the evidential base designed for the long term with year on year data inputs. In addition, the precursor charity of the MS Trust, ARMS, attempted to establish a register of PwMS who were willing to have their details used in research that in 1983 totalled 826 individuals (Monks and Robinson 1989). However, apart from two obscure papers by Robinson (1988 and 1991) little seems to have come of this initiative.

In South East Wales, an extensive database of patients with MS has been built up over the last three decades at the Department of Neurology at the University Hospital of Wales in Cardiff. It began with the population based survey of PwMS in South Glamorgan in 1985 reported in Swingler and Compston (1988). Since then an equivalent survey was carried out 20 years later (Hirst et al. 2009), and patient records on clinical and many demographic variables have been prospectively updated where possible but especially since 1999 (Hirst et al. 2008b). This has resulted in an information record of some sort on 2,050 PwMS in the area, thought to be approximately 90 per cent of the prevalent total (Hirst et al. 2008a, 281). It has been used in a number of seminal inquiries into MS incidence (Hirst et al. 2009), deaths (Hirst et al. 2008b), disability progression (Hirst et al. 2008a and 2008b), the validity of patient-derived data (Ingram et al. 2010) and the relationship between relapses and depression (Moore et al. 2012).

In other countries, however, a number of MS research visionaries did begin to develop suitable data sets for long-term purposes. Good examples of this work exist in London Ontario that began in 1972, British Columbia in 1980, New York State in 1996 and Lyons and Burgundy in France at the start of the twenty-first century. In addition, in the US the Department of Veteran Affairs has provided evidence on people in the armed forces who developed MS from 1998 and a national patient-led data-base, the North American Research Committee on MS (NARCOMS) began in the mid-1990s with by now as many as 17,000 active participants (Hurwitz 2011a and 2011b). However, the gold standard for such work is to be found in Denmark where a registration system for all citizens has permitted the creation of a national register of PwMS since1956 that can be directly linked with other morbidity and demographic data sets (Koch-Henriksen et al. 2001). While all these data bases suffer from problems of comparability because of different modes of ascertainment and diagnostic criteria, they have nevertheless produced a number of useful general observations on issues such as disability progression and life expectancy, to be discussed later in this book, that have enhanced the case for equivalent data sets elsewhere in the world such as in Germany and New Zealand. Unfortunately, in the UK a far-less coordinated approach has materialised with three different data bases under construction in the second decade of the twenty-first century: The South West Impact of Multiple Sclerosis Project (SWIMS), the Scottish MS Register and the UK MS Register project.

The Scottish MS Register is an incidence database that has attempted to amass evidence on all new cases of MS in that country since 1 January 2010 using the Poser or McDonald diagnostic criteria. As such a possible diagnosis of MS or a CIS designation is not included. The data collected includes demographic information, family history of MS, date of first symptoms, referrals, types of investigations, diagnosis and MS nurse involvement. The information is collected in a hospital environment and collated by the Information Services Division of NHS (National Health Service) Scotland where it is handled in accordance with the principles of the Data Protection Act (1990) to ensure confidentiality. No information on the number of cases collected by this register has yet been published on their website.

The UK MS Register, launched formally in May 2011, is in the process of being developed in pilot form for a set of five areas that will include NHS centres in Belfast, Edinburgh, Swansea, London and Nottingham, but in parallel includes a national trawl for evidence too (Ford et al. 2012). In the early stages of this project, the emphasis has been on the creation of computer systems that will store personal evidence anonymously and then link that data with their medical records (MS Society website). Eventually the aim will be to offer a national, efficient, sustainable and easy-to-use system for the long term, although the precise definition of MS to be adopted has not yet been made clear. For the most comprehensive picture possible of life with MS in the UK it would be advantageous if the Scottish and UK registers were compatible, but whether this will be possible seems not to have been established.

The UK MS Register collects evidence through an opt-in system in which PwMS of 18 years and above, once convinced it is a good idea to take part, must access a particular website to enter their details. This register project therefore ignores those PwMS who for whatever reason do not have easy access to a computer and those with MS of less than 18 years of age. The numbers of PwMS who may fall into these categories is unknown. In addition, there must be a serious concern that the PwMS who join the Register may be biased in some systematic way because this is a self-selecting form of data collection. Such biases may be in terms of, for example, membership of the MS Society (the sponsors of the project), highly likely since 77 per cent of the early participants heard of the project from this source (Osborne et al. 2012, 32), age (those with the time to fill out the forms) or level of education (those who can most easily appreciate its benefits and fill out the forms efficiently). Thus, the representativeness of the Register's evidence must be challenged. In one of the Register's initial projects, on anxiety and depression in PwMS (Jones et al. 2012), there appeared to be some confusion on this issue. At one point their research report stated (p.8) that 'Within the sample there were a broad range of ages and MS durations and our respondents were reasonably representative of the characteristics of prevalent MS cohorts reported elsewhere'. This may be so but, this is an inappropriate comparison because only one of the cited references was for a UK location, Cornwall and Devon in SW England. Yet, later on they accepted that 'The study was based on self-reported information and the respondents were not necessarily a fully representative sample of people with MS in the UK' (p.9). Why try to pretend otherwise? However, to resolve such concerns conclusively may require an attempt at the full enumeration of all PwMS in at least one of the UK Register's pilot regions. What does appear to be the case is that the UK Register project is enumerating more PwMS with a relapsing remitting form of the disease compared to other national or regional surveys that is more people with a relatively early form of the illness. For example, in the previous chapter (Table 2.1) it was estimated from various sources that RRMS accounted for approximately 45 per cent of PwMS in the UK, but the UK Register's sample reported 63 per cent of respondents with this form of MS. Yet, there was no major difference in the ages of the Register members and the average for the regional cohort evidence noted above; the mean age for the former being 50.8 years (Ford et al. 2012) and for the latter 49.7 years. This is another issue about the UK Register evidence that needs resolving.

One further serious concern of longitudinal data bases is the need to secure evidence from the members of the register on a regular basis (say annually) over the long term otherwise it will soon become moribund and irrelevant. This necessitates the data base organisers to accomplish successfully the formidable task of maintaining the interest of their subjects indefinitely. Whether this will be possible remains to be seen.

The SWIMS project is much smaller in scope than the other two initiatives, consisting of only the two counties of Devon and Cornwall in South West England, but is far more advanced in terms of evidence collected and in the publication of initial findings (Zajicek et al. 2010). This project also includes a regular informative newsletter that is available online. The SWIMS initiative has three clearly defined objectives:

1. To develop improved measurement instruments for clinical trials.
2. To evaluate the longitudinal performance of a variety of patient-reported outcome measures.
3. To develop prognostic predictors for use in individualising drug treatment for patients, particularly early on in the disease course.

Thus, this is very much about developing a longitudinal medical understanding of MS from a patient's perspective in which any useful social evidence will be initially of only marginal concern. This, however, does not negate the SWIMS database being employed in future social science research activity.

Since August 2004 PwMS have been asked to take part in the SWIMS project through four main mechanisms:

1. Patients attending neurology clinics, accounting for 63 per cent of recruits.
2. Patients identified from hospital case notes to be approached by a neurologist (21% of recruits).
3. GPs who were asked to approach patients not already taking part (6% of recruits).
4. Patients who self-referred after awareness campaigns through the MS Society, local media and the SWIMS website (6% of recruits).

The project is therefore heavily dependent on the neurology clinic for its contacts with PwMS that has the added advantage of helping to confirm formal MS diagnoses.

By the beginning of 2010, the SWIMS project had recruited almost 1,000 PwMS for which the baseline characteristics have been described in Zajicek et al. (2010) and of those approached to take part 75 per cent had agreed to do so. This is a remarkable achievement because the input demanded from each recruit was not trivial. For those individuals with a clinical diagnosis of MS, an initial set of nine separate questionnaires measuring different aspects of a person's disease, abilities and quality of life have to be completed, followed at six-monthly intervals by a follow-up questionnaire. What is more, by April 2008 only 88 individuals with MS (8%) had been lost to follow up, including 25 deaths and 15 moving out of the area, and 92 per cent of all questionnaire booklets had been returned (Zajicek et al. 2010, 4).

This database certainly has great promise for the future, but as described in Zajicek et al. (2010) raises three concerns. The first concern is a perennial one for these kind of samples, namely their representativeness of the wider population from which they were drawn. Ideally such a database should include all those with MS, but this would have been impossible to achieve for a number of straightforward reasons. These included, for example, PwMS not hearing about the project to those not wishing to take part. In this case too some PwMS were deliberately excluded, namely those with MS less than 18 years of age and those who were too cognitively impaired to complete the necessary paperwork. But, did some PwMS deliberately exclude themselves? Zajicek and colleagues believe they did not pointing out that 'The demographics of the SWIMS sample were similar to other surveys of MS in regions of the UK' (Zajicek et al. 2010, 6). Although only a limited range of characteristics is presented, this would appear to be true in terms of age at entry but not so clear cut for gender balance. The mean age at entry of PwMS into the SWIMS project was 51.6 years and the mean for the 21 regional studies in Table 4.3 was 49.7 years rising to 51.9 years for the four regions investigated in the 1990s which is exactly the same age as the mean for the 4 national surveys of MwMS (members of the MS Society with MS) in Table 4.1. The equivalent female/male ratio for the regional studies in Table 4.2 was 2.4 rising to 2.6 for those undertaken in the 1990s that is the precise figure for the national surveys of MwMS (Table 4.1). All of which were somewhat lower than for the SWIMS database at 3.01. Unfortunately, what was not considered were the characteristics that were most likely to lead to people taking part in this project such as their level of education, affluence and membership of the MS charities? Could it be therefore that the SWIMS project is principally a survey of MS charity membership in Devon and Cornwall, an issue already noted relating to the national UK register?

The second issue of concern is the arithmetic error in the calculation of the expected number of PwMS in their region based on the MS prevalence of 118/100,000 inhabitants obtained from epidemiological work in Plymouth in 2001 by Fox et al. (2004). If such a rate was applied to the population of Cornwall and Devon of 1.7 million people, then a figure of 2,006 PwMS resulted, not the 1,800 given in the text, and at a stroke the percentage coverage of their 967 recruits is reduced to less than 50 per cent. What is more, this issue escalates alarmingly if the MS prevalence rate for England of 199.9/100,000 obtained by Mackenzie and colleagues (2014) in their General Practice Research Database (GPRD) assessment of the number of PwMS in the UK were used to estimate the expected frequency of PwMS in the SWIMS region.

The final area of concern relates to the announcement by Zajicek and colleagues (2010, 3) that Devon and Cornwall were ideal for longitudinal study because 'the population is relatively stable and migration rates are low.' This is just not so. The South West of England as a whole, that admittedly is much larger than just Cornwall and Devon, revealed the largest net regional inflow of migrants in the UK at the end of the twentieth century and the beginning of the twenty-first century (National Statistics Online). For example, in 2001 there were 143,000 in-migrants to and 111,000 out-migrants from the South West to other parts of the UK (Regional Trends 2008, 95). For Cornwall specifically, the Demographic Evidence Base published by its county council stated that migration was the single greatest driver of population change with middle and older working age groups being the most active, not the retired (Cornwall Council 2009) and, although a similar analysis has not been undertaken for Devon, migration rates were very similar. For example, for the year after SWIMS began to recruit, 2005, inflow of migrants to Devon were 3.8 per cent of total population and outflows 3.2 per cent, while equivalent figures for Cornwall were 3.9 per cent and 2.9 per cent respectively.[2] Furthermore, at the larger spatial scale of the local authority district, Torridge in Devon recorded the highest net inflow of UK migrants of any equivalent area in England and Wales in 2006; a staggering 2 per cent of its population (Social Trends 2008, 9). This is not an area with a stable population through time.

Research on PwMS regularly requires the collection of personal information through surveys, registers and from medical records. However, in many countries the introduction of data protection and confidentiality regulations has generated considerable legal and ethical implications on such activities. In particular, they have made the whole process of the collection, storage and use of personal data much more legally worrying and administratively burdensome for the researcher. For example, there is often the expectation and legal requirement for informed consent for all personal information collected and stored during research work and the enduring worry that many members of the public will wish to keep their personal details private and not allow their use (Lawlor and Stone 2001, Baird et al. 2009). As a result, the notion that individuals and especially patients have a responsibility, as well as rights, to the wider societal benefits research can produce becomes irrelevant. For clinical research in the UK, however, the situation is even more onerous with ethical compliance required at the local health trust level, at the national level (National Research Ethics Service) and at the European Union level (the Clinical Trials Directive) too.

For one-off questionnaire surveys, individuals can exercise a choice not to allow their data to be used simply by not responding. For longer term projects, such as disease registers, however, where multiple responses or data inputs may be required over many years this issue is much more worrying. Fortunately this does not seem to be the case for MS in the UK or at least for England and Northern Ireland in which a very positive altruistic standpoint towards the use of personal data in an MS register was discovered in a series of 10 focus groups with 55 individuals who either had MS or were professionally involved in their care (Baird et al. 2009, 93). This confirmed the earlier findings for an existing register in Leeds where only 4 per cent of individuals refused consent (Ford 2006). However, such information philanthropy is far from universal. More generally 'a conflict appears to exist, with public enthusiasm for health research mixed with concerns and caution over the use of personal information' (Baird et al. 2009, 93). For example, in a Canadian inquiry 28 per cent of a sample of PwMS would wish to be asked for their consent for the release of even anonymised data to medical researchers (Page and Mitchell 2006), while in the UK in other disease contexts Baird et al. (2009) observed that minority proportions of up to 25 per cent have been reported refusing consent for the use of their data. At this level of non-compliance serious biases in analytical results must be a concern.

Information on PwMS in the UK have been extracted from two relatively recent morbidity data systems concerned with the use of hospital and general practice services, the first with hospital attendance or episode figures and the second with the GPRD, the latter to be considered in some detail because of its use in three significant reports on UK MS incidence and prevalence by Alonso et al. (2007), Thomas et al. (2009) and Mackenzie et al. (2014).

In Scotland hospital admissions frequencies for MS since 1997 from the Scottish Morbidity Records (SMR01) System were used by Handel et al. (2009b) for the 14 Scottish Health Board areas for the period from 1997 to 2009. The SMR01 System records all inpatient and day-care discharges from non-obstetric and non-psychiatric specialists in NHS hospitals in Scotland in which up to six different diagnoses can be recorded, the accuracy of which has been regularly audited by the Data Quality Assurance Department of the Information Services of NHS Scotland. Furthermore, data linkage systems were used to ensure that each person was identified only once irrespective of the number of admissions they may have had and allocated to the area of their first known admission. For the 28 English Strategic Health Authorities between 1998 and 2005, a file of linked hospital admission statistics built from the English Hospital Episode Statistics by the staff of the Oxford University Unit of Health-Care Epidemiology covering all NHS hospitals has been the data source in two geographical analyses linking MS admission rates with other diseases and ultraviolet radiation (Ramagopalan et al. 2011a and 2011b).

It has already been established in this chapter that hospital records will not account for all PwMS in a region, only a large proportion of them. In particular, people at both ends of the disability spectrum may rarely visit a neurologist and therefore be missing from this sort of evidence. As a result, such material may be of little use in establishing the magnitude of the MS burden in any area. However, it may be of use in a relative sense to indicate the ranking of places, the areas with the highest and lowest numbers of PwMS if admission practices could be shown to be similar across the regions. There may be a good case to be made for such a view if all health-care organisations followed similar protocols, and indeed Ramagopalan et al. (2011a) made a valiant attempt to demonstrate this for England by showing close correlations between different lengths of hospital stays. However, the empirical evidence on the medical care of patients with MS to be reviewed in Chapter 7 shows huge variation between places, a veritable post-code lottery. What is more, we have no idea of the degree to which hospitals in one health authority area actually care for the PwMS in their putative 'home' area. Could it be that a hospital with a good neurological reputation may develop a wide care hinterland stretching outside the boundaries of the health authority in which it resides? Thus, it is not at all clear that hospital admission biases were constant across either the Scottish or the English Health authorities and therefore their evidence must at best be thought of as merely indicative of trends and far from authoritative.

The collection electronically of GP evidence in the UK that would eventually lead to the GPRD began in earnest with the establishment of the venture capital company VAMP (Value Added Medical Products Ltd) in 1987 to recruit practices to generate a comprehensive observational database from clinical practice (Lawson et al. 1998, 445). Over time the intention was to produce a longitudinal medical record from primary care that included evidence by patient on: medical symptoms and signs; therapies and treatments; referrals, laboratory tests; demographics, lifestyle factors; registration and practice. The participating GPs agreed to be trained to provide this information in a standardised computer format and also agreed to provide photocopies of paper medical records if requested. In 1994 the Office of Population Censuses and Statistics (part of the Office for National Statistics) took over running the database on behalf of the Department of Health (Lawson et al. 1998, 445) and in the second decade of the twenty-first century was subsumed within the Clinical Practice Research Datalink at a time when it accounted for more than 4 million patient records, 8 per cent of the UK population in 2010 (Mackenzie et al. 2014).

For the pioneering VAMP database, Jick and colleagues (1991) investigated the degree to which diagnostic information sent by a consultant's letter was recorded onto patients' computer records. They discovered that for a sample of 1,191 cases 87 per cent (1,038 cases) had had the correct diagnosis transcribed onto their computer files and that for prescription drugs the success rate was higher at 90 per cent (Jick et al. 1991, 767). Similarly, van Staa and Abenhaim (1994) reviewing more than 500 discharge summaries discovered that the correct principal diagnosis was present in the computerised record in 90 per cent of cases. Whether these are acceptable proportions is a difficult question to answer. For a cohort of GPs who were supposed to be trained and willing to do such a task perhaps not, that may be mitigated by the fact that these studies were carried out in the early years of the computerisation process. However, this clearly is an important issue that must be regularly assessed if GP computer-based data is to be employed successfully for epidemiological, drug evaluation and health delivery research.

An evaluation of the use of GPRD information specifically for MS research was undertaken by Alonso et al. (2007) in an attempt to derive age and sex specific incidence rates for the UK; in other words rates of new cases of MS. This involved a two-stage process. First, for the period 1993–2000 all cases with a first diagnosis of MS and with at least one full year's worth of information on their record prior to diagnosis were identified. This generated 930 cases. Second, photocopies of all MS-related paperwork about these cases from GP surgeries were requested to try to confirm the diagnoses. This included consultation letters, specialist referrals, test results and hospital discharge letters. From this material 438 (47%) were confirmed as MS on review, 98 per cent of which had already been confirmed by a consultant neurologist in the UK (Alonso et al. 2007, 1737). The other 492 cases were not confirmed because of the following reasons:

1. They were prevalent MS (83 cases), that is, they already had MS and therefore could not be new cases.
2. A diagnosis of possible MS was given (59 cases).
3. They did not have MS (52 cases).
4. No medical records were available because the patient had transferred to another practice (71 cases).
5. The person had died (10 cases).
6. The GP did not collaborate (217 cases).

From this evidence the optimist might argue that, of the cases for which written paper evidence was available (632), the correct MS code had been given in both the incident cases (438) and the prevalent cases (83), that is 521cases or 82 per cent; the prevalent cases signifying a correct disease diagnosis but with the wrong stage of the illness; that is 82 per cent as the positive predictive value of an MS code in the GPRD. This was the view taken by Alonso et al. (2007) and by Thomas and colleagues (2009) in a later prevalence study of MS in the UK that formed the basis for the MS Society's view on the number of PwMS in the UK as 100,000. The super optimist, however, might go a stage further to argue that 'possible MS' is a perfectly acceptable element of the McDonald MS diagnostic system and therefore this group should also be included increasing the level of accuracy of the GPRD with an addition of 59 cases to 92 per cent. This would accord with the degree of predictive value of the GPRD for other conditions. As a counter the pessimist would be only too quick to point out that in the Alonso et al. (2007) exercise, that was supposed to identify incident cases of MS, only 438 (47%) could actually be confirmed from the material provided and only 580 (62%) cases of MS. Thus, it is difficult to accept that MS data in the GPRD has been properly validated by the Alonso et al. (2007) research other than to suggest that for any point in time more incident MS cases will be recorded than actually took place. There must, therefore, be a question mark over the degree to which aggregate data on MS from the GPRD can be believed.

Because of the extensive range of neurological codes on the GPRD, there has always been the possibility of an incorrect code for MS being entered accidently, never mind an unintentional misdiagnosis. Thomas et al. (2009) decided to adjust their prevalence estimates in two ways to try to take account of such possibilities, to offer two different estimates of the number of PwMS. First, they adjusted according to the proportion of definite MS cases with a record of a referral to a neurology department or with hospital feedback. This occurred in 75 per cent of female MS cases and 72 per cent of male MS cases to offer a minimum estimate of the number of PwMS. Second, they adjusted their figures according to the Alonso et al. (2007) proportion of 82 per cent to offer a maximum estimate. The argument, however, for 92 per cent accuracy of MS diagnoses would appear just as strong. By contrast, the investigation of GPRD evidence by Mackenzie et al. (2014) attempts to account for potential under-recording in a far from transparent way by using equivalent estimates from the 44 per cent of the GPRD entries to be found in Hospital Episode Statistics.

These observations reveal some awkward problems with this sort of analysis. First, and perhaps most seriously, that a large proportion of GPs may not take part in the provision of paper evidence although they have nominally agreed to do so. In the Alonso et al. (2007) example it was 23.3 per cent. As a consequence, an independent judgement of diagnostic veracity becomes impossible in almost a quarter of cases. If this issue is extended to include those individuals whose records were not available because they had either changed practice or died during the study period, then the proportion of unavailable paper records rises to 32.0 per cent! Indeed, this relative paucity of data validation is in Zajicek's (2007) view the principal weakness of this specific research and of the GPRD generally. He asks 'can we be sure that everyone with a label of MS has the diagnosis and people without a label do not?' (Zajicek 2007, 1742). Of course, no one ever shall be but, there is a need for some confidence in the vast majority of cases. In this research it would appear an acceptable proportion has not been reached. Finally, Alonso and colleagues' (2007) findings illustrate the degree of patient movement between practices, of 7.6 per cent, or 8.7 per cent if deaths are included too, at an annual rate of approximately 1 per cent.

Alonso et al. (2007, 1739) go on to observe that their study relied on two assumptions. Their first assumption was 'that the ascertainment of MS cases by GPs was complete.' From what we have already seen above from regional epidemiological studies in the UK, we know that was not the case, and in some cases could be less than 60 per cent. Their second assumption was that 'the proportion of true incident cases in practices that provide medical records was the same as in the others.' Their reasoning for this was that MS cases will hardly be wrongly identified by their general practitioners because they need such specialist care for the long term in which they, their GP, will play a pivotal role. This is a wholly unconvincing argument because in the early stages of the disease, when they are 'incident', the principal focus of this study, disability is often minimal and transient with medical needs limited; an easily disregarded situation. It is only much later in the disease when medical help may become increasingly necessary and needing a range of different specialisms that the disease becomes much more memorable for the GP.

There are two further issues concerning the GPRD data that require airing to be able to judge its usefulness in MS epidemiological work. The first issue revolves around the way chronic conditions were recorded and the second relates to its representativeness of the UK population. For the GPRD, a GP need only record a patient's diagnosis once on their computerised record, when the diagnosis actually occurs or perhaps again when a new drug is prescribed. Thus, for individuals with chronic conditions that have long periods of symptom and medication stability, such as MS, and especially the more benign or quiescent kind, an MS diagnosis may easily be missed if the GPRD is scanned for only a short period. As Hollowell (1997, 39) pointed out under such conditions prevalence will be underestimated because some patients with the chronic illness will not have the need to contact their GP during the period under scrutiny. It is also increasingly possible in the UK that PwMS may not consult their GP because their care is organised mainly via a hospital-based neurology unit or a specialist nurse. As Ford et al. (1998, 608) point out for the case of Leeds in which 20 per cent of prevalent cases in 1996 were 'apparently not known to their general practitioners', neurology services were seen as the main point of medical contact. In such cases GPs may not be directly informed of their patients' changing medical condition. These points have serious implications for the contemporary use of GPRD information for the study of MS and could easily lead to its estimated numbers being unnecessarily frugal.

On GPRD representativeness one must begin by arguing that because the UK National Health system provides a universal service for all citizens, no segment of the population should be excluded. Indeed, the correlations between the age/sex percentage distributions for England and Wales combined and the GPRD were extremely close (Lawson et al. 1998, 447). However, for regional populations there was substantial variation. For example, for the UK as a whole in the mid-1990s, the GPRD encompassed 6.0 per cent of the total population whereas for Scotland and Yorkshire the proportions were only 2.8 per cent and 3.0 per cent respectively. By contrast, the greatest regional coverage occurred in East Anglia at 12.2 per cent (Lawson et al. 1998, 447). The under-representation of Scotland for MS research purposes may be a particularly important observation because this area is known to have a relatively high prevalence of MS (see Chapter 5). This point was observed by Alonso et al. (2007, 1737) too, yet no deductions were drawn from it, not even that it would tend to depress estimates of incidence and prevalence below what they really should have been.

GPRD information has also been biased towards the larger GP practices such that in 1994 practices with one doctor accounted for only 18 per cent of GPRD contributing practices in England and Wales yet they were 31 per cent of all practices. Similar proportions for the biggest practices with 6 or more partners were 15 per cent and 11 per cent (Lawson et al. 1998, 446). And, single-doctor practices tended to be older male doctors significantly over-represented in inner-city locations (Gatrell and Elliott 2009, 135–6). Thus, the centres of London and Birmingham in particular may be poorly represented in the GPRD (Walley and Mantgani 1997, 1097; Hollowell 1997, 39). Is it possible to accept therefore that GPRD evidence is representative of practices in the UK? The jury must still be out on this issue.

3.3.3 Surveys of PwMS

For national survey work no complete list of PwMS exists and, therefore, proxies have had to be employed. Until recently the lists of national MS charities had been the principal realistic option. Now many PwMS may be contacted electronically through their participation in MS registers. But, as will be argued in what follows, it is crucial to realise that such research is usually of MwMS and not necessarily of all PwMS; these two populations may be different. Yet too often this issue is crudely glossed over with reference to a few demographic figures or virtually ignored altogether.

In order to draw inferences from a sample about the population from which it was drawn, and especially to be able to use powerful inferential statistical techniques, certain rules have to be followed. One of the most important of these, at least in terms of the chances of it being knowingly breached, is that each observation must be independent of all other observations. In other words no form of bias must enter the selection process. The accepted best way of achieving this result is by drawing a sample randomly so that each unit of observation has had an equal chance of selection. By contrast, allowing individuals to select themselves to take part in a survey, for example through an advert in a magazine or on a website breaks this rule. It directly allows a form of selection bias to enter the sampling process, creating an opportunity for particular subgroups of respondents to be over-represented such as the better educated, those good at filling out forms, those with most free time or those with the most serious grievance. Thus, in assessing the value of research findings, it is not just the veracity of the data sources that is important, it is also vital to understand the appropriateness of the methods to which they have been applied. Unfortunately, in what follows it will be shown that some of the most important and promising socio-economic research on PwMS undertaken in the UK in particular often presents significant methodological questions relating usually to sample definition that may limit the usefulness of its results. Three problem groups of approach can be identified. First, those that corrupted a random sample of MwMS with an additional self-selected group. Second, those with a confused sample, aiming for numbers of observations at the expense of the clarity of sample definition. And, third those that accepted too readily that MwMS were effectively the same as PwMS. Two good examples of the first group can be found in the UK research of McCrone et al. (2008) on the costs of MS and by Green and colleagues (2007 and 2008) on the social impact of MS and its congruence with wider social trends.

For the latter research a large stratified random sample of 1,200 was undertaken in 2003 of MwMS, producing a 67 per cent response (Green et al. 2007, 528). At this point a large representative sample of MwMS had been secured, reliable evidence about the MS Society's membership. It could then have been employed in numerous descriptive and comparative exercises with other socio-economic data. Unfortunately, such clear methodological waters became hopelessly muddied by the belief that this sample seriously under-represented younger PwMS and the newly diagnosed. An attempt to rectify this situation was made by trying to recruit these putative absentees on-line, via the MS Society's website and through chat rooms. Here an invitation to opt into the study was posted from which 133 usable replies were received. Thus, a self-selection process was added, and not just of MS Society members, but of anyone who consulted its website. And, crucially therefore the whole notion of a representative sample of MwMS broke down. We have no idea how the online sample related to the population of PwMS at all. Indeed, it is possible that some people could have been in both groups, random and online. Thus, the amalgamated sample used in this study's principal analyses was confused and compromised. The authors do accept their 'respondents are not representative of all people with MS' (Green and Todd 2008, 171) and 'were not necessarily representative of the general population of people with MS' (Green et al. 2007, 533). They never could have been. It also becomes difficult to conceptualise exactly to what they apply their subsequent sophisticated statistical analyses; at best a large amorphous set of people who probably have MS; important perhaps because of its size, not because of its representativeness.

The work of McCrone et al. (2008) began well with a massive randomly selected postal survey of MwMS totalling 4,000. At the same time an invitation to take part directly in the study was placed in the March 2005 issue of the MS Society's *Teamspirit* periodical that resulted in an unspecified number of replies. The results from these two groups were then added together for analytical purposes yet they were very different in character. The former was random and representative of its background population of MwMS; the latter self-selected, unrepresentative and corrupting of the joint group of which it became a part. Like in the research by Green et al. (2007), there was the possibility of people taking part in both groups to be counted twice and, once again therefore an amorphous group of putative PwMS resulted. The paper does accept that their group of respondents was 'probably not wholly representative of people with MS in the population' (McCrone et al. 2008, 858). Sadly it is difficult to work out what it might represent. Once again, if this research has any importance it is most likely because of its sample size and not because of its representativeness.

In terms of research making use of a confused sample of PwMS, the publication by the MS Society in 2002, *Are we being served? Health care experiences of people with MS,* offers a good example. This particular work was the result of the largest response from any self-selecting survey of UK MS charity members so far achieved of 16,400 from a questionnaire placed in an MS Society magazine for which a response rate of 35 per cent was claimed (MS Society 2002, 3). According to this study, 'The survey sample was taken from the MS Society data base of 45,000 people and from people with MS who were not members of the MS Society, who were targeted through primary and secondary care settings using comprehensive data bases of the NHS services likely to be used by people with MS' (MS Society 2002, 6). This is unintelligible gobbledegook that must have been designed to confuse more than illuminate. What in fact happened was that in addition to a complete trawl of the MS Society members through their magazine postings, this project distributed questionnaire forms to primary and secondary care establishments where interested PwMS, or with any other complaint and including the perfectly well, may pick them up to fill out if they so wished. Thus, the comprehensive data base of the NHS was not of PwMS but of places where they may possibly visit for treatment. This is a blunderbuss approach to data collection and like all such wide-bore weapons is indiscriminate in its victims with an uncertain outcome. The final sample used in the analyses therefore was a confusing self-selected one. How it was then possible to work out the denominator for the percentage response rate given in the document is a mystery? What is worse, the process annoyingly confused the background population; it is not just MwMS, it also included others who picked up a questionnaire form in any medical establishment and submitted it. If the analysis had included only MwMS, then it could have provided some clear evidence of their demographic characteristics and care needs. But it did not! This was a major wasted opportunity.

There are other good examples of jumbled samples too that did not involve the listings of MS charity members. For example, in a project on the usefulness of socio-economic variables as predictors of the health status of PwMS by Riazi et al. (2003), 500 of the responses to the Hobart et al. (2001) quality of life research were added to 150 attendees with definite MS at a weekly outpatient clinic at the NHNN, 97 PwMS admitted to the NHNN for either rehabilitation and/or IV-steroid treatment and a postal survey of 119 people with a confirmed diagnosis of PPMS. The reasons for grouping this jumble of different types of PwMS and different modes of selection were not explained. The result, predictably though was another amorphous collection of observations from which no deductions of any value or use could be made. Their conclusion therefore in the title of their paper, 'socio-demographic variables are limited predictors of health status in multiple sclerosis', cannot be drawn from their analysis, no matter how intuitively appealing.

The use of members of the main MS charities as proxies for the national population of PwMS raises the important question as to the degree to which the former may reflect the latter? Do the populations of members of the MS Society and members of the MS Trust differ demographically, medically or in any other way from the national population of PwMS that could make it unsafe to use them as suitable substitutes?

This issue has usually been tackled by comparing MwMS and PwMS on one or two demographic characteristics such as average age or gender balance. For example, in the MS Society's huge survey of its membership in 2012/3 that produced more than 10,500 self-selected replies dismissed the issue in a few disappointingly vague sentences: 'The demographics of those who responded are as we would expect. In the UK around three times as many women as men have MS, and our survey respondents reflect this. Our respondents were slightly older than the MS population, reflecting our membership, but people of all ages and all types of MS responded' (MS Soc 2013, 7). Meanwhile, in other published research it has just been assumed that members of an MS charity are the same as PwMS more generally as in the work on the quality of life of PwMS by Orme and colleagues (2007) using the circulation list of the MS Trust's Quarterly Newsletter. In this case it is simply asserted without any corroborative evidence that 'A cross-sectional study was performed in a large representative sample of the UK MS population' (Orme et al. 2007, 2).

However, if representativeness is to be based on demographic similarity, then there are a number of other attributes that may be of at least equal importance for behavioural explanation such as ethnicity, family and household composition, marital status, and especially employment, income and wealth. As Shakespeare and Watson (2001, 555) pointed out, 'access to economic and social power is a strong determinant of the life experience of disabled people.' For example, a disabled, unmarried, unemployed man with MS living alone may find it much more difficult to secure the care and support he needs than a disabled married woman living with her family. Furthermore, there is at least one other sense in which MwMS are definitely different from PwMS generally, an area, therefore, in which the former is knowingly biased, namely their membership of a support charity for which they made a conscious decision to join. The reasons for such a decision will have been varied and complex ranging from an altruistic desire to help others to perhaps a hope of helping themselves through better information and healthcare contacts. And, such decisions will potentially be immersed in very different lifestyles and views on the relationship MwMS wish to have with the society of which they are part. Nevertheless, the decision to join a disease specific charity or pressure group knowingly biases the results and may make them unsafe to be regarded as representative of the wider community of PwMS. Clearly, a great deal more comparative evidence is required to decide whether MS charity members are suitable surrogates for the national population of PwMS.

Finally, it must be emphasised that while there have been many examples of questionable methodologies in the research on PwMS, there have also been many examples of good practice too. For example, probably the clearest and most successful attempts to survey PwMS so far in the UK have been undertaken in the development and testing of patient-based quality of life measures by Hobart and colleagues (2001) and Ford et al. (2001a and 2001b) that is discussed in Chapter 6. In these cases large random samples of both MwMS nationally (1,530 individuals) and of PwMS from a local urban register (199 individuals) were carried out along with more detailed preparatory focus group work.

3.3.4 Small groups for qualitative analyses

In many areas of the study of people with disease easily quantified issues of 'how many', 'where' and 'when' are less important than concerns of why and how decisions were made, to investigate in detail what actions were taken and why, that is a concern with the processes of human behaviour. In such circumstances large random samples are less important and almost certainly prohibitively expensive. Instead, smaller groups of respondents are appropriate using in-depth interviews and focus groups to collect verbal evidence for qualitative techniques of analysis.

Traditionally a number of differences are often drawn out between quantitative and qualitative approaches to research. In the latter participant selection is purposeful rather than random or self-selected, its form of analysis contextual rather than reductionist, its concern for the impact of the researcher, its ability to cope with a variety of responses rather than a list of predetermined ones. However, in reality both types of approach are often used side-by-side; that is they may complement one another. And, therefore in this book, although the emphasis may be on the quantitative, qualitative approaches are used to aid explanation where appropriate.

The use of small group analyses in the study of PwMS began in the mid-1990s with two seminal pieces of research, the first in Canada by Dyck (1995) on the impact of MS on women's lives, while in the UK it began with Robinson and colleagues (1996) 'A view from the front line', an attempt to '...understand the needs of PwMS as far as possible from their own point of view' (Robinson et al. 1996, viii), accepting that: 'People are just different from each other in relation to their needs, and PwMS are no different.' (Robinson et al. 1996,32). This work was followed by a similar analysis of the views of people involved with the formal and informal care of PwMS, by Robinson and Hunter (1998) 'Views from the other side'. The first of these two studies was particular important because it was the first time the views of PwMS on their care were researched rather than accepting the handed-down wisdom of the medical professionals nominally responsible for their care. For this the foresight of the then Director of Welfare Services of the MS Society, Jan Hatch, deserves great praise for commissioning the work.

The research undertaken by Robinson and colleagues (1996) was based on what were regarded as radical research methods by the medical establishment at the time, qualitative techniques. In this case evidence was collected during 18 focus groups in 1996 at 6 different sites: London, Preston, Exeter, Coventry, Belfast and Aberdeen. At each location separate focus group meetings were held for PwMS, informal carers and medical professionals. In total 325 PwMS, 100 carers and 75 professionals took part in the meetings. The discussions in each focus group were recorded and transcribed, and it is these transcriptions that provided the raw material analysed for this research. About the focus groups Robinson et al. (1996, 174) made the curious observation that 'focus groups were as representative as possible of the kinds of PwMS.' Unfortunately, we are not told how this was achieved especially since there was a clear failure to represent the Welsh in the research. Indeed, a moment's reflection ought to have made it abundantly clear that this type of research can rarely be expected to be representative. It is not about securing a reliable sample of some wider population that can be used for inferential analysis. It is much more about seeking detailed understanding of peoples' actions and decisions. However, in this case generalisations were attempted by coding the transcripts for common themes, that is, the qualitative evidence transformed into the quantitative, merely as a way of being able to deal with, make sense of and present a huge amount of transcribed verbiage. The methodology for this research was more about purposeful sampling than any random selection of participants; that is arranging for informed respondents who had detailed knowledge of the subjects posed to be present in the focus groups.

Since that time the use of focus groups and in-depth interviews to collect evidence on the behaviour of PwMS has grown enormously to include topics as varied as vocational rehabilitation services (Sweetland et al. 2007), palliative care (Edmonds et al. 2007a and 2007b, Higginson et al. 2008 and 2009), lay person-led expert patient programmes (Barlow et al. 2009a), the availability of personal data for research (Baird et al. 2009), the adjustment of adolescents whose parents have MS (Bogosian et al. 2011), gender differences in the experience of MS Coyle (2005) and Jobin et al. (2010) and of caring for someone with MS (Courts et al. 2005).

3.4 Responses to interviews and questionnaire surveys

Obtaining useful information for research purposes from interviews and questionnaires depends on two important qualities of the target audience: their willingness to take part and their ability to provide reliable and accurate responses.

On the former the evidence is very strong indeed that PwMS are willing to be involved in research by responding in large numbers not only to questionnaires sent to them through the post but also to less personally targeted requests for data through inserts in magazines and online surveys for which the respondents have to make a determined effort to take part. For example, response rates to the surveys of MwMS by Green et al. (2007) was 67 per cent, by McCrone et al. (2008) 48.7 per cent and by Hobart et al. (2001) 78.6 per cent, and response rates for questionnaire surveys of patients attending neurology clinics have usually even been higher, with Ford et al. (2001b) reporting one of the highest response rates of all at 91 per cent (180 questionnaires returned). What is more, even the work of Greenhaigh et al. (2004, 578) that demanded the completion of a daily impact diary over a period of 12 weeks achieved a response rate of 82 per cent. Thus, there can be no doubt that PwMS are willing to give up their time to respond to information requests from research workers.

But, are their responses believable? Though there is very little evidence on this issue, it must be initially argued that if a person agrees to participate in a research project it is to be expected that they would try to provide accurate information. Not to do so would be wholly contrary, undermine the exercise in which they have agreed to participate and be a complete waste of their time. Thus, accepting that PwMS who respond to research requests for information try to supply accurate data, do they succeed? The accuracy of patient-derived disease information was tested on a sample of 79 PwMS for whom confirmed longitudinal clinical evidence was available for at least 20 years from the records of the Neurology Department of the University Hospital of Wales in Cardiff and who agreed to respond to questionnaire or telephone interviews on this evidence (Ingram et al. 2010). When tested on issues such as the occurrence of various disease milestones, relapses, disease course and type, questionnaire respondents were more accurate than telephone interviewees. For example, correlation coefficients between questionnaire and clinician-derived data on time to a set of four different disability states were all above 0.9. However, questionnaire responses were not so successful on issues of symptom description, relapse rates and course of disease at onset. Caution though must be attached to these results for a number of reasons. The first reason was because of the small sample size and the second was because of possible biases pulling in opposite directions. On the one hand, this study included only PwMS with a long-term clinical record who almost by definition must have been regular highly motivated clinic attendees. Such people would most likely develop a good understanding of their disease and stand an above average chance of completing their questionnaires correctly. On the other hand, the PwMS in this study all had a relatively high disability score and therefore may have had lower recall ability.

Unfortunately, it is not just with the accuracy of the patient-derived evidence that a reviewer of research on PwMS must be concerned, but with the way that information is presented and written about too; that is the bias, or 'spin', that is placed on the material. In other words, it must be accepted that different points of view come into play when different types of people are involved. Sometimes such effects are innocent and understandable. For example, the impact of MS on a person's life can be assessed differently by the different groups of people involved in that person's life and care, as discovered by van der Linden et al. (2008) using the MS Impact Scale (MSIS-29). In this case, compared to the assessment of the person with MS, health-care professionals tended to underestimate impacts probably because of their familiarity with the disease and close relatives tended to overestimated disease impacts. Another good example of the difference in point of view can come from the move into a wheelchair by a person with MS when walking becomes too difficult. The physiotherapist will view it as a functional necessity to aid mobility and limit orthopaedic damage to their patient. The person with MS may view it very differently, and resist the move for as long as possible, for it is a sign of 'giving in to the disease', of eventually accepting a defeat (Robinson et al. 1996, 29). A similar effect, of observable difference between patients and relatives this time, was described by Tripoliti and colleagues (2007) in assessing the usefulness of proxy assessments of the quality of life of PwMS. In this case 40 PwMS and the family relative who knew them best independently completed the Functional Assessment of MS (FAMS) instrument. In general the relative, or potential proxy, underestimated the quality of life score offered by their relative and that this was true for the six subscales of this device too: mobility, symptoms, emotional well-being, contentment, thinking and fatigue, family well-being. However, 13 of the respondents whose relatives with MS offered low quality of life scores tended to overestimate their scores. Could it be, Tripoliti et al. (2007) asked, that relatives may be conservative in their assessments of their relatives' quality of life, underestimating high scores and overestimating low ones? Of course, no answer was forthcoming, but it does suggest that considerable caution needs to be taken when using quality of life estimates from different groups of subjects.

It must also be understood that what people say and how they say it may vary according to whom they are talking and the circumstances in which they find themselves. In an interview situation therefore, with an 'expert' in front of them, it is highly likely that an interviewee will present, or at least try to present, a 'public face' in which things that are unpalatable, undesirable or rude are avoided and a socially acceptable form is attempted. This may be in sharp contrast to the 'private face' that would be offered to close friends/relatives of the same background and experience. In health-related research this may be a particular problem because of the way in which matters of health are often imbued with a moral component in which 'health' is good and 'unhealthy' is bad. Thus, even when a person's ill-health is accepted as no fault of their own but as a random product of nature, they may still lie about their state of health. This was discovered in a detailed set of interviews with 24 people in the East End of London about their health and health care in which Cornwell (1984, 124) was able to conclude that 'The initial statements people made about their health bore no relation to their medical histories.' It was only after multiple interviews with the same individuals that accurate information was obtained, after a trusting relationship had been established. Such an issue could easily manifest itself in interviews with PwMS because of the often unsavoury nature of many of its symptoms and be of serious concern for the newly diagnosed before they become more accustomed to their condition.

More alarmingly, however, even seemingly clear factual evidence can be written up in different ways to give quite conflicting meanings. For example, to take the Royal College of Physicians (RCP)/MS Trust (2008) Audit of MS services, in the report on this research in the MS Trust's magazine *Open Door* for August 2008 (p.9) it was stated that 'only 36% of PwMS had access' to neurological rehabilitation services. This 'fact' is also repeated in the *BMJ* in July 2008 News section by Lisa Hitchen (BMJ 2008; 337: a734) as 36 per cent of PwMS in England 'could access neurological rehabilitation services.' The clear conclusions that surely must be derived from this information could only be that, five years on from their publication, the NICE guidelines on the care of PwMS were not being met and that PwMS were receiving a bad service from the NHS in England and Wales. However, referring to the 35-page summary document available online, the actual report stated on page 16 that 36 per cent of respondents with MS in England 'thought that they could be seen by a specialist neurological rehabilitation service if needed.' Now, there may be a great deal of difference for many reasons between what PwMS thought was available and what actually was available. In fact, no reliable evidence at all was presented on the supply of neurological rehabilitation services in this report. At best this was inaccurate reporting. Also on page 16 of this audit report, it was stated that only 7 per cent of the respondents were 'very dissatisfied' with the service they received and 23 per cent 'very satisfied'. Not the results one would have expected from a profoundly disgruntled clientele!

3.5 Conclusion

This chapter reviewed some of the major challenges of undertaking meaningful research on PwMS that are crucial for an understanding of much of the research that has been published so far with particular emphasis on the UK. These difficulties stem from three main quarters. First the chronic nature of the disease itself and the way its diagnosis has changed through time. The second difficulty concerns the available information sources on PwMS while the third relates to problems with research methodologies. Selected examples of these challenges were then provided from four broad identifiable approaches to research on PwMS that have provided the main evidence for this book: regional counts of PwMS, the growth of registers and databases of PwMS, major surveys of PwMS and small group qualitative work. The chapter concluded by considering the veracity of the research evidence provided by PwMS.

4
What Type of Person Suffers from MS?

4.1 Introduction

The objective of this chapter is to investigate whether there are any demographic characteristics shared by people with Multiple Sclerosis (PwMS). Does the disease display a much higher preference for particular age, ethnic or social groups; does it prefer one gender to another? Or is MS socially non-discriminatory with no particularly vulnerable demographic groups, found with equal force in all social strata? The evidence with which this wholly descriptive exercise can be approached comes from two main sources: regional epidemiological enquiries of PwMS and various surveys of PwMS on a number of different social- and health-related issues. The first source of demographic evidence includes the 20 or so regional epidemiological studies of MS in the United Kingdom (UK) since the mid-1980s in which the total ascertainment of all cases of the disease was attempted. Here, with one major exception by Swingler and Compston (1990), the demographics of PwMS was not the main concern, but they nevertheless consistently reported in some detail on age and gender and to a much poorer degree on ethnicity and deprivation/social class. These four dimensions of human characterisation are reviewed in Sections 4.2 to 4.5. From reviews of the regional evidence up to 1993 both Mumford et al. (1992, 881) and Robertson et al. (1995, 74) observed common trends, the latter stating, 'One of the striking features of all these studies is the similarity in clinical aspects of disease including age and sex distributions, age at onset, disease course, disease duration and diagnostic classification.' Whether it still applies to later studies are tested in this chapter. Into these descriptions supportive evidence from the second source, the main surveys of PwMS (Table 4.1) undertaken recently, some of which were reviewed critically in the previous chapter,

Table 4.1 Surveys of PwMS

Lead author	Year and area of survey	No. of cases	Mean Age, years	Age range	Sex ratio, fem/male	% female	Survey subjects
Hobart	c. 2000 UK	766	51	23–87	2.8	74	MwMS
Hobart	c. 2000 UK	713	52	18–82	2.5	71	MwMS
Hobart	c. 2000 UK	602	51	23–87	3.3	77	MwMS who could walk
Ford	c.2000 Leeds	180	46		3.6	78	Leeds prevalence register
Freeman	c.2000 London	150	44.6	24–78	1.7	60	PwMS at the NHNN
MORI	2003 UK	4,620			2.6	72	MwMS
Riazi	2000 UK	638			1.7	63.5	Mixed
Orme	c. 2005 UK	2,048	51.4		2.9	74.5	MST
McCrone	2005 UK	1,942	54.5		2.6	72.2	MwMS
Green	2003 GB	787	M: 52.8 F: 50.4	22–84	3.3	76.6	MwMS
Holmes	1994 UK	672	50		1.9	65.6	MwMS
Forbes	England 2000	293	47.5		2.5	70	PwMS with an MSN
Forbes	England 2000	323	50.7		2.5	71	PwMS without an MSN
Hakim	1986–89 Hants.	441	48.3	19–82	2.1	67	All PwMS
MacLurg	N. Ireland 2001	149	51.0	24–82	2.8	74	PwMS
RCP and MST	England and Wales 2008	1,300	51 (median)		2.7	73	MST
Zajicek	Cornwall and Devon 2010	c.960	51.6		3.01	75	All PwMS
Ford et al. (2012)	UK 2011–2	7,279	50.8	18–95	2.4	70	All PwMS*
Jones	UK 2011–2	4,178	50.9	20–87	2.4	70	All PwMS*

Sources: Ford, Gerry, Johnson and Tennant (2001a), Freeman and Thompson (2000), Green et al. (2007), Hakim et al. (2000), Hobart et al. (2001 and 2003), Holmes et al. (1995), McCrone et al. (2008), MacLurg et al. (2005), MORI (2003), Orme et al. (2007), Riazi et al. (2003), RCP and MST (2008), Zajicek et al. (2010), Forbes et al. (2006a), Ford et al. (2012), Jones et al. (2012).

MwMS – members of the MS Society with MS

MST – members of the MS Trust's mailing list

MSN – MS Nurse

NHNN – National Hospital for Neurology and Neurosurgery

RCP – Royal College of Practitioners

* From the UK MS Register in which different numbers of respondents apply to each question.

are interwoven where appropriate. These surveys, mainly of members of MS charities, are also important because they provide evidence on three other demographic characteristics, employment, education and marital status that are discussed in Sections 4.6 to 4.8. Where possible this material is then placed in an international context.

It is important to realise that the majority of the material presented in this chapter comes from a number of snap-shots in time, for specific places in specific years. It is therefore static in nature and no attempt is made in this chapter to consider how individuals with MS and the way in which they may be described changes through time because of their illness. That task is considered in Chapter 6, 'The Impact of MS'. It is also not the direct objective of this chapter to ascribe a causal connection between MS and any demographic characteristic although in some circumstances the temptation has been too great to pass. They should, therefore, be viewed as potentially causal, consequential or coincidental with the potency of their relationship with the disease essentially undecided and unknown. Finally, by way of introduction, it may be worth considering whether any of the demographic categories considered of social class, marital status and age group may have changed in significance over the time period of this review? For example, with rising life expectancy individual and most certainly societal attitudes towards old age have changed substantially witnessed by the pressure in the UK during the early years of the twenty-first century to increase the age at which a state pension may be drawn. It is not known conclusively whether life expectancy for PwMS has kept pace with general population trends, nor is it known whether old age and retirement can be viewed in the same way by PwMS as people without MS. However, they are potentially important avenues for future research.

4.2 Sex

From the published writings on the regional epidemiology of MS in the UK since the mid-1980s, the distribution of the disease between the sexes has been characterised by two distinctive features. The first, and most important observation across all papers, must be that women developed the disease more frequently than men by at least a ratio of two to one (Table 4.2). Furthermore, in Jersey in 1991, Leeds in 1996, Tayside during the same year, central Glasgow in 2000 and Plymouth in 2001, the ratio was nearer three to one; evidence that in itself might lead to the suggestion that the female predilection for MS has been getting stronger during the recent past. While this point may be as yet contentious for

86 *People with Multiple Sclerosis*

Table 4.2 Female to male ratios in regional MS studies since 1985

Area	Year of survey	Fem/Male ratio
Sutton (south London)	1985	2.0
South Glamorgan	1985	2.0
South Hampshire	1987	2.0
South Glamorgan	1988	2.0
5 GP Practices in rural Suffolk	1988	2.4
Rochdale *	1989	2.1
South and east Cambridgeshire	1990	2.5
Guernsey	1991	2.6
Jersey	1991	3.0
Brighton and mid-Downs	1991	2.5
South and east Cambridgeshire *	1993	2.6
North Cambridgeshire *	1993	2.2
Lothian / Borders	1995	2.5
Leeds	1996	2.8
North Northern Ireland	1996	2.1
Tayside	1996	2.8
Fife	1996	2.4
Leeds	1999	N/A
Central Glasgow	2000	3.2
Plymouth	2001	2.7
North Northern Ireland	2004	2.0
South Glamorgan	2005	2.4
Aberdeen City, Shetland and Orkney combined	2009	2.5

*All cases with a Poser classification of MS.
Shaded areas indicate enquiries using definitions of MS other than Poser or McDonald.

the UK as a whole, what cannot be in dispute is that there were many more women with MS in the regions of the UK so far investigated than would have been expected from the natural population split between the sexes that for the period since 1970 has been ever-so – slightly in favour of women in all four countries of the UK.

The available evidence on the incidence of MS also supports the disease's preference for women. For example, in South Glamorgan between 1985 and 1988 the female to male ratio of all new cases was 2:1 (Hennessy et al. 1989). The equivalent ratio for Leeds between 1996 and 1998 was 2.3:1 (Ford et al. 2002) and for Tayside between 1970 and 1997 was 2.8:1 (Donnan et al. 2005). For central Glasgow between 1981 and 1998, the annual female incidence rate was 7.7/100,000 inhabitants compared with the male rate of 3.5/100,000 (Murray et al. 2004) while the equivalent rates for north Northern Ireland in 1996 were 10.3/100,000 and 8.3/100,000 respectively (Gray et al. 2008). The most comprehensive regional consideration of MS incidence, however, was carried out in South Glamorgan where, for the 515 new cases of MS between 1985 and 2007, 75 per cent were female and the female to male ratio increased from 1.9 to 4.6 (Hirst et al. 2009, 390) to become the principal motor behind this region's increase in MS prevalence of 45 per cent in the 20 years between 1985 and 2005. Thus, MS would appear to have been primarily a women's disease and probably increasingly so. However, the most recent evidence on the incidence and prevalence of MS in the UK from 1990 to 2010 using General Practice Research Database (GPRD) evidence challenges this view (Mackenzie et al. 2013). In this case the ratio of women to men remained constant over the 20-year period at 2.4 with the incidence of both men and women declining at a rate of 1.51 per cent per year. Unfortunately, no explanation was offered for this apparent aberrant result. Has the growth of new cases of MS in both men and women really come to end in the UK or are there problems with the information sources that could account for this result?

The second feature of the published descriptive epidemiological work on the sexual differences in MS frequencies was until very recently the disregard in the written record of female dominance to almost misogynistic proportions; the empirical evidence was before the authors' eyes and noted in their results but few commented on it in the discussion sections of their papers. There were a few exceptions. The most significant of these by far was in the work of Hirst et al. (2009) for South Glamorgan, already noted, because of its extensive longitudinal reach. A further four noted the gender imbalance in their discussions. Sharpe et al. (1995), for example, in their description of the number of people with MS in the Channel Islands observed not only a major difference between the gender prevalence rates in both Jersey and Guernsey, but more importantly recorded a significant difference between these rates for women between the two islands despite having virtually identical age/sex profiles. However, no adequate explanation was offered for these differences. Forbes et al. (1999, 1037) suggested unconvincingly that part of the excess in female MS numbers compared with men may have been due to a diagnosis bias in their favour 'in the presence of suggestive symptoms.' While it may be true that some women may be more 'in tune' with their bodies than some men, more prepared to report subtle changes in their bodily functioning to their doctors, it must be doubtful that women could have been preferentially diagnosed with MS by competent professional neurologists with just 'suggestive symptoms' under the strict guidelines of the Poser criteria. Gray et al. (2008,

885) suggested that the increasing female to male ratio of 2:1 in their study in 2004 of north Northern Ireland compared to the Allison and Millar (1954) work in 1951 for the whole of the province of 1.26:1 may be accounted for by a higher female incidence in 1996 of 10.3/100,000 (male rate = 8.3/100,000). And, a similar comparison was undertaken by Visser and colleagues (2012) in the extreme north east of Scotland. The rate for the Aberdeen City, Orkney and Shetland combined in 2009 was 2.5 compared to only 1.8 for the North East of Scotland in 1973. Gray et al. (2008) went on to list the many possible reasons for a disproportionate increase in female incidence rates, originally noted by Orton et al. (2006, 935) for Canada, of life style changes such as the changing roles of women in the workforce, outdoor activity, dietary habits, alterations in menarche, timing of childbearing and changes in contraception practices. They do not, however, consider whether these factors might vary between countries or their specific relevance to Northern Ireland society.

Given this paucity of comment on the gender division of MS frequencies, in only 4 of a possible 22 papers, it is not unexpected to find little comment too on this phenomenon in the review papers of this work. For example, in the survey of MS in the United Kingdom by Robertson and Compston (1995) covering the period from 1951 to 1993 the marked gender difference in MS frequencies was most surprisingly not listed as one of their identified trends. Similarly, in Compston's (1990a) 'dissemination of multiple sclerosis' celebratory lecture, the illness was disseminated in terms of race, place, genetics and families, but not by gender, with the only reference to this issue being the observation on page 213 that the milder form of the disease was typified by young onset in females with a contrastingly poor outlook for a late onset in males. This may seem doubly surprising because Swingler and Compston in a 1990 survey of the demographic characteristics of MS in South Glamorgan observed that the illness was most prevalent in middle-aged Caucasian women. By 1997 the issue had been reprieved by Compston to feature in an article entitled 'genetic epidemiology' in which it was stated that MS was almost always found to be more common in females than males at a rate of 2:1 irrespective of ethnicity. What is more, it was also observed that younger people diagnosed with MS were more likely to be female with the older ones more likely to be men.

It could be argued as disingenuous not also to report at this point that an earlier review of all available incidence, prevalence, morbidity and mortality statistics on MS relating to the UK from 1921 to the early 1980s by Swingler and Compston (1986) noted a number of gender differences in three important respects. First, standardised MS mortality rates 1921–80 for all the four countries of the UK were consistently higher for females than males, especially after 1951 (p.1119). Second, hospital discharge evidence 1968–78 for PwMS demonstrated significant increases over the period for both men and women, but with the latter being consistently much higher than the former (p.1119). And, third in terms of two national morbidity reviews in 1958 and 1974, much higher GP MS consultancy rates for women than for men were recorded: 70/100,000 compared to 50/100,000 and 80/100,000 compared to 40/100,000 respectively (p.1120). But, none of this was remarked upon in the discussion section of their paper.

The 19 surveys of PwMS (Table 4.1) provided supporting evidence for the high proportion of women in the MS population. In Table 4.2, 6 were equal to or lower than the mean for the 21 regions of 2.4:1 female to male ratio. The results for the Hakim et al. (2000) and Holmes et al. (1995) inquiries should perhaps be expected because they were earlier in date than the others. By contrast, the 1.7 for the work of Riazi et al. (2003) and Freeman and Thompson (2000) probably reflect the jumble of separate elements used in the former and the small sample size in the latter that both strongly indicated their unrepresentativeness. Similarly, the 2.4 for the two surveys emanating from MS Registry evidence stem from uncertain origins. The other surveys, all of MS charity members, no matter how imperfect methodologically, indicated a much higher female to male ratio than the regional work: Hobart et al. (2001) in 2000 2:8 and 2.5, MORI (2003) in 2003 2.6, Green et al. (2007) in 2003 3.3 and McCrone et al. (2008) in 2005 2:6. These consistent results may suggest that the MS Society in the UK in the early twenty-first century had a higher proportion of female members than the UK MS community as a whole. The equivalent ratio of 3:1 for the survey by Orme et al. (2007) and the 2.7 for the RCP/MST (2008) audit of MS services would tend to suggest this finding may hold true for the membership of the MS Trust too.

The female dominance of MS prevalence and incidence is not just a feature of the UK, it is now regarded as a prominent feature of the experience of many regions internationally. For example, Koch-Henriksen and Sorenson (2010) in an extensive survey of 178 prevalence and incidence research papers from around the world since 1965 written in English observed that within a general, although not ubiquitous, increase in MS prevalence and incidence through time for women, three important trends in female to male MS ratios can be detected: an increase with year and incidence and a decrease with latitude. For example, using the

Danish MS Register, the most complete national MS monitoring system in the world, while the incidence rate of MS in men had remained constant since 1950, in women it had doubled since 1970 resulting in an increase in the female to male sex ratio. Similarly in North America, female to male sex ratio increased substantially in the twentieth century: the Canadian Collaborative Project on Genetic Susceptibility to MS noted an increase from 1.90 for people born between 1931 and 1935 to 3.21 for those born between 1976 and 1980 (Orton et al. 2006) and the NARCOMS members ratio increased from 2 in patients diagnosed in 1940 to 4 for those diagnosed in 2000 (Cutter et al. 2007). The MS sex ratio also tended to increase if repeat surveys were undertaken for the same area, although there were three noteworthy exceptions, two in Norway and one in Olmsted County USA (Koch-Henriksen and Sorenson 2010, 527).

Again, it must be emphasised that even in the most recent authoritative reviews of MS in, for example, 'McAlpine's Multiple Sclerosis' (Compston et al. 2005) or 'Brain's Diseases of the Nervous System' (Donaghy 2009), while the gender ratio in favour of women is noted there is no comment on why this dominant demographic feature may have come about. Yet, it is difficult to believe that such a finding does not have an important causal function for the disease in biological terms or in social terms or even in both. However, by the second decade of the twenty-first century important genetic elements to the disproportionate number of women developing MS had been observed (Chao et al. 2011). First, it was found that PwMS who had a specific gene variant known to increase the risk of MS were three times more likely to be women than men. And, second women were more likely than men to inherit these susceptibility gene variants from a female relative; daughters more susceptible to MS than sons therefore. Thus, over time the proportion of women with MS would tend to increase. But, the relative increase in MS female incidence has taken place over too short a timescale to be explained by genetics, other environmental or behavioural factors must be at work too; factors that may interact with genes specifically in women to trigger MS.

Two aspects of recent societal change, prominent in the UK, that may have a bearing on gender trends in MS, and for which some empirical evidence is available are smoking and occupational change. On the former, it was suggested in Chapter 2 that smoking both directly and indirectly may produce an MS response in susceptible individuals. While at this level of the individual such a relationship may have some traction at a population scale any possible association is much more slippery. For example, there would appear to have been a steady increase in MS prevalence during the recent past but in smoking there has been a trend in the opposite direction. For example, according to factsheets produced by ASH (Action on Smoking and Health) in the mid-1970s almost 50 per cent of men and 45 per cent of women smoked regularly. By 2010, these proportions had reduced to 21 per cent and 20 per cent respectively. Similarly, as will become apparent later in this chapter, while MS appears to be more prevalent among the managerial and professional socio-economic groups than in the manual ones in the UK, smoking behaviour trends in the opposite direction. Approximately 29 per cent of men and 28 per cent of women in the routine and manual occupations regularly smoke compared with 14 per cent and 12 per cent respectively in the managerial and professional occupations. However, there are two aspects of recent smoking behaviour that may be relevant to the gender difference in MS prevalence rates. First, it is the relatively young adult age groups and marginally so among women that displayed the highest recent smoking rates of 29 per cent in the 20–24 age group with 28 per cent for men across the 25–35 age group. The greatest difference between the sexes though was to be found in teenage smoking habits. In this aspect girls recorded a higher percentage of regular smokers than boys from at least 1982. For example, when the difference was at its greatest in 1986, 27 per cent of girls aged 15 years regularly smoked compared with 18 per cent of boys. Could such behaviour help prime their bodies for an MS response later in life?

There have been some profound changes in the role of women in western society too since the Second World War that may have made them more likely to develop MS than men. For example, if it could be argued that MS was the result of a microbial infection in which proximity between individuals was important for its spread from one person to the next, then economic and social processes that brought people in close proximity to one another could be important in providing the conduits for the expansion of MS susceptibility. At the macro level of analysis of the nation state this could include industrialisation and urbanisation, the moving of people and especially women from domestic work in rural familial self-sufficiency to factories in urban settings. Such a scenario might, for example, help to account for the increasing sex ratio of MS with latitude.

Within the UK specifically increasing the recent opportunities for social interaction especially for women and therefore proximity for the spread of viruses can be inferred from two trends. The first trend is the rise in the proportion of women in the formal work force. For example, in 1971 the employment rate for women of working age was 56 per cent.

By 2007 this had increased to 70 per cent (Social Trends 2008, 49). Meanwhile, the equivalent rates for men had declined from 92 per cent to 79 per cent. The second trend involved the rise in the number of people, and especially of women, in higher education; a particularly important phenomenon if late onset EBV (Epstein-Barr virus) is to be regarded as one of the principal triggers for MS. Between 1970 and 1971 and 2005 and 2006, the number of men in higher education increased from 416,000 by 161 per cent to 1,085,000 while the number of women in higher education expanded more than 6 fold (205,000 to 1,456,000: 610%) to exceed the number of men (Social Trends 2008, 36). No matter how enlightening such ideas may be for the growth of the incidence of MS they would be difficult to test because people within the UK do not always live out their lives within one region; they often go to a higher education institution in a different region to their original home and begin their working lives in yet another region. Thus, in addition to a population level analysis of the development of MS in nation states, another at the individual level, following the lives of people, where they lived, their relationships, education, employment and health, may be of equal significance to understand the growth of MS.

It may not be just the rise of women in the workforce that could be important in a full explanation of the growth of MS in women over the recent past, but also the growth in the types of jobs women have tended to occupy over that period. McDowell (2009), for example, observed that as participation rates increased and time, especially for the more affluent, became increasingly precious, then tasks once carried out in the home such as child care, cleaning, care for elderly relatives, gardening, dog walking, catering, leisure, hairdressing and even sex have become increasingly provided through the market. And, many of these jobs, typically regarded as low-status occupations, poorly paid and part-time, often directly concerned with servicing the bodily needs of others have been taken up by women. As a result, the self-service economy of Gershuny (1978) in which household tasks were undertaken by family members using consumer durables and white goods is increasingly being replaced by bought-in labour using the same technologies. At the same time growth in service sector jobs that required close contact between the provider and the consumer in which good looks, personality and manners on the part of the provider were at a premium, such as in sales assistants (even telephone sales), restaurant and bar staff, nursing and caring have become another important source of growth in jobs for women. Thus, in Great Britain, for example, in 2001, 16 per cent of the workforce was employed in social and personal services compared with 10 per cent in 1980 and

7 per cent in 1950 (McDowell 2009, 37). Female employment in sales increased from 648,000 in 1951 to 834,000 in 1981 to 1,360,000 in 2001 (McDowell, 2009, 38), while over the same three points in time female employment in personal services rose from 621,000 through 813,000 to 1,549,000. What is more, McDowell (2009, 38) suggests that 10 per cent of the UK workforce in 2001 were in occupations that necessitated actual physical contact of the bodies of the provider and consumer, what she refers to as 'high touch occupations'. The growth of such jobs for women may well offer a mechanism for the transmission of potentially MS-promoting viruses and perhaps also with a female bias in MS incidence. But, to investigate whether such a mechanism had a role to play in the growth of MS in women over the last three or four decades would require much more detailed research at the individual level.

4.3 Age

Age, according to Bhopal (2002, 8), is 'the most influential and important of all epidemiological variables.' It is both a biological and a social factor to add to the existing environmental mix. In the case of MS in the UK similarity typifies the regional evidence by age (Table 4.3). Across all regions for which published material was available, the mean age of disease onset and the mean cohort age show remarkable unanimity. The mean age of disease onset, that is when the first overt clinical signs of MS became apparent, began on average early in the fourth decade of life, typically 32 to 34 years, with South Cambridgeshire reporting the lowest average of 30 years. Perhaps the large proportion of relatively young adults in this university dominated area may account for this result. Other countries of the western world have shown similar results. For example, in London Ontario mean age of onset was 30.5 years between 1972 and 1984 (Weinshenker et al. 1989), in Perth and Hobart in 1981 Australia peak incidence fell in the fourth decade of life (Hammond et al. 1988) and in Denmark mean age of onset between 1949 and 1996 was 34.7 years for men and 34.1 years for women (Bronnum-Hansen et al. 2004). Socially the actual average age of disease onset is a profound observation because it means that for most people with MS their diagnosis took place at about the same time as they were making some of the most significant decisions of their lives about relationships, starting families, careers and major investments such as buying a house. The possible impacts of an MS diagnosis on a person's life are considered in detail in Chapter 6.

The mean ages of regional cohorts of PwMS are also very similar at between 49 and 51 years. The exceptions in this case were at a higher age for Plymouth at 52 years and for the combined areas of Aberdeen City, Shetland and Orkney at 53 years. Perhaps the attractiveness of the South West of England to retired people, or people close to retirement age, might help to account for the former result with the relative inability of older generations to leave North East Scotland compared to the young helping to account for the latter. The survey research also supports a mean age for PwMS tending towards 51 years (Table 4.1) with the oldest cohort in the economic study by McCrone et al. (2008) at 54.5 years.

Table 4.3 The ages of PwMS: summary statistics from regional research

Area	Year of survey	Mean age (years)	Mean age at onset (years)	Mean duration to survey (years)	Age range
Sutton (south London)	1985	49	34	15	20–82
South Glamorgan	1985	49	32	17	10–85
South Hampshire	1987	49	33	16	18–82
5 GP Practices in rural Suffolk	1988	49	37	11	N/A
Rochdale *	1989	49	35	14	N/A
South and east Cambridgeshire	1990	49	30	19	17–83
Guernsey	1991	M: 50 F: 46	N/A	N/A	N/A
Jersey	1991	M:54 F: 44	N/A	N/A	N/A
Brighton and mid-Downs	1991	49	33	16	16–87
South and east Cambridgeshire *	1993	49	32	17	18–85
North Cambridgeshire *	1993	50	34	17	8–84
Lothian / Borders	1995	49	N/A	N/A	8–91
Leeds	1996	51	34	16	23–86
North Northern Ireland	1996	49	32	18	18–79
Tayside	1996	50	34	15	N/A
Fife	1996	50	N/A	N/A	N/A
Leeds	1999	N/A	N/A	N/A	N/A
Central Glasgow	2000	50	34	16	21–75
Plymouth	2001	52	35	17	23–89
North Northern Ireland	2004	50	33	18	N/A
South Glamorgan	2005	51	32	19	18–90
Aberdeen City, Orkney and Shetland combined	2009	53	32	19	N/A

N/A – not available.
* for all cases with a Poser classification.

There may be the slightest of hints in the regional evidence that the average age of regional MS cohorts increased over the 20 or so years of the review period by approximately one year. For men and women in England and Wales aged 45 years, the expected number of years of life remaining increased from 28.3 years in 1980 to 32.6 years in 2000, with the equivalent change for women from 33.7 years to 36.6 years (Office for Health Economics website). Despite alleged improvements in keeping chronically ill people alive over this period, the increase in the average age of regional cohorts of PwMS may therefore seem disappointingly small.

When the age ranges of regional cohorts are considered, the most senior individuals all fell within the range of 80 to 90 years with 2 exceptions at younger ages, north Northern Ireland in 1996 at 79 years and central Glasgow in 2000 at 75 years, both areas with high death rates compared with the rest of the UK. In the more recent work for the MS Register, however, a much older person of 95 years was recorded (Table 4.1). Unfortunately, a closer comparison of the age distributions of the surveys of PwMS was compromised by three of them using a different set of age categories from the regional work and four of them giving no age distributions at all. Only the MORI survey allowed a direct comparison with the regional work and in this case there was a much smaller proportion of observations in the under 35 years age group at 6 per cent of cases (Table 4.4) whereas in all the regional surveys it was never lower than 12.2 per cent and usually 3 or 4 percentage points higher. This finding may indicate that the MS Society had on average an older cohort of members with MS than the equivalent national population.

The lower level of age ranges is probably affected by the unwillingness of some neurologists to give, or even to recognise the possibility of giving, a diagnosis of MS to a child. Indeed, the Poser diagnostic scheme for MS specifically excludes children under the age of 10 years. Thus, some reports may have failed to include children in their results and this must lead to the questioning of the comparability of these regional inquiries into MS. The diagnosis of children with MS is not such an ethical problem in the early twenty-first century though with paediatric MS being a well-recognised phenomenon (Banwell et al. 2007) and children of only three and five years being recently diagnosed in the UK: Lucy Wood in Durham (*MS Matters* 2010, Issue 91, page 4) and Sam Blyth in Scotland (MS Trust, recent news story page) respectively. However, only three of the regional studies included here reported on children with MS for their lowest age of their ranges: South Glamorgan in 1985

Table 4.4 The distribution of PwMS and the population of the countries of the UK by age group

	SUTTON %	SOUTH GLAM 1985 %	SOUTH CAMBS %	SUSSEX 1991 %	SE SCOT' 1995 %	TAY SIDE 1996 %	FIFE 1996 %	N.N.I. 1996 %	N.N.I. 2004 %	ENG' 2001 %	SCOT' 2001 %	WALES 2001 %	N.I.I. 2001 %
0–14		0.2	0.8		0.2					19.0	17.9	18.9	19.8
15–24	2.6	4.8		1.2	1.4	1.5	1.0	2.0	1.1	12.1	12.5	12.2	14.2
25–34	15.4	15.9	11.5	13.5	12.8	10.9	11.6	11.0	11.1	14.4	13.8	12.6	14.4
35–44	22.6	19.7	34.8	27.8	24.9	24.8	24.6	24.8	23.0	14.9	15.4	14.0	14.7
45–54	25.1	22.7	19.5	26.9	26.2	32.7	31.1	26.0	30.3	13.2	13.6	13.5	11.9
55–64	18.5	22.0	15.5	15.3	18.2	17.2	19.7	20.1	20.3	10.5	10.9	11.4	9.6
65–74	11.8	11.3	13.6	11.6	12.3	9.4	8.5	14.2	9.7	8.4	8.8	9.1	7.5
75+	4.1	2.7	3.2	3.6	3.5	3.6	3.4	2.0	4.6	7.5	7.1	8.3	7.9

at 10 years of age and both North Cambridgeshire in 1993 and Lothian and Borders in 1995 at only 8 years. In the future therefore it is likely that the age distributions of PwMS will be stretched in both directions as more children are diagnosed with the disease and existing PwMS are helped to live longer. This will make future comparisons through time of the ages of PwMS just as problematic as they are now.

Another way of analysing the age distribution of PwMS would be to decide if it differed in any important way from the age distribution of all inhabitants in the UK. In other words, were there any age bands in which PwMS were more or less frequent than would have been expected from the age distribution of all people. Information to help with such an inquiry can be found in Table 4.5 where area populations are expressed in percentage terms across eight age bands for nine regions and the four countries of the UK. For all the MS regional data the distributions are remarkably similar emphasising in particular few PwMS in the first 25 years of life at less than 5 per cent of observations. This result becomes dramatically more apparent when compared with what would have been expected from the age distribution of all people in the UK at almost 30 per cent. The unusually high percentage of young people in Northern Ireland at 34 per cent is worthy of special mention given the regular use of the population age structure of this region as a basis of inter-regional standardisation techniques. What is clear from these figures, however, is that in aggregate terms MS is not a disease of childhood or early adulthood. This evidence also shows that MS is not a disease of old age either. The proportion of PwMS over the age of 75 years was half the proportion of the whole population of that age; an observation that could be indicative of PwMS on average tending to die earlier than the rest of the

Table 4.5 Distribution of PwMS by age group and female/male ratios for selected regions

	SUTTON 1985	SOUTH GLAM 1985	SOUTH CAMBS 1990	SUSSEX 1991	SE SCOT' 1995	TAY SIDE 1996	FIFE 1996	N.N.I. 1996	N.N.I. 2004
0–14									
15–24	0.7	6.0	∞	3.0	1.8	4.5	4.0	∞	∞
25–34	2.8	3.4	3.8	3.3	2.9	3.9	4.4	2.5	3.6
35–44	1.8	1.9	2.7	2.3	3.3	3.3	2.0	3.9	1.4
45–54	2.5	1.5	2.5	2.0	2.8	2.3	2.5	1.8	2.4
55–64	2.0	1.6	1.8	2.8	1.7	2,7	2.5	1.7	2.1
65–74	2.8	1.6	2.0	2.9	2.9	3.3	1.5	2.3	1.4
75+	7.0	∞	5.0	3.0	3.1	2.3	2.8	1.5	1.8

∞ indicates there were no men with MS in this category.

population. Given the relative paucity of cases of MS in these age ranges it is only reasonable to expect relative excesses in others. This occurred in the 45 to 54 years age range with almost twice as many PwMS than would have been expected. It was only in the 65 to 74 age range that the two age distributions showed any signs of accord.

Given the close congruence across all the regional studies of MS of the mean cohort age and the mean age of onset, it may be tempting to suggest that this indicates MS is fundamentally a life-course illness in which similar disease events occur at similar times in individuals across their disease careers irrespective of place or year; that is disease onset, significant disabling events, functional deficits and even death taking place at similar ages. If so one would expect the ages of such events to be tightly packed around their mean ages with low standard deviations. In terms of age of onset at least the available information does not support such a view. For example, in Hampshire in 1987, the mean age of disease onset was 32.6 years with a range of 10 to 60 years and a standard deviation of 9.9 years, that is a relatively wide spread about the mean (Roberts et al. 1991). Similarly, for north Northern Ireland in 1996 the mean age of onset for women was 31.0 years and for men 33.0 years both with a standard deviation of 10.1 years (McDonnell and Hawkins 1998). Finally, for Sutton in 1985 the age of disease onset was described in 5-year age bands from 14 to 19 years in which there were 10 cases to 60–64 years in which there was just 1 case. In between these more than 20 cases fell in each of the age bands 20–24 and 45–49 years (Williams and McKernan 1986). Thus, while disease onset in this case may have been infrequent in the under 20s and over 50s, it was relatively evenly spread between these age extremes with no marked concentration. In South Glamorgan, however, age of onset was more temporally concentrated with 33 per cent of all incident cases in the model class 25–34 years and 21 per cent in each of the 10-year age bands on either side (Swingler and Compston 1988, 1523).

Were there any important age differences between men and women with MS? Table 4.5 presents female/male ratios for each of the regions for which comparable age-specific evidence was available. In every case, except for Sutton in 1985 for the 15–24 year age band, there were more women with MS than men. Indeed, for 4 of the cells at the age extremes where female/male ratios tended to be at their highest, there were no men at all; 3 in 15–24 year age band and 1 in the oldest group. These results seem to be indicative of four enduring features of MS gender differences by age. First, women tend to develop MS at an earlier age than men. Second, men with MS tend to die earlier than women with

MS. Third, male MS prevalence tends to peak at a higher age than women. For example, in Rochdale in 1989 male prevalence peaked in the 45–54 year age band whereas women peaked between 35 and 44 years (Shepherd and Summers 1996). A similar finding was discovered by McDonnell and Hawkins (1998) for north Northern Ireland in 1996. In South Glamorgan, by contrast, in 2005 the highest prevalence occurred in higher age ranges: 45–54 for women and 55–64 for men (Hirst et al. 2009). Meanwhile in South Cambridgeshire in 1993 both men and women recorded their highest prevalences in the same age band, 45–54 years (Robertson et al. 1996b). And, the final age/gender trend would be that women tend to have longer MS careers than men.

4.4 Ethnicity

There appears to be a consensus in the academic literature that MS prevalence varies between ethnic groups, at its highest in the Caucasian peoples, much lower in people from the Orient and Asia and according to Compston (1990b, 822) of legendary rarity in Africans. Thus, it would be a reasonable hypothesis to suggest that if these relationships held true, then places where non-white ethnic peoples are well represented would have relatively low rates of MS and vice versa. As shown in the following chapter, this relationship would appear to hold true at the international level and perhaps it could have some usefulness at a larger scale too. For example, within the UK the areas where non-white ethnic communities are concentrated such as in major cities and the industrial towns on the Pennine fringe would have relatively low rates of MS and, by contrast, where rates of non-white people were low, such as in Northern Ireland, Scotland and rural Britain, MS prevalences would be relatively high. The regional epidemiological evidence on MS would tend to support such a view. However, in all cases very few people of non-white ethnic origin were recorded to make one seriously question the reliability of the evidence and, therefore, whether the hypothesis had been adequately tested. Indeed, the evidence provided by the UK regional studies of MS on the disease's relationship with ethnicity is sparse, inconsistent and confusing.

In the two areas investigated in northern England where large concentrations of people of Indian subcontinent origin are known to exist, Leeds and Rochdale, few people of non-white ethnic origin with MS appear to have been recorded by either the institutions of the NHS or disease support groups that were the main sources of evidence for these inquiries. Ford et al. (1998, 609), for example, for Leeds in 1995 observed that MS prevalence was not consistently lower in areas of non-white ethnic concentrations suggesting that other factors such as economic status may be operating as confounding factors. However, and perhaps most significantly, over the next 4 years of the 176 MS incident cases recorded only 2 (1%!) were of non-white ethnic origin and both were born in the UK (Ford et al. 2002, 262). Similarly, in the study of MS in Rochdale in 1989, the strong impression was given that few people of non-white ethnic origin developed the condition because this demographic characteristic was not even mentioned apart from obliquely by noting that only 5 cases (2%) were born outside the UK (Shepherd and Summers 1996, 417). In areas where the proportion of people of non-white ethnic origin were relatively low such as in Cambridgeshire in the early 1990s and in Scotland during the next decade the number of PwMS from these communities was commensurately small. In North Cambridgeshire in 1993, only 4 people out of a prevalent total of 449 were of non-white origin: 2 Asian, 1 Afro-Caribbean and 1 Mauritian; 3 of whom were British born and 2 with white ancestry (Robertson et al. 1995, 74). Similarly, in central Glasgow in 2000 only 2 of the 245 prevalent MS cases were of non-white (Asian) origin (Murray et al. 2004, 103). Finally, in South Glamorgan between 1985 and 2005, the number of PwMS of non-white ethnic origin although increasing appeared to be substantially under-represented again supporting the view that MS is predominantly a disease of 'white' people. At the beginning of this period, the proportion of PwMS of non-white origin was 1.7 per cent whereas the proportion of non-whites in the whole of South Glamorgan was 4.4 per cent. In 2005, the equivalent proportions were 3.5 per cent (just 22 individuals) and 6.7 per cent respectively (Hirst et al. 2009, 389).

The surveys of members of the MS national charities support the above findings on ethnicity and MS too. For example, the surveys by Hobart et al. (2001 and 2003) both reported that 98 per cent of their cases of MS were of 'white' origin, the research by Green et al. (2007, 530) reported that 98.4 per cent of their respondents were 'white' while the early results from the UK MS Register indicated 93.8 per cent of respondents regarded themselves as 'white British' (Ford et al. 2012). Interestingly, the survey by Green et al. (2007) also observed that for individuals in the General Household Survey of 2001–2, 93 per cent were of 'white' origin suggesting, as in South Glamorgan, that there were fewer people of non-white ethnic origin in GB with MS than would have been expected from the national proportion of people in this racial group. But, are such low proportions of people of non-white ethnic origin with MS indicative of real trends in the UK, or are they more likely to be symbolic of powerful cultural forces that restrict PwMS from these communities being treated in the health services of the British state? The answer to this question is not yet known but needs to be sensitively researched.

There are two important confounding factors of relevance to this discussion that concern the changing MS propensity of people of ethnic origin over time that will alter the all-too-easy assertions made at the start of this section. First, as a result of inter-racial relationships it may be becoming increasingly difficult to be clear about what race people belong. Thus, the categorisation of people into ethnic groups and most certainly by outward appearance may be becoming increasingly less certain. Second, if the research findings of Elian and colleagues (Elian and Dean 1987, Elian et al. 1990) are to be believed, then whatever the initial benefit of a lower propensity to develop MS non-white racial origin may imbue in people in the UK, it will be lost in their future generations born in the UK. They will become increasingly subject to the same likelihood of developing MS as their 'white' neighbours. In other words racially determined risks of developing MS were either modified by the environment or, perhaps more controversially, were an artefact of the environment from the very start (Compston 1997, 556). Thus, the relationship between ethnicity and MS prevalence suggested at the beginning of this section should not be expected to persist indefinitely especially in communities where people of non-white origin have become well established over more than one generation. Indeed, this may have been one of the reasons why in a multiracial population in southern California between 2008 and 2010, the white ethnic communities recorded 140 per cent more new cases of MS than would have been expected from their heir background population and the black community more than twice as many (Langer-Gould et al. 2013). By contrast, the Hispanic peoples recorded 60 per cent of what would have been expected and the Asians 30 per cent. As a result, in this place at this time it was the black community that was most at risk of developing MS, a result almost entirely due to an excess of MS in black women.

Unfortunately, the rise of MS in black communities comes with major health-care consequences for both the individual and the communities in which they live because evidence from both sides of the Atlantic in London and New York strongly suggests that people of black ethnic origin tend to develop an aggressive form of MS more often than other ethnic groups (Koffman et al. 2013, Weinstock-Guttman et al. 2003).

4.5 Deprivation/Social class

The link between deprivation and illness along with its usual concomitants of lack of material resources, poor housing, weak educational achievement, poor nutrition and adverse health behaviours has been well established especially in the British research literature both for the individual and ecologically for small census areas (Carstairs and Morris 1991, Shaw et al. 2000). Thus, deprivation is now seen as a definite risk factor for many diseases. This has not been the experience for MS, however, where the complete opposite seems to have held sway for the limited evidence that is available. For example, in the early research of Phadke and Downie (1987) on North East Scotland almost two thirds of the 839 patients with an MS diagnosis in 1980 belonged to social classes I to III (professional, managerial and skilled occupations)[1] and for which the authors remark (p.8): 'This preponderance of high social class is highly significant when compared to the distribution of the general Scottish population'. Murray et al. (2004) echo this observation for central Glasgow in 2000 in which the Carstairs and Morris (1991) deprivation measure was used at the scale of the post-code sector. In this case four census-based variables, overcrowding, car ownership, male unemployment and the social class (IV and V) of the head of household, were amalgamated into a single index. For the most deprived areas of central Glasgow the standardised MS prevalence and incidence values were 57 per cent and 56 per cent respectively whereas for the most affluent areas they were much higher at 150 per cent and 170 per cent (Murray et al. 2004, 102). A similar finding was reported by Visser et al. (2012, 723) for the combined areas of Aberdeen City, Orkney and Shetland in 2009 in which the lowest socio-economic group recorded an MS prevalence rate 2.5 times lower than the other groups; that is 103/100,000 compared to 244/100,000 for PwMS living in the least deprived areas. In other words, in this part of the world in the early twenty-first century the most multiply deprived areas were the best places to live to avoid developing MS.

If there was any value in this latter relationship, then it would be difficult not to reach for the hygiene hypothesis for a possible explanation (Fleming and Cook 2006), that the early immune system needs to be challenged to develop properly to allow it to beat threats later in life, with modern antibiotics, vaccines and quarantine behaviours tending to prevent this. Unfortunately, research evidence from outside Scotland and especially from Denmark and Canada does not support this view (Giovannoni and Ebers 2007). While this hypothesis is concerned with the environmental conditions that may lead to the development of MS, what has not been considered anywhere in the literature are the environmental conditions that may be related to the progress of the MS disease once contracted. Does, for example, material wellbeing or living in an area with easy access to appropriate health care reduce potentially harmful comorbidities and slow the disease's progress? It is known that certain lifestyle choices such as smoking (Hernan et al. 2005) may have adverse effects on PwMS. But, could it also be true that certain 'therapeutic landscapes' (Gesler 1992) known to have a positive impact on health generally could also improve the life chances of PwMS? The relationships between material conditions, life style choices of PwMS with the progress of their disease is a virtually unexplored territory that needs to be colonised with some urgency to help people develop coping strategies for their condition.

The national survey results of PwMS in the UK on deprivation were also suggestive of an inverse relationship with MS prevalence, the most persuasive coming from the work by Green et al. (2007, 530) where it was observed that 86.1 per cent of PwMS involved were home owners compared to only 74.8 per cent of members of the 2001–2 General Household Survey. In other words, more MwMS than would have been expected from general population trends could afford to own their own home. At first glance this may appear counter-intuitive given, as shown in Chapter 6, most PwMS have some form of disability, and disability and poverty in the UK are closely related (Parcker 2008). However, this relationship relates to the ability to own a house of the household in which a person with MS lives and not to them alone. It will depend on their partner's circumstances as well as their own.

4.6 Employment

One of the important components of wellbeing is employment, not only through the income it may generate, but also through the personal identities it creates and the social interaction it engenders. Evidence on the employment status of PwMS across all parts of the western world investigated so far has shown that many of them of working age are unemployed and often according to Simmons (2010, 607) at a rate higher than 50 per cent, much higher than for the regional or national populations of which they are part. For example, using the NARCOMS database to survey almost 9,000 PwMS in the United States (US), 60 per cent of working age were unemployed over the previous 18 months. In addition, 6 per cent had lost their jobs and only 3 per cent gained employment (Julian et al. 2008, 1359). In a survey in Australia of more than 2,300 PwMS in 1981, only 50 per cent of men and 27 per cent of women of working age reported being employed (Hammond et al. 1996). And, using the Danish National Registry for 10,849 PwMS and 43,396 controls, the employment rate of the former was only half of the latter (Jennum et al. 2012). The survey work of PwMS in the UK also shows the low rates of employment among PwMS. For example, in the McCrone et al. (2008) sample only 21.3 per cent were in work (full time, part-time, self-employed or student) with 21.3 per cent retired due to illness (presumably their MS but not necessarily so). The work of Hobart et al. (2001) presents very similar figures with 18.0 per cent employed and 54 per cent retired due to MS. Meanwhile, the two surveys in the research by Forbes et al. (2006a, 990) paint a similar picture too with 49 per cent and 48 per cent of their respondents retired due to MS. However, using different terminology, Green et al. (2007, 530) suggest rather more PwMS may be in work by reporting 29.9 per cent of their sample in paid employment. Nevertheless, this research also indicated that the proportion of people in work with MS was much smaller than the proportion of all people in the UK in work at 59.6 per cent. The UK MS Register research also reports this disparity in that 41.9 per cent of respondents with MS of working age (16–64 years) were in employment compared to a national equivalent of 76.9 per cent. Furthermore, 32.7 per cent of the Register's respondents of working age said that they were sick/disabled compared to the national equivalent of 24.5 per cent (Ford et al. 2012).

It may, therefore, seem reasonable to conclude that PwMS have a much lower rate of employment than would be expected from national trends and have been denied many years of income from their lost years of employment. For example, in a study of more than 2,200 Danes with MS, with disease onset on average in their mid-30s and an average disease duration to retirement about 13 years, many PwMS would have lost about 15 years of gainful employment if normal retirement age was in the mid-60s (Pfleger et al. 2010a). This would almost certainly have had a negative impact on their future income, pensions and quality of life. Similarly, in a much smaller questionnaire inquiry in South East Wales, of 169 people who were employed at diagnosis 43.3 per cent had left employment at a mean time since onset of 11.9 years and only 6.5 per cent had retired at the national age for their gender (Moore et al. 2013), suggesting many years of lost employment. But, we have no evidence on just how important this employment loss may have been to family incomes and affluence. For example, there was no indication in most of this type of work of the degree to which the person with MS who is without employment was once the principal earner of a family. In fact, this is impossible to judge because despite the relatively high proportions of women and married individuals in these samples it is not known the degree to which they approximated to traditional early twentieth century families of the male being the main source of income. Much more research in this area is required to discover the effect of MS-induced unemployment on personal and family incomes and wellbeing.

The issue of employment loss and maintenance for PwMS will be considered again in Chapters 6 and 7 but at this point it is important to be aware of the main reasons for PwMS changing their employment status. Some are very direct and clear such as growing physical disability that may affect mobility and dexterity leading to problems of getting to, accessing and using the workplace safely. As a result, manual occupations will be less likely to sustain the employment of PwMS in contrast to clerical/office-based jobs. It also follows in part that educational attainment may become a good predictor of the ability of a person with MS to remain in work (Simmons 2010, Pfleger et al. 2010a, Moore et al. 2013). However, work even in these occupations may be compromised if the person with MS begins to suffer the externally less obvious symptoms of problems with cognition and fatigue, the most common symptom of the condition.

4.7 Education

Most of the limited evidence on this attribute tends to support the view that PwMS tend to be well-educated and often to a higher level than the community in which they reside. The early evidence on this issue reviewed by Hammond et al. (1996) for a number of different countries supports this assertion as does their own material for Australia at least in terms of the age of leaving school. Most of the recent survey work of PwMS in the UK was supportive too. For example, Orme et al. (2007, 4) for members of the MS Trust discovered that 39.8 per cent of respondents had at least a university or polytechnic qualification and for the early UK MS Register respondents 33 per cent said they had a university bachelor or postgraduate degree and 34 per cent an occupational diploma or certificate. Meanwhile, the Forbes et al. (2006a) surveys indicated that 60 per cent and 63 per cent of PwMS had been in education for more than 14 years, while the McCrone et al. (2008, 850) survey of MwMS noted 22.5 per cent with a university degree or above, but a lower figure of only 16.2 per cent was reported in the survey by Green et al. (2007, 530). Tellingly, however, this latter inquiry also observed that 15.1 per cent of the General House hold Survey (GHS) members fell into this category. Perhaps, therefore, the difference in educational attainment between those with and without MS had not been so great after all. It is also not difficult to suggest from this material that the major difference in educational attainment may not necessarily be between those with and those without MS but between those with MS who join an MS support charity and those with MS who do not and, furthermore, have the time, interest and competence to fill out questionnaires and surveys. It may also more worryingly indicate that there are certain sections of the MS community in the UK that its support charities have not yet managed to persuade to join.

4.8 Marital status

Most of the national surveys of PwMS in the UK offer information on the marital status of their respondents but the categories used are often irritatingly different and so prevent precise comparisons. The most reliable results by Hobart et al. (2001) reported that 66 per cent in their first sample of PwMS and 70 per cent in their second sample were married. The McCrone et al. (2008, 850) results also attest to the majority of their respondents being married but in terms of 'living with a spouse or partner' at 70.3 per cent and the two surveys of Forbes et al. (2006a, 990) note slightly higher married/with partner proportions of 77 per cent. By contrast, Green and colleagues (2007, 530) reported on this issue in terms of the percentage of PwMS who were divorced by gender: 7.0 per cent for men with MS and higher at 10.1 per cent for women with MS. Why there should be a 3 per cent point difference between the sexes on this attribute is unknown. However, it may be of interest to note that a similar difference existed in the divorce proportions for members of the GHS at this time too at 4.5 per cent for men and 7.4 per cent for women, but in both cases 3 per cent points less than their MS counterparts. Does this suggest that MS is associated with an elevated divorce rate as observed in the Introduction of this book? The research by Hakim et al. (2000, 290) in Hampshire suggested it may not. Their trawl of all PwMS between 1986 and 1989 discovered that only 9 per cent of their regional total was divorced compared with what they call a divorce rate for England and Wales of 13 per cent. Unfortunately, that rate actually referred to the annual number of persons divorcing per thousand married and is not at all comparable to their MS divorce figure which relates to the number of divorced PwMS as a proportion of their sample of PwMS. Thus, this unexpectedly positive evidence is irrelevant. However, according to Green et al. (2007, 530), the difference between the divorce percentages for men with MS in their survey and men in the GHS was not significantly different statistically at the 5 per cent level whereas the difference for women was highly significant at the 1 per cent level. Thus, there may have been serious sexual differences in the likelihood of being divorced for PwMS in the UK. But, from a multivariate analysis they (Green et al. 2007, 533) concluded that gender divorce rate differences for MS populations 'would appear to be attributable to confounding factors such as age.' Thus, no matter how intuitively reasonable it may seem, there is no convincing evidence for the UK that PwMS have a higher divorce rate than the general British population. And, it therefore follows that the comment by Amor and van Noort (2012, 21) in their book 'MS: the facts' that for PwMS: 'The rate of divorce is double that of the population', was wrong for the UK at the start of the twenty-first century.

But, could it have been correct elsewhere? The available limited evidence is far from directly supportive. For example, most cross-sectional analyses from Germany, Australia and Denmark indicate that the majority of PwMS, usually at approximately 75 per cent, were married at the time of their surveys (Pfleger et al. 2010b, 878). Furthermore, relationship failure seemed to have been related to level of disability (Hammond et al. 1996), female gender (Glantz et al. 2009) and having no young children (Pfleger et al. 2010b) but, only the latter study tracked PwMS through time to estimate relationship failure. In this case, using the Danish MS Registry, of the 1,804 PwMS with onset between 1980 and 1989 who had a partner, the probability of remaining in the same relationship for 5 years was 86 per cent for PwMS and 89 per cent for a set of matched controls that declined to 33 per cent for PwMS and 53 per cent for controls at 24 years (Pfleger et al. 2010b, 879). Thus, while it is possible that in some countries PwMS may have a higher divorce rate than the population of which they are part, there is no indication here that this rate could always be twice as high.

One of the important qualities that marriage brings is companionship, someone with whom to converse and share one's daily life that may be vital in avoiding loneliness and social isolation, especially so for the physically disabled with limited mobility. In this context, therefore, it is reassuring to note that most PwMS appeared to be either married or in a long-term relationship and had some opportunity in this context for social interaction. The depressing view presented in the

'Introduction' of PwMS being doomed to living alone does not appear to be the general case. This is also borne out by the fact that in the surveys by Forbes et al. (2006a, 990) only 14 per cent and 16 per cent of their 2 samples lived alone. Even so this may still imply that a large number of PwMS may be experiencing serious problems of loneliness and isolation and steps must be taken by the relevant social and charitable organisations to try to overcome them. It is also possible that such problems may be most acutely felt by the most seriously disabled because in their research on a palliative care service in South East London, Higginson and Hart (2006, 160) discovered that even in their small sample of 51 PwMS with a mean EDSS (Expanded Disability Status Scale) score of 7.8, 18 per cent lived by themselves with formal care coming to their place of residence to help them. Much more needs to be known about this potentially seriously disadvantaged group to discover what may be realistically done to help them in the ways in which they want to live their lives.

4.9 Conclusion

The regional epidemiological studies of MS in the UK and in other places too suggested six important demographic features:

1. The gender balance was heavily in favour of women with female to male ratios being in excess of 2:1 and for the more recent years somewhat higher.
2. The mean age of regional cohorts was no lower than 50 years with mean age of onset being between 30 and 35 years.
3. There were far smaller proportions of PwMS in the youngest and oldest age bands compared to general populations. The relative paucity of mature PwMS may be suggestive of a lower average age of death for PwMS than for the general population.
4. For whatever reason, few people of non-white ethnic origin with MS were recorded by any of the MS surveys, regional or national, implying their proportion of all PwMS to be relatively small at the start of the twenty-first century.
5. There was no convincing evidence that divorce rates for PwMS were higher than would have been expected from general population trends.
6. There appeared to be the tentative suggestion that MS and deprivation were inversely related to both the individual and small area scales.

Thus, to answer the major question posed by this chapter, MS did appear to be definitely demographically discriminatory, in favour of women, the middle-aged, white ethnic origin, relatively well educated, married and the relatively affluent.

However, this chapter must conclude with three important notes of caution. First, much of the evidence presented was for the late twentieth century and therefore perhaps losing its relevance for the contemporary world. Furthermore, probably the least reliable material was the most recent. In particular, it must be considered that some of the more favourable findings for the MS community such as home ownership rates may relate to a particularly fortunate group of people who were born within 10 to 20 years of the end of the Second World War, to live through a time when housing and higher/university education was relatively cheap. It was also a period of very high inflation, peaking in 1975 in the UK at 24 per cent that quickly diminished acquired debts. There must now be an urgent need to source up-to-date evidence on the demographic nature of PwMS to discover how these relationships may have changed for more recent cohorts of PwMS. The second note of caution comes from the fact that there are major areas of the lives of PwMS about which almost nothing is known; housing, occupations, incomes, social status, relationships, lifestyles, social and recreational activities to name some of the more obvious attributes. Yet, if society wishes to help affect their lives for the better some of this information is vital and properly organised research must be set in progress to collect it. Finally, it must be remembered that it is unrealistic to study demographic characteristics individually, they inevitably operate together in bundles to form an individual; the middle-aged, Caucasian women of Swingler and Compston's (1990) research, for example. What is more, they often operate individually and collectively to reinforce one another to make living with MS more difficult than it should be and probably directly contributing to making MS itself worse! Such multivariate research is considered in Chapter 6 in terms of the impacts of MS on peoples' lives.

5
How Many People Have MS? A Case Study of the UK

5.1 Introduction

This chapter is concerned primarily with establishing an estimate of the number of people with Multiple Sclerosis (PwMS) in the United Kingdom (UK) and the ways in which that number may change through time, the 'components of change'. It begins by placing the UK in an international context, demonstrating it is a country with one of the highest MS prevalence rates in the world; a finding that of itself helps to justify the geographical emphasis of this book. It then reviews the various estimates for the number of PwMS in the UK before considering first how MS varies within and between its four constituent countries and, second how the separate components of change have influenced these numbers.

5.2 The components of change

The components of change in the number of PwMS for any region between two points in time may be considered to be made up of three elements: 'stayers', those who are present in the region at both the beginning and the end of the period, additions and deletions. Additions have three different elements: incident cases (the newly diagnosed), migrants into the area already with MS and the rediscovered (PwMS who had been lost temporarily from the accounting system). Following a similar rubric, deletions include the following elements: PwMS who died, PwMS who moved out of the region and those with MS who had been lost from the accounting system. It is shown in what follows that repeat surveys of areas regularly discover cases of MS that should have been recorded for an earlier point in time. The reasons for this are varied, numerous and usually peculiar to the individual case. They should therefore be acknowledged as an unavoidable element of this sort of analysis irrespective of the care and believed universality of the adopted system of ascertainment. The corollary of this situation is also possible that PwMS may become untraceable to review with no evidence of death or out-migration. Furthermore, given the difficulty of diagnosing MS, it is inevitable that if cases are reviewed over time some reclassifications will take place in and out of either the McDonald or the definite and probable Poser diagnostic schemas.

5.3 International context

According to the Atlas of MS (MSIF 2013, 8), there were approximately 2.3 million PwMS in the world in 2013 and that this total had increased from 2.1 million in 2008. Unfortunately, the degree to which this represents a real increase in the number of people with the illness rather than increased awareness and diagnostic capability is not known. The 2013 estimate was calculated from a global median prevalence of 33/100,000 people from the 92 countries that took part in the exercise that collectively represented 79 per cent of the world's population. Now, the most widely quoted estimate for the number of PwMS in the UK for the early years of the twenty-first century was 100,000 (Thomas et al. 2009) or roughly 4 per cent of the world's total. However, at this time the UK's share of world population was much lower at approximately 1 per cent that suggests the UK had approximately 4 times the number of PwMS that would have been expected from its population. And, as can be seen in Figure 5.1, on MS prevalence by country in 2013, the UK was placed in the highest category of 100 PwMS/100,000 population and above along with much of Europe, Canada and the United States (US). Thus, the UK is one of the countries of the world where the chances of a person developing MS has been, and still is, at its zenith. In fact parts of Scotland have consistently recorded the highest prevalence rates for large population areas anywhere in the world (Pugliatti et al. 2002, 182).

The two recent atlases of MS (WHO and MSIF 2008, MSIF 2013) both demonstrated that while MS appeared to be present in all nation states, its prevalence varied hugely between them, from more than 100/100,00 population in most of western Europe and North America to less than 5/100,000 in most of Africa and south east Asia (Figure 5.1). Thus, MS appeared to be concentrated in relatively high-income countries where mainly 'white' people lived, findings that follow directly from the

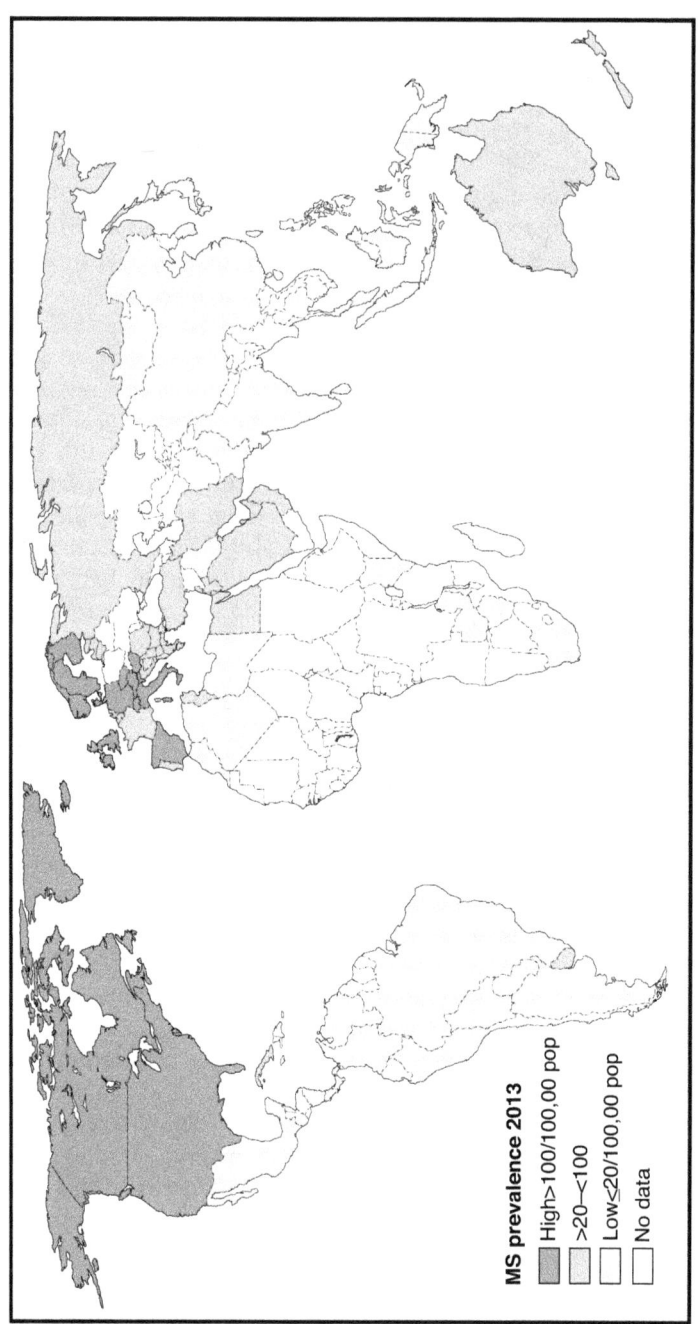

Figure 5.1 Worldwide prevalence of MS by nation state
Source: MSIF (2013) Atlas of MS 2013, p.8.

demographic depiction of the illness in the previous chapter that imply both genetic and socio-economic factors in its aetiology.

Observing the geography of MS among nation states and at the larger regional scale has led to some authors suggesting a gradient of both MS incidence and prevalence with latitude (Mayer 1981, Simpson et al. 2011). For example, in Australia Hobart had a higher MS prevalence than either Perth or Newcastle (Hammond et al. 1988), in the UK Shetland was higher than Hampshire (this chapter), in the US Minnesota was higher than Texas (Evans et al. 2013) and in France Picardie higher than Provence (Vukusic et al. 2007), with Simpson et al. (2011) in a major review of more than 320 peer-reviewed papers from 59 countries demonstrating a strong positive relationship globally between MS prevalence and latitude that directly implicated an environmental factor in the chances of someone developing MS. In this case exposure to ultraviolet radiation with its important role in the production of vitamin D has received most attention as discussed in Chapter 2. Some authors have not been convinced that the gradient in MS incidence will endure through time especially in the northern hemisphere with increased incidence rates in lower latitudes leading to its decline and ultimate elimination (Koch-Henriksen and Sorensen 2010 and 2011, Alonso and Hernan 2008). Meanwhile an increased life expectancy of PwMS may have helped to preserve the prevalence gradient in recent times. Simpson et al. (2011) accept that in extreme northern latitudes MS incidence and prevalence do decline but argue that this is probably the result of genetic differences among the indigenous peoples of these areas and the result of a relatively high intake of vitamin D through their diet. However, as explained in Chapter 2, untangling the genetic and environmental impacts in MS aetiology are fraught with difficulties because of the ways they most likely interact with one another in complex ways; an 'obsolete' endeavour now according to Koch-Henriksen and Sorensen (2011, 62).

5.4 The number of people with MS in the UK

Despite the UK being one of the places in the world where the chances of developing MS were at their highest, no effective surveillance or enumeration strategies were established within its international boundary. This has led to a series of questionable national estimates. The MS Society, for example, claimed for the decade up to 2009 there were at least 85,000 people in the UK with an MS diagnosis, although the origins of this figure are as mysterious as the aetiology of the illness itself. Interestingly, Holmes et al. (1995, 184) claimed a similar figure of 87,873 (quoted as

88,000 in Kobelt et al. 2000, 7) for 1993, again of unspecified methodology although allegedly derived by consultants working for Schering Health Care Ltd. Blumhardt and Wood (1996, 108) in their analysis of the economic burden of MS offered somewhat lower figures of 60,000 for the mid-1990s for England and Wales and 8,300 for Scotland with no estimate for Northern Ireland.

For the start of the twenty-first century Thomas and colleagues (2009) using General Practice Research Database (GPRD) evidence produced a much higher range of estimates of the number of PwMS in the UK in 2007 from a minimum of 88,760 after adjustment for neurological referrals to a maximum of 98,110 following the confirmed diagnostic proportion of 82 per cent. However, this investigation is only available as a three-page briefing note on the MS Society's website; the original project report still confidential five years after its production.[1] Furthermore, it has not been published as an academic paper and therefore not subjected to the rigours of independent peer review that must lead to the questioning of its value and integrity. In fact, some of the limitations to this form of analysis were offered in Chapter 3, all of which would have led directly to increases in the estimated numbers of PwMS in the UK probably by up to 10 per cent. This would result in a figure much closer to the most recent estimate of the number of PwMS in the UK by Mackenzie et al. (2014) of 126,669 for 2010. Thus, the figure of 100,000 eagerly quoted by the MS community for the number of people with the condition in the UK, while a definite improvement on what went before, may have already begun to perform a disservice to its client group by substantially underestimating the true figure.

All these estimates of the number of PwMS in the UK and its constituent countries by Mackenzie et al. (2014) in Table 5.1 were higher, and sometimes to a substantial degree, than those suggested a decade or so earlier by other commentators. For example, Compston (1990a, 207) stated boldly without explanation or citation that there were 60,000 PwMS in Great Britain (i.e., the UK without Northern Ireland). The possibility of the total doubling in 20 years to match the most recent estimate seems unrealistic and therefore these totals cannot be easily reconciled. Similarly, the work of Richards et al. (2002) to calculate the number of patients with MS in England and Wales for the end of the 1990s does not rest well with the results of Thomas et al. (2009) or Mackenzie et al. (2014) either. Their analysis, commissioned by National Institute for Health and Care Excellence (NICE) to aid deliberations over the therapeutic use of disease modifying drugs (DMDs) for MS, was based on regression models of regional MS prevalence rates against latitude.

Table 5.1 Estimates of the number of PwMS in the four countries of the UK in 2010

Country of UK	Population in thousands	Estimate of the number of PwMS	Prevalence (Number/100,000)
England	52,233.9	104,451	199.9
Northern Ireland	1,799.8	3,838	213.2
Scotland	5,222.3	13,328	255.2
Wales	3,006.3	5,052	168.0
UK	62,262.3	126,669	203.4

Source: Mackenzie et al. (2014, 83).

These were generated across both areas within the UK and internationally to include places of similar latitude both north and south of the equator in North America and Australasia. As the authors themselves somewhat ruefully admitted 'the exact applicability of this relationship to the UK context remains unclear' (Richards et al. 2002, 21), yet they persisted to produce estimates much lower than the work of Mackenzie and colleagues (2014), of between 58,000 and 63,000 for the number of PwMS in England and Wales. It is not known the degree to which this tawdry piece of research was used to underpin resource allocation for MS in any part of the UK. One can only hope it never was. But, in their document on the management of MS in primary and secondary care of the same year, NICE (2002, 3) offered an even lower figure of between 52,000 and 62,000 for the number of PwMS in England and Wales. By contrast, the estimate of Mackenzie et al. (2014) for the number of PwMS in Scotland, 13,328, was much higher than other suggested totals for the country. For example, the Scottish Needs Assessment Project (2000, 4) quoted a figure of 10,400 while the website of MS Scotland (accessed in October 2009) stated that 10,500 people had MS in their country.

5.5 Prevalence rates in the UK

As the decade of the 1990s began to unfold, two important transformations emerged in regional enquires into the prevalence and incidence of MS in the UK. First, the diagnostic criteria used to define the disease shifted to the more restrictive and precise Poser standard. Second, the geographical emphasis shifted southwards, not only within Scotland via Tayside to south of the Clyde-Forth axis but also away from Scotland altogether to places in England. At the same time a number of trends detected in earlier regional work in the reviews of Swingler and Compston

(1986) up to the early 1980s and Robertson and Compston (1995) for the next decade persisted. First, the research in the more northerly parts of the UK continued to record much higher prevalence rates than those in the south. By now though the formerly all-pervasive search for a latitudinal gradient in MS prevalence in the nation had been replaced by an acceptance of a step change in rates between Scotland and Northern Ireland in the north and England and Wales in the south. As Robertson and Compston (1995, 5) admitted, 'the evidence for a systematic change in prevalence of people with multiple sclerosis with latitude in the United Kingdom now seems less secure.' It is also important to observe what this change in geographical emphasis meant for possible disease causation; no longer was there a search for a biological agent that necessarily changed systematically with latitude, but an acceptance that a political or cultural border may be in place that tended to keep those with a relatively high propensity to develop MS to the north of it and those with a lower propensity to its south, namely the political and cultural boundary between Scotland and England (see Figure 5.2).

The second pervasive trend in UK MS prevalence studies, with one possible minor exception, was that where repeat surveys had taken place in the same region over time increases in prevalence were discovered. Here four very different regions, South Cambridgeshire, Leeds, north Northern Ireland and South Glamorgan, offered diverse examples.

Finally, many of the problems of analysis that shackled comparative regional prevalence studies in the past persisted: different interpretations of the MS diagnostic criteria (e.g., the age of inclusion criteria); different primary data sources; different types and sizes of region; different socio-economic characteristics of regional populations. Over time there could also have been important changes in the disease phenotype at play and therefore the characteristics of people that may put themselves at risk of developing MS. And, the lack of commonality or standardisation of approach in these studies necessitates any putative conclusions to be regarded as little more than speculations. Hirst and colleagues (2009, 386) emphasise this point by stating a 'simple comparison of disease expression in geographical and temporally distinct populations is problematic.'

The principal regional prevalence studies in the UK since the end of the 1980s are listed in Table 5.2 and mapped in Figure 5.2. There are two main reasons for beginning this review at this time. The first reason is because it was at this time that the rather liberal interpretation of MS by Allison and Millar was replaced by the more demanding Poser criteria; the second because the regional research up to that point had been

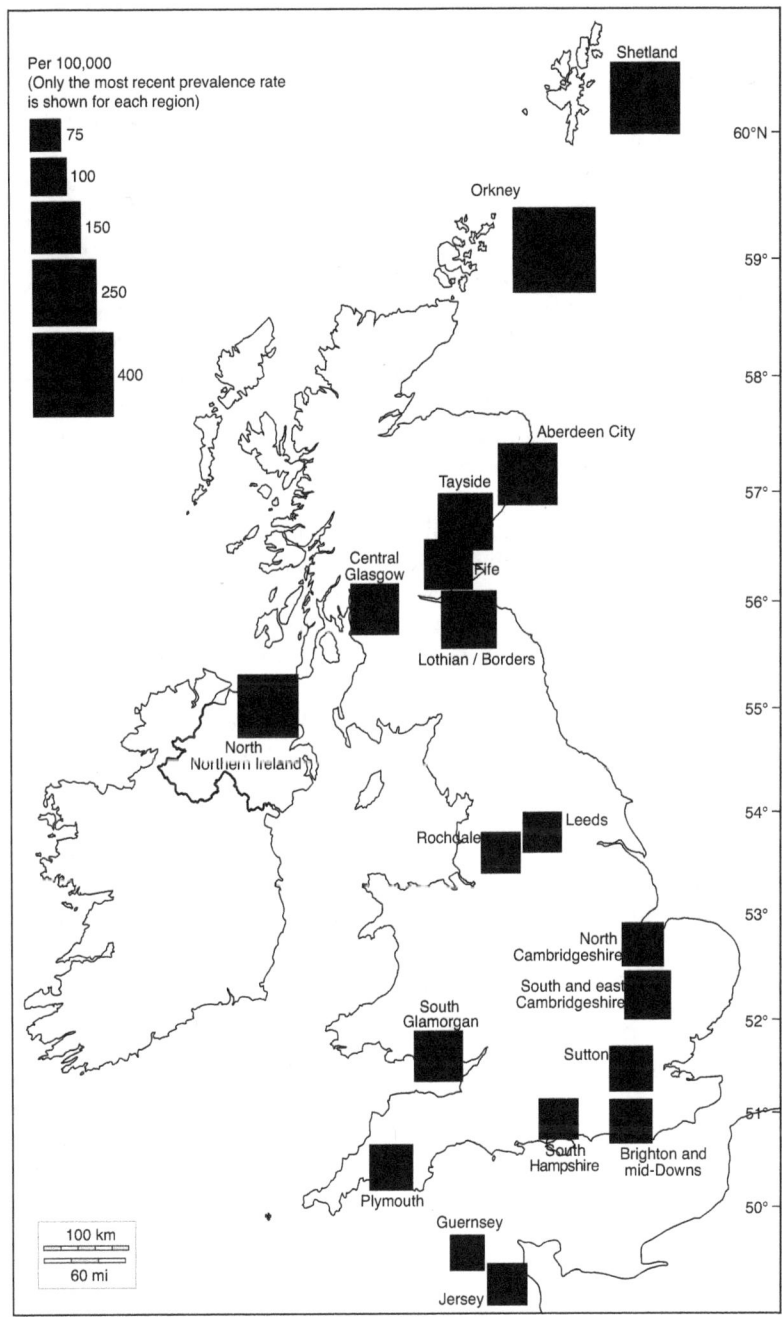

Figure 5.2 UK regional MS prevalence rates

thoroughly reviewed elsewhere by Swingler and Compston (1986) and Robertson and Compston (1995). While allowing for a modest overlap between their work and this one, there seemed little to be gained from repeating their clear descriptive analyses.

The areas studied vary hugely in type and size from boroughs of major cities such as Sutton in London to Rochdale in Greater Manchester to whole urban areas such as Leeds and Plymouth and to individual island clusters such as Orkney and Shetland. But, mainly the areas investigated have been defined in terms of health authority districts and authorities, not an unexpected situation given the focus was on a disease and the main information sources were from medical establishments. The size of these units of study relating to their populations have been as small as 20,000 for the islands of Orkney and were at a maximum for the Lothian and Borders Health Boards at 850,000. However, it is the smaller study areas, especially the general practitioner (GP) catchment areas that revealed the greatest variation in prevalence rates. For example, Markby (1987, 505) observing the MS prevalence rate for his own practice was as high as 500/100,000 was moved to survey his fellow GPs in the New Forest to discover much lower rates of 143 (twice), 145 and 154. A decade later in Fife against this 'kingdom's' overall prevalence of 143/100,000 inhabitants individual GP practice areas ranged in MS prevalence from zero where no PwMS lived to 464 at its highest where 18 PwMS lived (Grant et al. 1998, 46–7). Similarly, in South Glamorgan where Swingler and Compston (1990) carried out an ecological analysis across its 64 communities, as they called them, MS prevalence rates ranged from zero in nine areas to 435/100,000 in Sully, one of the four having significantly high results. The other three were Heath (219), Llandaff (253) and Radyr (386). It is possible that some of these spatial concentrations of PwMS in very small areas could represent the purposeful clustering of people with the disease at some time after diagnosis such as in regional rehabilitation centres or in residential homes for the significantly disabled run by charities such as Cheshire Homes or John Grooms (now Livability). Indeed, this was the case in two of the significant spatial concentrations, Llandaff and Radyr, identified by Swingler and Compston (1990) in South Glamorgan. However, it is unlikely that such clear clustering of PwMS in certain places represented a geographically specific causal factor. It was much more likely simply to reflect the geographical outcome of the vagaries of the housing market relative to people's constraints and choices and differential migration by age group. For example, the relatively high prevalence of MS in a small number of Suffolk GP practice areas (Lockyer 1991) was probably the result of the out-migration of the relatively young, leaving behind an excess of the age groups most likely to have MS. Such differential migration by age may also have had a role to play in understanding the high prevalence rates in Orkney and Shetland too.

While the discovery of local spatial clusters of PwMS may have been the motivation for epidemiological work in the New Forest, Suffolk and Fife and the output of the spatial ecological work in South Glamorgan, a specific search for them took place in Tayside between 1970 and 1997 (Donnan et al. 2005) in the belief that their presence might indicate an infectious agent in local MS aetiology. During this research, 772 cases of definite and probable MS were recorded at the high annual incidence rate of 7.2/100,000 with a clear temporal periodicity of 2–3 years. Furthermore, their spatial scanning techniques identified 2 spatio-temporal clusters between 1993 and 1995 at an incidence rate of 17.1/100,000/year, the first in a rural area to the south west of Perth and the other in part of central Perth itself. Unfortunately, Perth was not identified on their accompanying map. Nevertheless, with the empirical evidence at their disposal they were able to discount possible susceptible groups such as young women, ascertainment changes, deprivation and migration as possible explanations. Thus, they concluded an infectious agent was the most likely cause of their identified spatial and temporal clusters.

There was no consensus among the authors of the regional prevalence studies in Table 5.2 on the optimal size of study area with some unashamedly suggesting their chosen region to be about right or even optimal. Swingler and Compston (1988, 1523) for example, from their work in South Wales, argued that a study area with a population of approximately 500,000 would be suitable for adequate precision and remaining manageable stating 'under-ascertainment and error in diagnosis will contaminate studies based on a very large population, whereas confidence limits for prevalence estimates will widen if too small a denominator is used.' By contrast, both McDonnell and Hawkins (1998) and Gray et al. (2008) claim optimality for their much smaller area in north Northern Ireland of less than 150,000 inhabitants at the end of the twentieth century.

Manageability though is not just about the population of the study area, it is much more about the number of cases of MS that have to have their diagnoses checked and verified by clinical staff; that is the available resources for the research required. With two neurologists each perhaps the studies in South Wales and north Northern Ireland were not that

120 *People with Multiple Sclerosis*

Table 5.2 The principal regional MS prevalence studies published since 1985

Area	Year of Survey	Year of Publication	Type of Region	Size: Population
Sutton (south London)	1985	1986	London borough	169,600
South Glamorgan	1985	1988	County	376,718
South Hampshire	1987	1991	Health Board	417,000
5 GP Practices in rural Suffolk	1988	1991	GP Practice catchments	31,379 patients
South Glamorgan	1988	1989	County	376,718*
Rochdale	1989	1996	Metropolitan borough of Greater Manchester	207,600
South and east Cambridgeshire	1990	1992	Health District	288,410
Guernsey	1991	1995	Island	61,164
Jersey	1991	1995	Island	84,085
Brighton and mid-Downs	1991	1995	Health District	596,594
South and east Cambridgeshire	1993	1996	Health District	290,700
North Cambridgeshire	1993	1995	County District	378,959
Lothian / Borders	1995	1998	Health Board	864,300
Leeds	1996	1998	Health Authority	732,061
North Northern Ireland	1996	1998	Ballymena, Moyle, Ballymoney and Coleraine Districts	146,066
Tayside	1996	1999	Health Board	395,600
Fife	1996	1998	Health Board	354,273
Leeds	1999	2002	Health Authority	728,840
Central Glasgow	2000	2004	3 local Health-Care Cooperatives	169,000
Plymouth	2001	2004	Plymouth and surrounding area	341,796
Tayside	2002	2005	Region	383,405
North Northern Ireland	2004	2008	Ballymena, Moyle, Ballymoney and Coleraine Districts	160,446
South Glamorgan	2005	2009	Cardiff and Vale of Glamorgan unitary authorities	424,633
Aberdeen City	2009	2012	City	205,446
Orkney	2009	2012	Island group	20,000
Shetland	2009	2012	Island group	22,656

*The population total given for South Glamorgan in both 1985 and 1988 appears to be the same. Actually the one given for the latter in the text (Hennessy et al. 1989, 1087) is 3,766,718, an order of magnitude too big.

Note: The shaded areas indicate studies that used neither the Poser nor the McDonald criteria to diagnose MS.

dissimilar because with widely differing prevalence rates, both areas had similar numbers of confirmed cases of MS, 370 and 381 respectively.

One of the least convincing reasons, however, for choosing a particular region for study comes from Fox et al. (2004, 56) for the Plymouth area, namely low migration rates, simply because, as was shown in Chapter 3, it was not true. This study was also infuriating for two other reasons. First, because the population quoted for the area of interest of 342,000 for 2001 conformed neither to the census population of Plymouth of 241,000 for that year nor to the population of Devon of 706,000 which makes relating this work to other demographic information problematic. The second reason for irritation was because it was one of the few research papers that claimed in their title to be presenting evidence for a much larger area than was actually the case. Their paper states that it was a study of the epidemiology of MS in Devon whereas in reality it was more likely to be mainly concerned with Plymouth, 37 per cent of that county's population. A similar example relates to Northern Ireland by McDonnell and Hawkins (1998), where the title implied total provincial coverage and therefore comparability with some of the early seminal work by Allison and Millar (1954). However, the actual research only covered 9 per cent of the province's population in the districts of Ballymena, Ballymoney, Coleraine and Moyle. It is not the modest deception itself that is of concern, but that authors reviewing the material quote results for the smaller areas as if they were for the much larger ones stated in the titles of the papers, as evidenced by Hirst et al. (2009, 390).

What perhaps became clear, however, from these regional studies of the prevalence of MS in the UK was the dominance of pragmatic reasons for the choice of area studied, no matter how erudite the authors tried to make them appear. In every case it was the region in which the neurologists practiced their craft that was chosen for study. This is a perfectly understandable state of affairs. It was the area the researchers knew best, had most insight into the potential information sources and the issues concerning their patients. Only in the case of the study of south east Scotland by Rothwell and Charlton (1998) did the authors claim a sample size calculation was undertaken to allow a statistically significant difference to be derived between their work and equivalent research elsewhere. They suggested this would necessitate a study area of at least 500,000 people which could have been achieved by just concentrating on the Lothian area. Surprisingly, therefore, these two authors failed to act on their own calculations because they went much further to include the Borders area as well. This made their analysis the largest modern regional MS prevalence study so far undertaken in the UK to encompass more than 850,000 people. However, this example also served to highlight the point that so far no one has suggested any compelling theoretical reasons for the choice of a region or regions for MS prevalence studies in the UK and acted upon them. And, the reason for this was most likely because the aetiology of the illness at a population level was, and still is, so poorly understood.

The results from the principal regional MS prevalence studies since the mid-1980s are presented in Table 5.3 by year of survey and in Table 5.4 by the magnitude of the result. The latter includes only the 19 truly comparable studies using similar rubrics and MS definitions. A number of important points become clear from these arrays.

The first must be the collapse of interest in UK regional MS prevalence studies during the first decade of the twenty-first century. There were only 6 papers published in this area during this time period, with 12 during the 1990s and 8 in the decade before that (Robertson and Compston 1995, 4). A cascade of three reasons may begin to account for this change. First, the cost and effort of constructing, or even updating, a provisional list of PwMS in an area whose diagnoses then need to be reviewed must have been a major disincentive to research continuing in this area, especially when, and this is the second reason, the intellectual return has been of questionable value, or 'tantalisingly vague' as Robertson and Compston (1995, 2) put it. The final reason for UK regional prevalence studies having only a brief favourable airing during the 1990s by UK neurologists may have been that by that time they had something much more satisfying with which to get involved, therapies that for the first time may actually slow the MS disease process; inquiries into the background dynamics of MS would not be able to compete successfully with getting involved in clinical trials of DMDs.

The second important observation from Tables 5.3 and 5.4 must be the large range of prevalence scores recorded, from a maximum of 410/100,000 in Orkney in 2009 to a minimum of just 76/100,000 in Guernsey in 1991. Thus, it becomes remarkably clear that the UK cannot be typified by a single prevalence rate. Three important conclusions follow from this observation. First, in order to derive a reliable national estimate of the number of PwMS much more detailed regional evidence is needed to begin to understand this geographical variation. A national register of PwMS could greatly assist such an endeavour. Second, until such an exercise is completed, national estimates of MS load must be treated with caution. However, the third and probably most important conclusion of the major variation in MS prevalence must be from a resource

Table 5.3 UK regional MS prevalence rates by year of study

Area	Year of Survey	Size: Population	Cases	Prevalence/ 100,000
Sutton (south London)	1985	169,600	195	115
South Glamorgan	1985	376,718	381	101
South Hampshire	1987	417,000	395	95
5 GP Practices in rural Suffolk	1988	31,379 patients	62	153
South Glamorgan	1988	376,718	379	100
Rochdale	1989	207,600	232	96
South and east Cambridgeshire	1990	288,410	322	112
Guernsey	1991	61,164	45	74
Jersey	1991	84,085	84	100
Brighton and mid-Downs	1991	596,594	665	111
South and east Cambridgeshire	1993	290,700	380	131
North Cambridgeshire	1993	378,959	404	107
Lothian / Borders	1995	864,300	1,613	187
Leeds	1996	732,061	617	85
North Northern Ireland	1996	146,066	254	168
Tayside	1996	395,600	727	184
Fife	1996	354,273	508	143
Leeds	1999	728,840	680	93
Central Glasgow	2000	169,000	245	145
Plymouth	2001	341,796	402	118
Tayside	2002	383,405	905*	236
North Northern Ireland	2004	160,446	370	231
South Glamorgan	2005	424,633	620	146
Aberdeen City	2009	205,446	442	215
Orkney	2009	20,000	82	410
Shetland	2009	22,656	66	291

* Not actually given in the text; calculated from other evidence.

Note: The shaded areas are for studies that used neither the Poser nor the McDonald criteria to diagnose MS.

provision perspective. Such variation means that different regions will need different amounts of MS support; they cannot all be expected to adhere to a national average. Only when a much better knowledge of this variation is achieved can the geography of MS resource provision ever be expected to match the geography of MS need.

The third important conclusion to be drawn from Table 5.4 is that the highest MS prevalence rates in the UK have all been found in Scotland and Northern Ireland (Figure 5.2) and dramatically so for the northern

Table 5.4 UK regional MS prevalence studies ranked by prevalence rate

Region	Year of Survey	Prevalence per/100,000
Orkney	2009	410
Shetland	2009	291
Tayside	2002	236
Aberdeen City	2009	215
North Northern Ireland	2004	231
Lothian Borders	1995	187
Tayside	1996	184
North Northern Ireland	1996	168
South Glamorgan	2005	146
South and East Cambridgeshire	1993	131
Plymouth	2001	118
South and East Cambridgeshire	1990	112
Brighton and Mid-Downs	1991	111
North Cambridgeshire	1993	107
South Glamorgan	1985	101
South Glamorgan	1988	100
Jersey	1991	100
Rochdale	1989	96
South Hampshire	1987	95
Leeds	1999	93
Leeds	1996	85
Guernsey	1991	74

islands of Orkney and Shetland in 2009. Indeed, Orkney's MS prevalence of 410/100,000 was according to Visser et al. (2012, 719) the highest regional rate in the world. After these islands Tayside in 2002 at 236/100,000 in Scotland and north Northern Ireland in 2004 at 231/100,000 were the next highest MS prevalence rates, at a similar level to the 215/100,000 in 2009 for Aberdeen City. Interestingly, after the earlier study of north Northern Ireland in 1996 that recorded a prevalence rate of 168/100,000 the next highest was also in western Britain, for South Glamorgan in 2005 at 146/100,000. Furthermore, all the prevalence rates in the English regions, apart from South and East Cambridgeshire in 1993, were substantially lower than this. There may therefore appear to be a good empirical reason to treat the four countries of the UK separately in the first instance. There is also a good policy driven reason for this in that each separate country of the UK is now responsible for the organisation and delivery of its own health services.

The fourth important observation to be made from Tables 5.3 and 5.4 is that, in all but one minor case, when repeat surveys were undertaken for the same area the prevalence rate increased. In the Northern Ireland example this was by an astonishing 38 per cent in 8 years. For South Glamorgan it was by 45 per cent in 20 years between 1985 and 2005. However, for the earlier and shorter period from 1985 to 1988 the smallest of possible declines took place from 101 to 100/100,000. In South and East Cambridgeshire, the increase was by an impressive rate of 17 per cent in just 3 years, the time it took for the prevalence in Leeds to increase by only 9 per cent.

For the four regional studies that could not be transcribed onto Table 5.4 because of methodological differences two important observations can be made. First, the two case studies at either ends of the Scottish central lowlands recorded very similar prevalence rates indeed and both higher than for all the other English regional studies with one exception, the 153/100,000 for 5 GP surgery areas in Suffolk in 1988. This latter result may seem particularly alarming because of the use of patient numbers as the denominator for the prevalence calculation. This was at a time when patient counts for GP practices tended to be higher than population census equivalents due to the tardiness of the former in recording deaths and out-migrants. Thus, all other things being equal, such exercises would have tended to produce relatively low prevalence estimates and that was definitely not the case here. It is, of course, possible that the area Lockyer (1991) surveyed was a genuine MS hotspot but, as already suggested, it is more likely to represent a chance result of the housing market and differential migration by age than any local causal MS factor.

5.6 The countries of the UK

5.6.1 Scotland

Scotland is of fundamental importance to the epidemiological study of MS not only in the UK but internationally too for at least five reasons.

1. It is the location of the first formally diagnosed person with MS in the British Isles, an Orcadian who died in 1898 (Robertson and Compston 1995, 3).
2. It has consistently included the region with the highest recorded prevalence rate in the world. This was in Orkney that had a prevalence of definite/probable MS of 258/100,000 during the 1970s (Swingler and Compston 1986, 1118–9) and in 2009 an MS prevalence of 410/100,000 (Visser et al. 2012, 722).

3. It is one of the few countries to include a number of regions, such as Orkney, Shetland, Grampian and Tayside, to be serially reviewed to show increasing prevalence through time. For example, the MS prevalence in Orkney grew from 111/100,000 in 1954 to 309/100,000 in 1974 and to 410/100,000 in 2009. Meanwhile Shetland for the same points in time it grew from 134/100,000 to 184/100,000 and then to 291/100,000 ((Robertson and Compston 1995, 3; Visser et al. 2012, 722).
4. The Scottish people have been regularly proposed to be one of the principal vectors for the spread of MS susceptible genetic material (Rothwell and Charlton 1998, McDonnell and Hawkins 1998 and 1999). Indeed, this will be suggested in the following section on Northern Ireland and has been used elsewhere too as in the tracing of allegedly Scottish surnames in New Zealand (Skegg et al. 1987). However, this so far has been on a much too simplistic level. Scottish ancestry is a great deal more than the distribution of Scottish sounding surnames (Shepherd 1999). A much more careful understanding of the origins of the Scottish people and how they then might have led to the spreading of MS is needed to move this question forward.
5. Scotland was the first of the four nations of the Union to begin to construct an MS Register.

While this may all appear to be superficially positive for the epidemiologist, in reality it presents more frustration than excitement for two reasons. The first reason, concerned with the construction of the UK MS Registers, has already been discussed in Chapter 3, while the second reason concerns the changing MS diagnostic criteria over the last 40 years. Much of the earlier Scottish MS epidemiological work adopted the Allison and Millar diagnostic criteria and that compromises any meaningful comparisons with more recent research. Of course, this is not a criticism of previous research; it is simply the result of changes in best practice. Nevertheless, it seriously devalues the usefulness of much of the pioneering epidemiological scholarship on Scotland by, for example, Fog and Hyllested (1966), Cook et al. (1985) and Poskanzer et al. (1980) on Orkney and Shetland and Sutherland (1956), Shepherd and Downie (1978) and Phadke and Downie (1987) on North East Scotland (the Grampian region); all of which should be read by the diligent student of this area of inquiry. However, for this analysis primarily of the post Allison and Millar era little of this work was directly relevant.

The four studies that meet the inclusion criteria in Table 5.4 were all for either the east and or the extreme north of Scotland; two for Tayside to the north of the Dee estuary by Forbes et al. (1999) and Donnan et al. (2005), one for Lothian and Borders in the south east by Rothwell and Charlton (1998) and one that considers Aberdeen City, Shetland and Orkney (Visser et al. 2012), all of which produced relatively high prevalence rates ranging from 184/100,000 in 1996 for Tayside to 410/100,000 for Orkney (Table 5.3).

For the beginning of the twenty-first century the Scottish Needs Assessment Project (2000, 4) suggested that the MS prevalence for the whole country should be of the order of 180 to 200/100,000 calculating a total of 10,400 PwMS, substantially less than the estimate by Mackenzie et al. (2014) of 13,328 PwMS at a prevalence of 255.2/100,000. In addition, they went on to argue that this rate would almost certainly increase; a conviction borne out by the Tayside evidence where prevalence increased by 28 per cent in just 6 years (Donnan et al. 2005, 407) and the huge increases in prevalence reported for the northern isles by Visser et al. (2012). The reasons for the rise in prevalence in Tayside were not given in any components of change terms other than to suggest the rates of out-migration had been low and the detection of new cases of MS had been gradually improving; the latter producing the extremely high annual incidence rate of 17.1/100,000 between 1993 and 1995 compared with an average for the whole 1970–97 period of 7.2/100,000. Whether this temporal spike in the incidence of MS in Tayside was anything more than a temporary phenomenon, the possible impact of an infectious agent, as the authors suggest, superimposed on a much longer oscillating secular rise has yet to be determined.

For the substantial increase in MS in the northern isles and Aberdeen, Visser and colleagues (2012, 723) considered the following seven possible proximate explanations.

1. Random variation that may have a particular marked impact on small island populations.
2. Improved case ascertainment.
3. Altered diagnostic criteria, yet moving away from the Allison and Millar criteria should have introduced a downward trend in the results.
4. Improved diagnosis.
5. The migration of high-risk individuals into the area, although there were few higher risk areas they could have come from.
6. Longer survival times.
7. Increases in incidence.

Visser et al. (2012) went on to argue that increased incidence was the most likely direct cause of the rise in MS prevalence in their areas of study with in-migration accounting for only 5 per cent of prevalent cases.

The geography of MS in Scotland in terms of hospital admission statistics for its 14 Strategic Health Authority areas between 1997 and 2009 was considered by Handel et al. (2009b) that encompassed 11,094 individual patients at an age-standardised admissions rate of 16.87/100,000 inhabitants. Among the Health Authority areas a contiguous group of 5 in the north of the country including Orkney, Shetland, Highland, Western Isles and Grampian can be observed in Figure 5.3, all with more than 20 admissions per 100,000 inhabitants. At the same time the lowest rates of MS admissions were to be found in the Borders and Forth Valley authorities. From these data a significant relationship of MS-patient admissions with latitude was discovered, reaffirming the more general relationship discussed in Section 5.3 and perhaps suggesting ultraviolet radiation, or vitamin D deficiency, as an important explanatory factor for the geographical distribution of MS in Scotland. However, the existence of a further contiguous group of heavily urban areas including Lothian, Lanarkshire and Glasgow towards the lower end of the admissions rate distribution may also indicate an inverse association with this attribute that perhaps may be measurable in terms of population density. Could this imply that living in cities may tend to confer some protection from developing MS? If such a view had any value one would have expected the rural Borders area of Scotland to have had a higher MS prevalence than its more urban northerly neighbour the Lothian region. But, this was not the case. The Lothian region MS admission rate per 100,000 people was 16.10 compared to a lower 13.84 for the Borders region. However, in the earlier prevalence research of Rothwell and Charlton (1998) for this area the position was reversed, with the Lothian region recording an MS prevalence of 185/100,000 and the Borders a higher prevalence of 201/100,000. The evidence in the Handel et al. (2009b) research was also at odds with the work of Shepherd (1999) for the Western Isles; the latter suggesting it should have a relatively low MS prevalence and the former indicating it did not. It is, of course, possible that where PwMS live may be different from where they have to go to hospital for major clinical events in their care, especially if they inhabit remote sparsely populated places. It may also be true that some data sources for different places at different points in time are fundamentally irreconcilable.

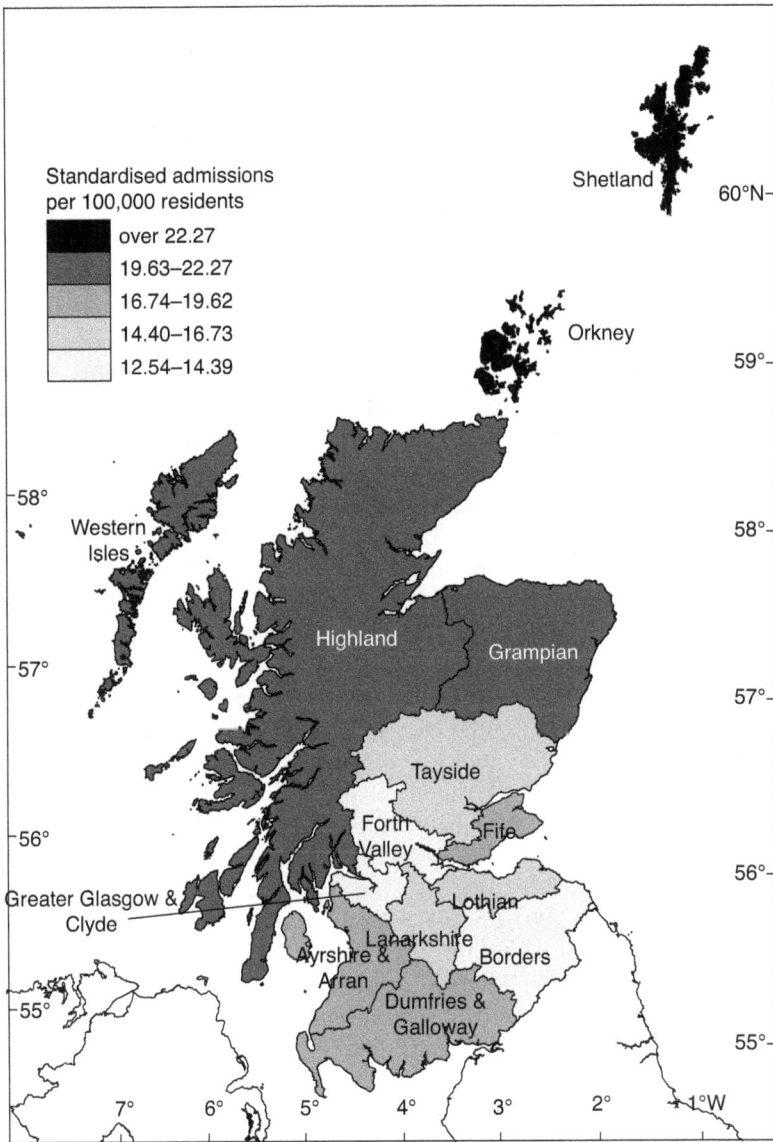

Figure 5.3 MS admissions to NHS hospitals in Scotland 1997–2009 by Health Board Area

Source: Derived from data given in Handel et al. (2009b).

5.6.2 Northern Ireland

To date there have been five epidemiological studies of MS in Northern Ireland. The first two undertaken by Allison and Millar (1954) and Millar (1980) attempted to survey the whole of the province and therefore according to later commentators (Gray et al. 2008, 884) by virtue of the size of their study may have missed cases and underestimated the true prevalence. To some extent this may have been mollified by the use of their more liberal eponymous definition of the disease. Nevertheless, they reported an increase in MS prevalence from 51/100,000 in 1951 to 80/100,000 in 1961, all exceedingly modest by the standards of the early twenty-first century. The third prevalence study by Hawkins and Kee (1988) considered only three administrative districts in the north of the province, Ballymoney, Coleraine and Moyle to which a fourth area, Ballymena, was added for the last two investigations by McDonnell and Hawkins (1998) and Gray et al. (2008). In all these three smaller studies prevalence increased through time from 137/100,000 in 1987 to 191/100,000 in 1996 for the first two studies using the Allison and Millar definition of MS and in Poser definite and probable terms the last two inquiries became 168/100,000 to 231/100,000. While this suite of investigations of MS in Northern Ireland clearly revealed an increase in prevalence through time, they were for three different areas and two different diagnostic schemas and are therefore not strictly comparable. Furthermore, it would be quite wrong to infer from these studies that their prevalence rates applied to the whole of Northern Ireland without strong evidence that the districts of Ballymena, Ballymoney, Coleraine and Moyle could be thought of as representative of the province as a whole. This can be usefully considered with the range of social variables arrayed in Table 5.5 from the 2001 Census of Population that includes ethnicity, gender, age structure,[2] limiting long-term illnesses and educational qualifications, all of which may be related to MS prevalence as shown in the previous chapter. To this has been added religious affiliation because in the Northern Ireland context Protestantism may be a good indicator of Scottish ancestry that in turn may be a good indicator of a raised propensity to develop MS.

During the seventeenth century more than 100,000 Scots, primarily Protestants from the west and central lowlands of their country were encouraged to move to Ireland. For the British state the reason for this migration was to begin to counteract the Catholic majority in Ireland; for the individual Scot the motivation was the promise of land and

Table 5.5 Population of Northern Ireland and the north Northern Ireland MS study area: selected characteristics in 2001

	Total Population	% Male	Ethnicity: %White	% Catholic	Mean Age	% 30-44 years	% Limiting Long-term illness	% born in Northern Ireland	% persons aged 16-74 with high ed' qualifications*
N. Ireland	1,685,267	48.74	99.15	40.26	35.83	22.22	20.36	91.04	4.87
Ballymena	58,610	48.75	99.31	18.96	37.39	22.04	17.69	93.88	5.46
Ballymoney	26,894	49.54	99.62	29.55	36.05	22.43	19.62	94.97	2.72
Coleraine	56,315	47.73	99.11	24.14	36.83	21.77	18.29	90.12	5.71
Moyle	15,933	49.15	99.69	56.61	36.96	20.45	21.18	91.87	3.79
	157,752								

Source: Census of population for Northern Ireland 2001: online tables.

* higher degree or NVQ level 5 or above.

a better life (Bardon 1992). These new peoples settling especially in Ulster brought with them not only a seemingly irreconcilable form of worship and later industrialisation through linen manufacture but perhaps also the genes that would enable Northern Ireland to become one of the world's MS hot spots (Pugliatti et al. 2002, 182).[3] In this province in modern times there are effectively only two religious forms, catholic and protestant, with the two tending to keep themselves territorially very much apart (Boal 1969). For example, in the 2001 census of population only 0.3 per cent claimed that they practiced a non-Christian religion, with another 13.9 per cent stating that they either had no religion at all or failed to state a religion (i.e., unwillingness, for whatever reason, to answer the question). Therefore, the geographical distribution of catholic worshippers, which is the easier of the two groups to consider because Protestantism is subdivided in the census into numerous subsets, would be, ceteris paribus, inversely related to the propensity to develop MS. Indeed, this potentially genetic difference between the north and the south of Ireland has already been suggested to explain the large disparity in MS prevalence rates between Wexford at 121/100,000 in the extreme south east and Donegal at 185/100,000 in the far north west observed by McGuigan et al. (2004, 573). This form of analysis was used again to try to account for the MS prevalences in these two areas of Ireland at the end of 2007 along with South Dublin. By this time the crude MS prevalence in Wexford had increased to 173/100,000 and in Donegal to 329/100,000 while the rate for South Dublin was 130/100,000 (Lonergan et al. 2011, 318). Unfortunately, attempts to explain these spatial differences in terms of latitude, MS-susceptible genes or serum vitamin D levels did not prove successful, although it may be worth noting the low prevalence rate for the major urban area. Nevertheless, this study did report an unexpected decline over the six-year period in female to male ratios in both Donegal and Wexford: from 2.2 to 1.5 in the latter and from 2.48 to 2.1 in the former for reasons that were not at all clear.

Most of the social dimensions shown in Table 5.5 for the four small districts of the north Northern Ireland used in recent MS prevalence research are very similar to their equivalents for the province as a whole with differences of just one or two percentage points. In gender terms for example, 48 to 49 per cent of all persons were male in all 5 areas. In ethnic terms 99 per cent and above were white with 90 per cent and above being born in Northern Ireland. Clearly this was, and still is, socially a very insular and homogenous part of the UK, at face value therefore ideal for epidemiological research. Furthermore, age structures across the study regions would appear to be similar with the average age at approximately 36 years and in terms of long-term limiting illness the percentage varied from only 17 to 21 per cent indicating perhaps only minor differences between them in terms of affluence, their need for medical services and their ability to work. However, when it came to the percentage of Catholics by area there are major differences. Three of the districts, Ballymena, Ballymoney and Coleraine, had much lower proportions of Catholics in them than the province as a whole at 40 per cent, while Moyle, the smallest district, had a much larger proportion. In fact collectively these four districts of Northern Ireland had a much lower percentage of Catholics at 26.42 per cent than the whole province at 40.26 per cent. If indeed religious affiliation is directly related to the chances of developing MS in this province, then the four districts chosen for close scrutiny by McDonnell and Hawkins (1998) and Gray et al. (2008) cannot be thought of as representing the province as a whole and should not be thought of as comparable with the earlier work of Allison and Millar. Indeed, given the relative paucity of Catholics in the areas concerned the last three studies of MS in Northern Ireland should be thought of as overestimates. This is borne out by the fact that if the prevalence of 231/100,000 from the research of Gray et al. (2008) was applied to the population of the province in 2010 of 1,799,800 then the total number of PwMS in Northern Ireland would be greater than the estimate for 2010 suggested by Mackenzie et al. (2014). It may also be of interest to observe that Ballymena, the area with the smallest proportion of Catholic residents, reached a prevalence rate of 174/100,000 in 1996 (McDonnell and Hawkins 1998, 425) higher than for all the four smaller districts combined of 168/100,000. This adds some evidence in support of an association between MS prevalence and religious affiliation that needs to be much more carefully researched in the province.

Because the incidence and prevalence of MS has been shown to vary by gender and age, many investigations have attempted to try to hold these affects constant by standardising the age/sex distributions using the 1961 population of Northern Ireland as a standard (Mumford et al. 1992 for South Cambridgeshire in 1990; Sharpe et al. 1995 for Jersey and Guernsey in 1991; Robertson et al. 1995 for north Cambridgeshire in 1993). According to Robertson et al. (1995, 75) the effect of this approach 'has been to eliminate all significant difference in prevalence except those between the southern England studies and Aberdeen where the contemporary rate is the result of serial surveys.' That would not appear necessarily to be true with the 95 per cent confidence range around the standardised prevalence ratio for the island of Guernsey in 1991 (70–121) falling outside the equivalent ranges for both South East Wales in 1985 (126–50) and North Cambridgeshire in 1993 (127–51). The regional work of Fox et al. (2004) for the Plymouth area in 2001 bucks this trend arguing that the use of the 1961 age/sex population distribution was both arbitrary and out of date, preferring instead simply to argue for specific age/sex prevalence rates to be compared between regions. The use of any age/sex distribution for standardisation purposes would by definition be arbitrary but the 1961 Northern Ireland one, in a sort of homage to the pioneering work of Allison and Millar, is a peculiar one to choose because the age distribution of people in this province tends to be different from the rest of the UK in that a higher proportion of young people were to be found in Northern Ireland than in any of the other countries of the UK. For example, in 2001, 20.2 per cent of the population of the UK was below the age of 16 years whereas in Northern Ireland the proportion was much higher at 24.0 per cent (Population Trends 2001, Vol. 106, 42).

It should also be pointed out that while age/sex standardisation may be of help in trying to understand why the numbers of people with MS may vary between regions, it does not aid with decision making on health-care provision for the disease. In these circumstances it is observing the very differences between places that are important not their statistical elimination.

The evidence presented so far on Northern Ireland may suggest a true increase in the prevalence of MS in this province and therefore a real increase in the number of people with the illness over time. However, what was not clear from this body of work was how this increase came about in terms of the components of change. For example, was it primarily the result of an increase in the incidence of the disease? The researchers clearly think this was one of the important elements of change but inadequately compared in support the incidence rate of 4.4/100,000 for 1961 (Gray et al. 2008, 885) for the province as a whole with the 1996 rate of 9.3/100,000 (Gray et al. 2008, 883) for the collection of northern districts. In addition, both Hawkins and Kee (1988) and McDonnell and Hawkins (1998) suggested increased survival times of PwMS as a reason for the increase in prevalence, but no attempt was made to rank or measure the relative importance of these two elements of change. Yet such an evaluation of the different components of change is necessary if some of the important biological and social factors favouring MS development are to be understood and the appropriate health-care services are to be organised to meet changing demands.

5.6.3 Wales

Although the first serious attempt to define the prevalence of MS anywhere in the UK took place in north Wales by Allison (1931) in 1929 discovering a rate of 25.8/100,000, it was in south Wales where a series of important epidemiological analyses for the same region have taken place in South Glamorgan (Swingler and Compston 1988, Hennessy et al. 1989) that became the rather more prosaically named Unitary Authorities of Cardiff and the Vale of Glamorgan (Hirst et al. 2008b and 2009). The first attempt at a comprehensive trawl of the relevant sources for PwMS for this area was undertaken by Swingler and Compston (1988) to record a total MS burden for the area on the 1 January 1985 of 381 definite and probable cases under the Poser diagnostic regime. This resulted in a prevalence of 101/100,000 (Swingler and Compston 1988, 1522). When the area was resurveyed and the existing cases reviewed for a new prevalence estimate for the 1 January 1988, the total number of people with the illness for 1985 was revised up to 382, a net increase of just one, giving a prevalence of 100/100,000 (Hennessy et al. 1989, 1085–7). However, this apparent stability was in fact the net result of substantial change. Though 320 PwMS (83.8%) remained in the area with the illness (stayers), there were 66 entries and 67 exits. The entries included 8 PwMS reclassified within the Poser rubric, 6 PwMS who moved into the area and 52 new diagnosees. Of the exits, there were 34 deaths, 24 PwMS who moved out of the area, 2 people who were diagnosed with another condition and 7 who could not be traced (Hennessy et al. 1988, 1085–7). What is more to emphasise the possible high rate of change of PwMS, of the newly diagnosed 1 had died and 4 had moved out of the region by 1988.

This 'components of change' analysis was in general terms extended to the first decade of the twenty-first century by Hirst and colleagues (2008b and 2009) but for some elements the time periods unfortunately did not match. For example, in terms of the total number of people with definite or probable disease, a value of 620 was given for 2005, that is a net increase of 238 cases since 1985, or 62 per cent, lifting the prevalence rate to 146/100,000. For incident cases the period from 1985 to 2007 was used, in which 582 were recorded with the annual rate per 100,000 increasing from 4.25 to 9.65 (Hirst et al. 2009, 389). However, when the mortality of PwMS in the area from January 1985 was considered the time period up to October 2006 was used (Hirst et al. 2008b). In this case, of the 379 cases of MS included in the study in 1985, 148 (39%) remained alive throughout the 262 month period (stayers),

10 (3%) were untraceable and 221 died (58%) although it was not at all clear how many of these individuals died in the study area or had moved out and then died. However, it is also important to observe what was not discussed in this work. First, the movement of people with MS in and out of the area during the 20 or so years after 1985 got no mention other than the implication that 8.9 per cent may have been in-migrants (Hirst et al. 2009, 388). This was because it was noted that such a proportion were diagnosed by a consultant neurologist outside the regional service on which this study was based. We have already seen from the work of Hennessy et al. (1989) that for as little as 3 years at least 5 per cent may leave, so for a time period 7 times as long this could be substantially more than 8.9 per cent. Second, no comment was made on the stability of the new diagnosees in the area. How many moved out or died before the end of 2005? It is clear from what has been presented so far that many must have done so and probably more than 300. And, how do these deaths and departures compare with the ones from the 1985 cohort?

Three conclusions follow from these observations. First, the complete evidence on the components of change of PwMS in the area has not been presented for the 1985–2005 era and therefore their absolute and relative importance cannot be assessed and the rate of turnover of people with the condition in the area is not known. Second, Hirst et al. (2009) point to the importance of the growing numbers of incident cases in generating the increase in the number of PwMS during their 20-year study. To account for the deaths that were also taking place, their assessment of the role of new diagnosees would appear to be understated. Finally, these research exercises demonstrate clearly the difficulties of setting up and maintaining a register of PwMS for any area because of the possible rate of change of its members that must be accommodated.

There are no major deductions that can be made from the above MS research in South Glamorgan about the likely trends in the whole of Wales. What is important to note, however, is that this epidemiological work in south east Wales forms just part of a large and growing body of research on the condition and care of PwMS in the area, introduced in Chapter 3 that are discussed in a number of different contexts in the remainder of this book.

5.6.4 England

There have been nine truly comparable regional epidemiological studies of MS carried out on the English mainland since the mid-1980s. They range from major cities such as Leeds where the lowest prevalence rate of 85/100,000 was recorded in 1996 to rural north Cambridgeshire just south of which the highest prevalence of 131/100,000 was discovered in South Cambridgeshire in 1993. At this superficial descriptive level of analysis, England would seem to be characterised more by diversity and difference than similarity. This point is exemplified by contiguous regions in both space and time providing very different results. For example, the MS prevalence in South East Cambridgeshire in 1993 was 131/100,000 whereas in North Cambridgeshire for the same year it was 107/100,000. Similarly, in South Hampshire in 1987 the rate was 95/100,000 compared to Brighton just to the east 4 years later where it was much higher at 111/100,000. Perhaps in this context the Channel Islands of Jersey and Guernsey could be added with very different MS prevalence rates of 100/100,000 and 74/100,000 respectively.

The only area in which common ground can be found in these studies was in the two cases of repeat surveys where increases in prevalence were reported, a phenomenon that has been observed elsewhere in the UK. For example, in South East Cambridgeshire MS prevalence increased by 17 per cent from 112/100,000 in 1990 to 131/100,000 in 1993 while in Leeds over a similar period it increased at only half that rate from 85/100,000 in 1996 to 93/100,000 in 1999.

These last two pairs of papers are worthy of closer scrutiny because of their detailed descriptions of change over time. The survey in South East Cambridgeshire began with the optimistic view (Mumford et al. 1992, 881) that 'it may be the case that initial surveys are now achieving more complete case ascertainment due to improved methodology.' Embarrassingly though, when the repeat survey was completed just 3 years later in 1993, 58 patients (16% of the original total) who should have been included in the earlier study were discovered. Two important conclusions follow directly from this observation. First, even with the best of intentions, attempts at universal coverage of PwMS at that time could be substantially wide of the mark. The second conclusion must be that the prevalence rate of 112/100,000 in 1990 becomes an underestimate, but by how much is unclear because this result applied to all cases that fell within the Poser classification of MS and not just the definite and probable categories. By contrast, it was also reasonable to assume that the 1993 prevalence rate for this area was a modest overestimate because the latter's rate was based on a population denominator for 1991 at a time when the area was growing rapidly due to the 'Cambridge Phenomenon' (Segal Quince and Partners 1985) that is expansion in the high technology, service and information sectors. Thus, in reality the growth in MS prevalence in South East Cambridgeshire in the early 1990s may not have been as great as first appeared. Indeed, this is assured given the observation by Robertson et al. (1996b, 274) that the prevalence increase 'mainly resulted from improved case ascertainment.' Nevertheless, the repeat survey of South East Cambridge in 1993 provided a detailed example of the way in which change may take place in the number of PwMS in an area, devalued for this analysis because it included all cases for which some form of Poser classification could be given and not just for those with definite and probable disease.

For 1990 Mumford et al. (1992) identified 374 patients with MS. By 1993 this number had increased to 441 patients (Robertson et al. 1996b, 276). Over this 3-year time period 303 patients (81%) remained in the area (the stayers), 138 were added to the total and 71 were deleted creating a net increase of 67 PwMS. Of the additions, 60 were entirely new diagnoses (43%), 58 (42%) were previously omitted cases, 8 (6%) were in-migrants and 12 (9%) came from an undefined source. Of the losses, 29 (41%) had died, 29 (41%) had moved out of the area, 6 (9%) proved not to have MS and 7 (10%) were lost to follow up. Interestingly, these were all remarkably similar degrees of change to those recorded above for another 3-year period from 1985 to 1988 in South Glamorgan by Hennessy et al. (1989).

In 1993 a complementary survey of PwMS was also undertaken for North Cambridgeshire for which the rather lower prevalence rate of 107/100,000 was reported (Robertson et al. 1995). The authors suggested that a significant difference in ethnic mix between north and south Cambridgeshire may have helped to account for this difference. This may well have been the case at the start of the 1990s but by the 2001 census was no longer the case. The three districts of North Cambridgeshire, Fenland, Peterborough and Huntingdonshire, recorded proportions of white ethnicity as 98.6, 89.71 and 97.15 per cent respectively while the equivalent figures for the 3 districts of the rest of the county, South Cambridgeshire, East Cambridgeshire and Cambridge City, were very similar at 97.06, 97.89 and 89.44 per cent respectively.

The two epidemiological enquiries into MS in Leeds in 1996 (Ford et al. 1998) and 3.5 years later in 1999 (Ford et al. 2002) provided another example of change over time on the basis of all people with a Poser MS categorisation that were not at all dissimilar to the results from the other two areas already discussed. In April 1996 there were 712 PwMS enumerated (including suspected cases). Over the next 42 months, 13 cases were discovered that should have been in the original 1996 population giving a grand total of 723. Of these, 656 (90%) remained in Leeds with MS (the 'stayers'), 50 died (7%) and 19 moved out (3%). In addition, 136 incident cases were recorded (19% of the 1996 total) that grouped together new diagnosees and in-migrants. The net result of these components of change was that the prevalence of MS in Leeds for definite and probable cases increased from 85/100,00 in 1996 to 93/100,000 in 1999, helped to a modest degree by a declining population denominator over the same period of time of 0.4 per cent.

Ford and colleagues (1998, 609) suggested that the relatively low MS prevalence in Leeds compared to other areas of the UK may in part be due to the above average proportion of ethnic minorities in the city that stood at 6 per cent when the 1991 population census was taken. While this may have indeed been the case at this spatial scale, at a larger scale within Leeds itself it was not so. For example, the Harehills district with a high proportion of non-white ethnic residents (30%) had the anticipated low MS prevalence rate of 42.3/100,000 for all Poser categories, and Otley with 99 per cent indigenous white residents had the relatively high rate of 142.8/100,000, but, Chapel Allerton and Wetherby with non-white ethnic proportions of 34 per cent and 0.5 per cent respectively recorded the counter-intuitively high prevalence rates of 100.1/100,000 and 105.5/100,000. Thus, there must have been other factors at work to account for these differences in MS prevalence in addition to ethnic affiliation. Ford et al. (1998) suggested that both enumeration difficulties in the inner city for the 1991 census and social class may have played their part.

In an exercise similar to the one noted earlier for Scotland, Ramagopalan and colleagues (2011a and 2011b) were able to analyse evidence on MS frequencies across the whole of England in the form of hospital admissions for the 28 Strategic Health Authorities (SHAs) between 1998 and 2005. As can be seen in Figure 5.4, this research demonstrated that the highest annual admission rates per 100,000 inhabitants were in Cumbria and Lancashire (20.3), North East Yorkshire and North Lincolnshire (19.9) and Northumberland, Tyne and Wear (19.7) with the three lowest all in Greater London (North West London 11.4; North East London 12.0; with North Central London and South West London both at 12.3). Such findings may begin to imply a gradation of disease rates with latitude and therefore directly with UVB radiation. However, the correlation coefficient between these two attributes discovered in this study was only 0.46 (Ramagopalan et al. 2011b, 1412) suggesting the relationship was much more complicated with a great deal more to be explained and understood. Indeed, an inspection of the spatial distribution of MS admission rates in England by latitude revealed a far from straight forward pattern. For example,

140 *People with Multiple Sclerosis*

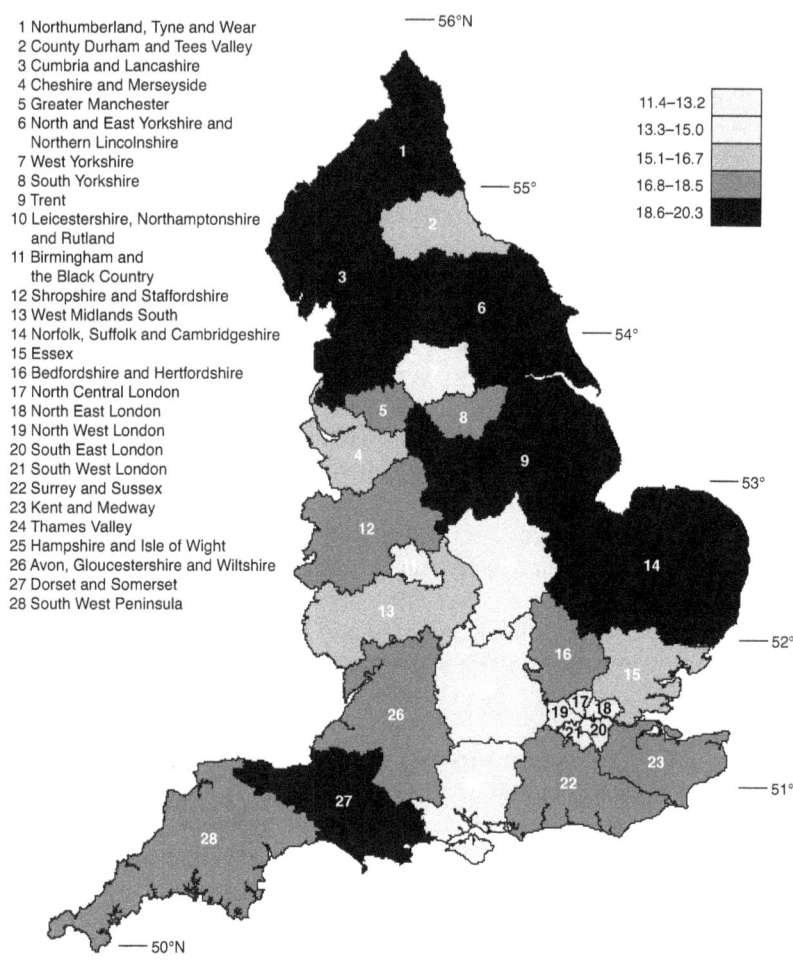

Figure 5.4 MS admissions to NHS hospitals in England 1998–2005 by Strategic Health Authority Area

Source: Derived from data given in Ramagopalan et al. (2011b).

in the south of England the Dorset and Somerset SHA recorded the sixth highest admission rate while Birmingham and Black Country SHA much further north recorded the sixth lowest. But, what stood out most of all from this geographical distribution were the relative low rates of hospital admission for MS across all five SHAs in Greater London. Indeed, a visual inspection of the map of hospital admission rates for MS would tend to suggest that all the major conurbations had relatively low rates of MS admissions compared to their surrounding territories. This would appear to be true for Birmingham, Teeside and West Yorkshire (Leeds) and perhaps also for Merseyside, Manchester and South Yorkshire (Sheffield). It would also seem to be the case that some of the most rural SHAs such as Dorset and Somerset, North East Yorkshire, Trent and Norfolk, Suffolk and Cambridgeshire had the highest rates of hospital admissions for MS.

If there was a rural propensity towards higher rates of MS what could possibly be the cause? Three possible approaches may be appropriate, concerning the distributions of ethnic minorities, deprivation and people with resilient immune systems (a variant of the hygiene hypothesis). But, first of all it is important to ask whether relatively fewer hospital admissions in cities could be function of the collection of the original evidence such that health organisations might systematically under record hospital admissions for MS in large urban areas. Given most major neurological centres in England are to be found in the big cities this would seem highly unlikely. Indeed, the opposite might be thought to be more likely because rural GPs may refer their patients to city hospitals for more expert assessment.

It has already been shown in Chapter 4 that MS prevalence varies between ethnic groups with those from an African or Asian origin least likely to succumb to the illness. It is also known that geographically the non-white population of the UK is heavily concentrated in the major cities with 45 per cent in London in 2001 (where they made up 29% of the residents) and 13 per cent in the West Midlands (National Statistics online). Thus, a relative paucity of MS cases would be expected in the big cities, to form part of a possible explanation for their relative lack of MS hospital admissions. It has also been observed that MS was less common in people of low socio-economic status, or in those living in the most deprived areas. Here again the big cities dominated the map of deprivation (Carstairs measure) in England and Wales in 2001 with, for example, 42 per cent of people in London living in the most deprived fifth of wards (Morgan and Baker 2006, 31). This may add another element of the explanation of relatively low hospital admissions for MS in the larger cities. However, what may also have been important was that urban areas are places where many different types of peoples come in close contact with one another. Could it be that in such environments more robust immune systems develop among their inhabitants with the strongest ability to resist the sorts of infections that may trigger MS? If so, then this may also have been yet another important reason why people in rural areas may have had a greater chance of developing MS than those in urban areas.

5.7 Components of change

5.7.1 Incident cases

This category relates to those unfortunate individuals who have received a diagnosis of MS for the first time, that is 'incident' cases of MS. It may be initially reasonable to assume that all new cases of MS recorded for a particular place or region result directly from people being newly diagnosed with MS. Unfortunately, it is possible that PwMS newly moving into a region, or in-migrants, may in some cases be classified as incident cases too because they are new cases of MS for that region. Indeed, in Leeds, for example, between 1995 and 1999 (Ford et al. 2002) this was the case. The degree to which this phenomenon corrupts regional evidence on incident MS more widely is unknown. However, it needs to be pointed out that the medical resource implications of these two different interpretations of incidence could be significant; the completely new case may qualify for relatively expensive DMDs whereas an in-migrant with MS may be at any stage of an MS career with appropriately variable medical needs. Where new cases of MS have been recorded for a number of years for a particular place prospectively then it is possible relatively easily to calculate a time series of annual incident rates as in the case of Hirst et al. (2009) for South Glamorgan and Donnan et al. (2005) for Tayside. However, when all that is available is a prevalent set for a particular year along with year of disease onset, then in some cases this series has been doubled to fill in the missing data for earlier years, allowing an annual series of incident rates to be estimated. This technique, that came to be known as the Poskanzer method after Poskanzer et al. (1963) on Northumberland, has been employed by for example, Rice-Oxley et al. (1995) for Brighton and mid-Downs and Swingler and Compston (1988) for South Glamorgan. However, as Ford and colleagues (2002, 262-3) observed such retrospective analyses in England have tended to generate somewhat lower incidence rates than prospective ones; they miss a great deal of the short-term detail in particular of PwMS who had relatively short lives. In other words they tend to overestimate survival times. More formally the Poshanzer method assumes that for any patient prevalence day is a random event and therefore the time from onset to prevalence day will be half the duration of the disease. Unfortunately, as Martyn and Osmond (1989) made clear only in the extremely unlikely event of all patients surviving for the same length of time would this method be valid and would lead in all cases to estimates of mean survival times from onset to death being considerably over optimistic.

The trends in incident cases in the UK, as one might have expected, tend to follow quite closely those of prevalence, although it should be noted that fewer regions of the UK have had evidence on this component of change published. Thus, the highest rates of MS incidence, with one notable recent exception, have tended to be reported for northern parts of Britain (Table 5.6). For example, Lothian and Borders reported an average annual rate between 1992 and 1995 of 12.0/100,000 (Rothwell and Charlton 1998), Tayside 7.2/100,000 between 1970 and 1997 (Donnan et al. 2005) and north Northern Ireland 9.3 in 1996 (Gray et al. 2008). At approximately the same time the rates of MS incidence in England were much lower at approximately 5.0/100,000/year including Rochdale and Leeds in the north through Cambridge more centrally located to Brighton and Hampshire on the south coast. All were above the 3.6 cases per 100,000 Alonso and Hernan (2008) calculated as an overall average from a meta-analysis of 36 published case studies, but

Table 5.6 Regional MS annual incidence rates in the UK

Area	Period of survey	Incidence rate: per 100,000
Sutton (south London)	1976–84	5.0
South Glamorgan	1947–84	5.4
South Glamorgan	1985–7	5.4
South Hampshire	1976–82	4.7
Rochdale	1985–9	5.4
South and east Cambridgeshire	1989–91	5.9
Brighton and mid-Downs	1978–84	5.0
South and east Cambridgeshire	1990–4	5.0
North Cambridgeshire	1990–3	4.8
Lothian / Borders	1992–5	12.0
Leeds	1995–6	4.4
North Northern Ireland	1996	9.3
Tayside	1976–7	7.2
Leeds	1996–8	6.1
Central Glasgow	1989–8	5.7
South Glamorgan	2007	9.6

Sources: Williams and McKernan (1986), Swingler and Compston (1988), Hennessy et al. (1989), Roberts et al. (1991), Mumford et al. (1992), Rice-Oxley et al. (1995), Shepherd and Summers (1996), Robertson et al. (1995), Robertson et al. (1996b), Rothwell and Charlton (1998), Ford et al. (1998), Ford et al. (2002), Murray et al. (2004), Donnan et al. (2005), Gray et al. (2008), Hirst et al. (2009).

surprisingly similar to the 5.5/100,000/year between 1993 and 2000 offered by Alonso et al. (2007) for the whole of the UK using GPRD evidence that by definition obfuscates the important geographical differences in MS incidence between its separate countries.[4]

The second clear trend in incidence work in the UK was that, where serial observations have been undertaken through time, rates have tended to increase. For example, in Leeds MS incidence rose from 4.4/100,000/year between 1995 and 1996 to 6.1 for 1996–8 (Ford et al. 2002) and in South Glamorgan it rose from 5.4/100,000 in 1985 to 9.65 in 2007 (Hirst et al. 2009). The exception in this series was in South East Cambridgeshire where the incidence rate declined from 5.4/100,000 to 5.0/100,000 during the early 1990s (Robertson et al. 1996b).

The third clear trend in recent UK incident rates was the difference between men and women in which the latter have been considerably higher than the former. For example, in north Northern Ireland for 1996 the MS incidence rate for men was 8.3/100,000 whereas for women it was 10.3/100,000 (Gray et al. 2008). In Leeds, for the 176 incident cases between 1995 and 1999, the female to male sex ratio was 2.3:1 (Ford et al. 2002, 261). Similarly, in Glasgow between 1989 and 1998, the average annual rate for males was 3.5/100,000 compared with females at 7.7/100,000 (Murray et al. 2004). And, in South Glamorgan between 1985 and 2007, the rates for men and women at the start of the period were 1.03/100,000 and 2.65/100,000 respectively, both climbing to 2.50/100,000 and 7.30/100,000 by the end of the period (Hirst et al. 2009).

Two of the above incidence studies that demonstrated the value of keeping long-term registers of PwMS are worthy of further comment. First, the research by Donnan et al. (2005) on spatial and temporal clusters of incident cases in Tayside between 1970 and 1997. In this case a general increase in the rate of MS incidence was observed for the whole period with a periodicity of every two to three years that the authors interpreted as evidence of an infectious agent at work. Furthermore, they observed an increase in the mean age of onset of MS from 33.2 years between 1970 and 1979 to 38.1 years for 1990–7 (Donnan et al. 2005, 404). This was a counter-intuitive result because with the increase of awareness of MS among medical staff and the public along with increased diagnostic sophistication one would have expected a decline in the age of onset. Could this have signalled a change in character of the MS disease?

The second piece of important research in this area had as its background the secular increase in MS incidence in South Glamorgan between 1985 and 2007 listed in Table 5.6 and the astonishing dominance of new cases of MS for women in this change (Hirst et al. 2009). The authors of this work diligently and meticulously considered all the possible methodological, diagnostic and accounting procedures that could have made this result a function or an artefact of the way the research had been carried out rather than a real finding to conclude it was substantially true. Unfortunately, the sort of environmental factors, behavioural changes or shifts in disease phenotype that could have produced such a large and sustained increase in the number of new cases of MS in South Wales at that time were not suggested. This question still remains to be answered. On observing that in South Glamorgan in the mid-1980s, incidence and mortality rates for MS were in equilibrium Swingler and Compston (1988, 1524) stated that 'prevalence is unlikely to rise substantially as serial studies are performed, unless there is a steady increase in disease duration.' At that time the profound increase in MS incidence among women would appear to have been unimaginable.

5.7.2 Deaths

The available published evidence on the mortality of PwMS in the UK is exceedingly sparse and substantially out of date. Since 1980 it includes only two nationwide evaluations of death certificate evidence, a two-page description in an atlas of mortality in GB, a brief note on death certificate evidence for England and Wales, three perfunctory mentions in regional components of change work, two descriptions of the decay of cohorts of PwMS through time as the people in them died and a matched analysis of GPRD evidence. The scene was set for mortality studies of PwMS by Williams et al. (1991) who reviewed death certificate evidence for the 30 years between 1953 and 1983 for England and Wales together, Scotland and Northern Ireland. They identified five main trends:

1. An overall reduction in death rates by 25 per cent.
2. An increase in the estimated median age of death from 52 to 59 years that, *ceteris paribus*, would lead to an increase in MS prevalence.
3. Better results for men than women: the latter's death rate declined by 23 per cent while the former's dropped by 30 per cent.
4. This better outlook for men was also noticeable geographically in the annual mortality rates across all the four countries of the UK (Williams et al. 199, 105). At this broad population level of analysis it would appear that mortality rates matched prevalence rates with Scotland having the highest, Northern Ireland the second highest and England and Wales somewhat lower. Indeed, this pattern was

confirmed by Swingler and Compston (1986, 1118–9) using standardised mortality rates for the four UK nations between 1976 and 1980 with Wales consistently recording the lowest regional rate between 1951 and 1975. No explanation was offered for this phenomenon.
5. A reduction in the mortality gap between Scotland and England and Wales.

The death certificate material collected by Richards et al. (2002, 24) for their inquiry into the epidemiology of MS in England and Wales portrayed a particularly bleak prospect for those with the condition. For the period from 1993 to 1997, approximately 3,428 death certificates were completed citing MS as the primary cause of death for which the mean age at death was 59.1 years for men and 60.4 years for women. This was at a time when the mean age at death for all causes for those who reached 20 or more years of age were 73.3 years for men and 79.1 years for women. Very similar results were reported by Shaw et al. (2008) from a descriptive analysis of almost 15 million recorded deaths between 1981 and 2004 in GB. Here the deaths noting MS as the main cause totalled 21,275, or 0.14 per cent of the total, of which 64 per cent were women at an average age of 59.4 years. Given the average age at death for all cases was 74.4 years, this material provided more evidence that PwMS may die at an earlier age than people generally in GB. What is more, as an estimate of the years of life lost because of MS, if PwMS had lived to the national average age of 75 instead of dying earlier, then 35,000 extra person-years of life would have occurred, 22,000 for women and 13,000 for men (Shaw et al. 2008, xxix).

Age/sex distributions of deaths by neurodegenerative diseases have recently been released by the National end of life care Intelligence Network (NEoLCIN 2010) for England for the years from 2002 to 2008 inclusive. Over this period there were 6,359 deaths in which MS was recorded as the underlying cause and 9,966 cases in which MS was mentioned on the death certificate. The distributions of these deaths by year clearly indicated an increase of death with and by MS with time as one may have expected from the general increase in the number of PwMS in the country. Furthermore, as one would also have anticipated there were more female deaths than male deaths over the 6 years at a ratio of 1.87 to 1. However, when the age of death histograms by gender were observed, and that was all that was given in the text, the distributions were very similar with the majority of deaths occurring in 'early older age' (NEoLCIN 2010, 10), the modal 5-year band occurring between 55 and 64 years, with both distributions skewed towards the older ages.

However, it must be remembered that the PwMS who died from their condition and therefore had it noted as the cause of death on their death certificate were most likely those with the most severe manifestations of the disease. PwMS with less severe disease tend to live longer, die from all the other common causes of death and often do not have MS noted anywhere on their death certificates. Nevertheless, this material provided further evidence that PwMS may experience shorter lives than the population generally.

The three short-term regional analyses of the components of change of the number of PwMS that included evidence on mortality came from South Cambridgeshire (Robertson et al. 1996b) between 1990 and 1993, Leeds from 1/10/1996 to 31/10/1999 (Ford et al. 2002) and South Glamorgan for the much earlier time of 1/1/1985 to 1/1/1988 (Hennessy et al. 1989). For the former, the annual mortality was 3.3/100,000 with a mean age of death at 64.2 years (range 40 to 85) and with a mean annual survival time from diagnosis of 28.2 years. In the earlier study in South Wales the mortality rate was a similar 3.1/100,000. In this study it was observed that the cause of death was directly related to MS in 54.1 per cent of cases and usually due to pneumonia, indirectly related in 5.4 per cent and not related to MS at all in 37.8 per cent with the cause of death not recorded in one case. For the West Yorkshire investigation two death rates were given of 1.9/100,000 in 1997 and 3.2/100,000 in 1998 being of the same order as the other death rates so far observed. Of the 57 deaths investigated through death certificates, 30 cases or 52.6 per cent could be directly attributable to MS, that is mentioned in Part 1 of the death certificate, 14 (24.6%) indirectly related (noted in Part 2) and with MS not being mentioned at all in 13 cases (22.8%). Of all these deaths, 28 per cent were directly due to conditions unrelated to MS and, where MS was directly implicated, respiratory disease, notably bronchopneumonia, was the principal culprit. In this latter set of deaths there were also two suicides.

More detailed inquiries into the causes of the deaths of PwMS were carried out in the two cohort studies by Phadke (1987) in the Grampian region of Scotland in which a deliberate effort was made to define personal attributes that led to a better or a worse prognosis and Hirst et al. (2008b) for South Glamorgan where they were not. These two investigations were very different from the above regional work in two important respects. First of all because they were only concerned with the cohort of PwMS at the start date of their studies and how that number declined through time. They therefore took no notice of new cases of MS that may be diagnosed in their areas after that point in time, or in-migrants, and whether any of these may subsequently have perished. In other words, they missed out on possible short-term change that may take place during their overall study periods and therefore could underestimate the importance of PwMS who had relatively short lives. The second important issue with these two cohort studies was that they brought into particularly sharp relief the proximate causes of the deaths of PwMS. In particular, they demonstrated that PwMS not only died from their condition and the medical complications it generated, they also died from many other causes too just like members of the general population.

The early research of Phadke (1987) followed a group of 1,055 PwMS in Grampian in 1970 prospectively for the next 10 years. Of the 216 people who died during this time, their ages ranged from 25 to 80 years with unfortunately no average given. Survival in this cohort was inversely related to age at onset and most assured for those with a single demyelinating event at onset either in the brainstem or in the optic nerves causing retrobulbar neuritis. By contrast, those whose initial event involved the cerebellum survived less well. Of all deaths, 62 per cent were directly related to MS with bronchopneumonia being the most common terminal event. Perhaps of greatest importance was the observation that life expectancy for PwMS was reduced across all age groups compared to Scottish controls and especially marked for those with age of onset of 40 years and above (Phadke 1987, 525–6). But, in terms of survival times there was some relatively good news for women because 17.1 per cent of them survived more than 40 years from disease onset compared with only 10.5 per cent for men (Phadke 1987, 527).

The most recently published regional MS mortality work by Hirst et al. (2008b) related to South Glamorgan and in essence was a continuation of the Swingler and Compston (1988) and Hennessy et al. (1989) research discussed above for 20 years into the beginning of the twenty-first century. From the original cohort of 441 PwMS in 1985, 221 had died during the 20-year surveillance period for which copies of their death certificates were secured. The mean age of death of this whole cohort was 65.3 years with perhaps surprisingly very little difference between the sexes: women 65.3 years, men 65.2 years. The age range of deaths of PwMS was from 25 years to 101 and, while the former is exactly the same start age as the Phadke (1987) research in Grampian almost a decade earlier, the upper age far exceeds their's by more than 20 years and represents the oldest person with MS noted in published UK MS research so far.

According to Swingler and Compston (1988, 1522), who undertook the first inquiry into this cohort of PwMS in South Glamorgan, the mean age at symptom onset was 32.2 years which strongly implied that many of the deaths investigated by Hirst et al. (2008b) would have been of people born during the 1950s or immediately after the Second World War, that is baby boomers. Now, according to the UK Government's Office for Health Economics, life expectancy in England and Wales at that time was 66.5 years for males and 71.2 years for females. Although it must be admitted that these were very broad average figures with no regard given to careful case-controlled matching, they did nevertheless indicate that life expectancy in South Glamorgan for those people with MS was less than for the general population in England and Wales and that the position was relatively worse for women than men; they lost more of their expected lives than men. In a much more sophisticated yet equally discordant way, Hirst et al. (2008b, 1019) using age-specific mortality rates make the same point. Of all the deaths in South Glamorgan investigated 57.9 per cent were related to MS with the most frequently cited terminal event being respiratory disease for both sexes, 50.3 per cent for women and 41.9 per cent for men (Hirst et al. 2008b, 1018), as in the earlier Scottish example. However, what cannot be inferred from this evidence is the direct involvement of life-style factors such as tobacco smoking, diet and exercise that have the potential to be changed.

Both of these two cohort studiers have problems with the definition of an expected distribution to compare to their observations. In the Phadke (1987) case, the comparator distribution was people living in Scotland aged between 10 and 20 years in 1930–2, a full 40 years before the series of deaths began in 1970. Unfortunately, no explanation was given for this choice. With disease at onset normally when people are in their early 30s, this would seem to be much too soon. However, given the secular upward trend in life expectancy choosing a later time series would only have tended to increase the difference between what was observed and what could have been expected, that is lowering the life chances of PwMS compared to the general population of Scotland.

In the Hirst et al. (2008b) analysis, the discordance came from using English evidence alone, and again without justification or explanation, for the expected disease distributions rather than ones from Wales to compare with their observations for South Glamorgan; in other words the geographical areas compared did not match, and did not even overlap. The degree to which PwMS in South Glamorgan should have their chances of dying from various conditions compared to people in England is open to serious conjecture. Nevertheless, in these terms while death rates generally were somewhat elevated with a Standard Mortality Ratio (SMR) of 279, the rates for respiratory disease (SMR 1,170) and infectious diseases (SMR 2,960) were substantially higher than trends in England, trends that would appear to have international resonance in the reviews and research of Bronnum-Hansen et al. (2004) and Ragonese et al. (2008). Thus, it is in these two disease areas where perhaps a preventative information programme needs to be put in place by National Health Services and the MS disease charities. By contrast, deaths from cancer (SMR 86) and cardio vascular disease (SMR 106) were relatively similar to English trends (Hirst et al. 2008b, 1020) and therefore the national preventative advice is as appropriate for PwMS as it is for the general public. What is more, earlier in their paper Hirst et al. (2008b, 1026) claim that their analysis 'has enabled accurate contemporary estimates of survival and disease duration for patients with MS in the UK.' This may not have been the case.

Research on the cause of death of PwMS by Lalmohamed et al. (2012) that links GPRD evidence with Hospital Episodes Statistics and National Death Certificates between 2001 and 2008 for the 211 participating British practices supports the above regional findings in two important respects. First, the death rate among the 69 PwMS who died was higher than among the controls without MS by 3.5 times. The second important similarity was that the main causes of death identified were very similar. Infections and respiratory diseases were the main cause in 58.0 per cent of cases, Cardiovascular in 30.4 per cent, Cancer in 20.3 per cent and MS itself in 30.4 per cent (Lalmohamed et al. 2012, 1011). However, these figures were difficult to compare accurately with the South Glamorgan material because the primary causes of death and other significant contributions to death had been amalgamated together, making their quoted proportions total far more than 100 per cent.

5.7.2.1 Suicide

In the regional epidemiological evidence on PwMS so far reviewed death by suicide was only mentioned twice. Once for Leeds where two cases occurred between 1996 and 1999 (Ford et al. 2002) and a second time by Hirst et al. (2008b) for the 1985 cohort of PwMS in South Glamorgan they monitored for two decades where there were none. Furthermore, in the analysis of GPRD evidence by Lalmohamed et al. (2012, 1011), deaths by accidents and suicide were found to account for a much lower proportion of total deaths than their matched counterparts (2.9% compared with 8.5%). These may seem surprisingly low results, especially when suicide has been a topic of such morbid fascination in the popular press and MS magazines for which recent examples would include the late Debbie Purdy's fight to clarify the law on assisted suicide, the activities of Dignitas in Switzerland (Fischer et al. 2008) and the suicides of famous, or perhaps more infamous, individuals with MS such as Cari Loder. It is also true that less notorious PwMS sometimes kill themselves too, such as Angela Harrison reported on the MS Trust website (18/05/2009) who decided she wanted to die before her condition became completely debilitating. Indeed, it may well be that many PwMS make such a pact with dying after receiving an MS diagnosis. The novelist M J Hyland (2012), for example, soon after her diagnosis decided she would commit suicide after living the high-life for two weeks at the Ritz in New York. But, like many other such individuals she changed her mind after realising there was a perfectly rewarding existence available even with her MS. However, such hyperbole and anecdote do not confirm that in the UK the suicide rate among PwMS was any higher than among the population as a whole. Certainly there was some evidence from other countries reviewed by Pompili et al. (2012), and most notably for Canada (Sadovnick et al. 1991) and Denmark (Bronnum-Hansen et al. 2005), for an elevated propensity of death by suicide among PwMS. In addition, the international review of the subject by Hawton and van Heeringen (2009) made this point too relating to a number of physical disorders of which MS was one along with cancer, HIV/AIDS, Huntington's disease, spinal cord injury and Lupus. However, they also mischievously concluded their essay by stating that many of these studies had methodological problems (Hawton and van Heeringen 2009, 1375), a point stressed by Feinstein (1997) over ten years earlier reviewing similar research. Thus, there was no empirical evidence to support the view that in the UK PwMS had a higher suicide rate than the general population. In fact the available evidence suggested the relationship was in the opposite direction.

There was nothing useful to be inferred from national statistics on the subject either. Suicide rates have tended to be lower for women than men: age-standardised for people more than 15 years was 17.4/100,000 for men and 5.3/100,000 for women. It has declined substantially for both older men and women since 1980 (over 45 years). On the one hand, while suicide rates for young men have tended to go up those for females have remained relatively stable. The biggest difference was for men over 15 years and by area of deprivation 1999–2003. The rate for men in deprived areas was 25.4/100,000 more than twice those in the least deprived areas at 11.9/100,000 (Social Trends 2008, 103). But, such a finding does not rest easily with the observation in the previous chapter of an inverse relationship between deprivation and MS prevalence. It also runs counter to the suicide risk factors for PwMS identified by Pompili et al. (2012) in an international review of the published evidence, namely depression, disease severity, social isolation, younger age, progressive disease, lower income, earlier disease course, higher levels of physical disability, not driving and to have suffered significant personal loss such as the death of a spouse or a divorce.

5.7.3 Migration

The available evidence on the role of migration in shaping the regional disposition of MS in the UK was both scarce and enigmatic; enough to show it could quite possibly have been important, but not enough to demonstrate it actually was. And, one of the reasons for this was the all too common practice noted above of treating in-migrants with MS as new diagnosees.

In the prevalence study of MS in South Glamorgan between 1985 and 1988, of the 442 cases at the start of the period, 20 (4.5%) had moved out of the area and 6 (1.4%) had moved in (Hennessy et al. 1989, 1038). This may imply migration was of very limited significance but for the same set of PwMS Swingler and Compston (1990, 68) observed that the disease was 'most prevalent among middle-aged married or divorced Caucasian women, *born in England rather than Wales*' [my italics]. This certainly implies some serious movement of place of residence of a number of women with MS at some time during their lives.

In South Cambridgeshire again, for three years, between 1990 and 1993, of the 344 PwMS at the start of the period, 29 (8.4%) had moved out and 8 (2.3%) moved in by the end of the study period. This investigation included the university city of Cambridge in which a large number of highly mobile students would reside temporarily, many of whom could be below the age to show the first signs of MS, who may nevertheless, add to a population denominator in an incidence or prevalence calculation. It was also clear that in a non-university town such as Rochdale in the late 1990s migration must have been important too in shaping the number of PwMS in the area because, according to Shepherd and Summers (1996, 417) 48.2 per cent of them were born outside the study area. Finally, in terms of the local movement of people within the UK, the change of place of residence of PwMS to benefit from a new nationally rationed therapy should be considered. There was most certainly hearsay evidence that during the 1990s and early twenty-first century some people changed their place of residence to be located in a health authority that had a more liberal policy on offering the new DMDs to people newly diagnosed with MS. There has been no systematic inquiry into this phenomenon, however.

At a broader international scale, Britain has often featured in MS migration discussions either as a destination for people carrying MS susceptible genetic material or as a departure point for people who may carry this material further afield. Poser (1995), for example, in his persuasive hypothetical essay argued that the Vikings in their raiding and colonial behaviour during the eighth and ninth centuries may have been an early vector for the genes that conferred MS susceptibility into eastern Britain and especially into Scotland. It was also possible that such genetic material could have come into England and then spread northwards by the Normans after their successful invasion of 1066; they were themselves, of course, descended directly from the Norsemen. Much later, as has already been noted, the migration of the Scots into the north of Ireland in the seventeenth and eighteenth centuries may have helped to increase the prevalence of the disease in that part of Britain. And, finally, Britain's colonial activities during the following two centuries, along with similar activity by other European powers, in South Africa, the Americas and Australasia may have helped to export the condition to those countries especially among their Caucasian residents.

It must be realised that in this latter discussion there is no suggestion that people who were actually suffering from MS took part in these migrations, especially if they were showing signs of disability. Indeed, chronic illness is usually regarded as a major disincentive to migration; such activity instead being associated with the young, healthy and successful. Of course, there have been exceptions to this that internationally would include the transportation of criminals to penal colonies, the emigration of peoples from places of famine and conflict such as in Ireland during the mid-nineteenth century potato famine and the slave trade, while much more locally would embrace the movement of older people to retirement places and the chronically sick to residential care facilities. And, one of the methodological difficulties that such observations pose is that migrants can in no way be thought of as representative of the populations of either the areas from which they departed or the destination areas where their journeys terminated.

The more recent investigations of MS and migration that involved the UK and its peoples have been primarily concerned with the impact of differing environments on increasing or reducing the chances of someone developing MS; the way in which the risk of developing MS changes according to race, age of migration and whether the move took place to or from high or low prevalence areas. Such evidence was included in an extensive international review by Gale and Martyn (1995) from which a set of four important conclusions were derived. And, although some of these are now in need of revision, each can be usefully employed to aid this discussion.

1. *Migrants who move from an area where MS is common to an area where it is rarer show a decrease in the rate of the disease.* For example, Hammond et al. (1988) for age standardised cohorts of PwMS in Queensland discovered that immigrants from England had a much higher MS prevalence than Australians in 1981; 26.1/100,000 compared to 17.8/100,000, both of which were substantially lower than all the English regional prevalence rates of MS reported above. Similar evidence was also reported for Perth and Hobart (Hammond et al. 1988, 10) in which age-standardised rates were 27.6/100,000 and 69.7/100,000 respectively for Australian born PwMS and much higher at 44.1/100,000 and 141.1/100,000 respectively for English born PwMS. However, in a later review of equivalent evidence for PwMS born in the British Isles compared to those born in Australia across five regions studied in a similar manner the relationship was not so unequivocal. As can be seen from Table 5.7 the prevalence of MS in New South Wales and South Australia was not higher among people born in the British Isles compared to those born in Australia (Hammond et al. 2000). No explanation for this finding was offered in the text.
2. *Migrants who move from an area of low prevalence to an area where it is more common tend to retain their lower propensity.* For example, the work of Elian and Dean (1993, 455) purported to demonstrate that deaths from MS among new commonwealth immigrants identified in hospitals in Greater London and the West Midlands were much less frequent than would otherwise have been expected from

Table 5.7 Prevalence of PwMS /100,000 in 1981 by region in Australia and place of birth

	Born in Australia	Born in the British Isles
Queensland	17.7	24.7
Western Australia	23.4	25.9
New South Wales	42.2	36.6
South Australia	31.9	23.0
Hobart	68.4	121.5

Source: Hammond et al. (2000, 971).

death rates in England and Wales. There were 12 deaths among those born in the Caribbean when 59 should have been expected; 6 deaths among Asian immigrants when 82 would have been expected and one from an Asian born in Africa when 12 expected. But, the numbers involved were extremely small for any firm conclusions to be derived.

3. *The chances of developing MS can change markedly between generations, with the offspring of migrants or second generation immigrants, tending towards the prevalence of their host region.* For the research undertaken by Elian and Dean (1987) and Elian et al. (1990) attempts were made to identify the UK offspring of people born in Asia, Africa and the West Indies who subsequently attended a hospital in Greater London or the West Midlands to receive a diagnosis of MS. For the identification of such cases they relied heavily on the records and memories of hospital staff and especially the consultant neurologists, registrars and secretaries. As a result it was unlikely all possible cases were identified. For the period from 1976 to 1984, only 16 cases were identified in Greater London (Elian and Dean 1987), and when the West Midlands was included (Elian et al. 1990) only 28 cases were relevant for a count on 1 April 1980. Although the numbers were exceedingly small, the authors claimed that they could be usefully compared with the research findings from Sutton in south London in 1985 (Williams and McKernan 1986) to show similar prevalence and incidence rates. If this was so, then the offspring of people who had moved to England from areas where MS was rare would have become much more likely to develop the condition than if they had been born in their parents' countries.

4. *A person's risk of developing MS may be established during the first two decades of their life.* The work of Dean and Elian (1997) on MS in migrants to England from India and Pakistan tended to suggest a 'critical age' of migration above which the migrant's chance of developing MS would be similar to their destination area; below which to their area of origin. And, Dean and Elian (1997) believed this 'critical age' was 15 years. Their work using evidence from hospitals in Greater London, the West Midlands, Leicester, Bradford, Halifax and Huddersfield revealed 36 people with MS from Indian and Pakistani backgrounds in January 1990 who had migrated to England before the age of 15 years when 20 would have been expected from the size of this age cohort (Dean and Elian 1997, 566). This, of course, built on much earlier work by Dean and colleagues (1976) on the incidence of MS in Greater London where it was argued that immunity

to MS developed in childhood. Now, according to Gale and Martyn (1995), research from South Africa, Israel and the US would tend to put this age somewhat higher at 20 years although for methodological reasons they were sceptical of any substantive relationship in this area. Research on immigrants from the UK and Ireland to Australia has attempted to answer this issue directly as part of an extensive array of investigations following a major point prevalence study of five regions of that country in 1981 (Hammond et al. 1996). If the 'critical age of migration' hypothesis had any explanatory value, then one would have expected those who migrated to Australia (an area of low prevalence) from the British Isles (an area of high MS prevalence) after the age of 15 years to have a higher prevalence of MS than those who migrated before the age of 15 years. Unfortunately, the available evidence on this point did not trend in the expected direction (Hammond et al. 2000, 971). But, as the authors pointed out such material may be contaminated by substantial bias by duration of residence. This was because those who had been in Australia longest would have had the greatest chance of developing MS. Therefore, a case controlled exercise was performed in which each migrant was matched by age and state of residence to 20 controls. However, in this case also any putative relationship between age of migration and the development of MS failed to materialise. Thus, the authors concluded that the risk of developing MS spanned a wide age range and was not determined either side of 15 years. It also followed that a much greater proportion of the British Isles-born migrant population was subject to the lower risk of developing MS in Australia than their non-migrating countrymen (Hammond et al. 2000, 973). Regrettably, though, the first of these two conclusions has now been over-turned by a reassessment of the evidence especially in terms of new denominators for the prevalence calculations better to denote those migrants into Australia at risk of developing MS (McLeod et al. 2011). As a consequence, the absolute risk of developing MS showed a marked difference between those immigrants from the British Isles entering before and after the age of 15 years. For the former, the prevalence was 22/100,000 in the 4 states of New South Wales, Queensland, South Australia and Western Australia, significantly less than for the 15 years plus age group at 45/100,000 (McLeod et al. 2011, 1147).

One of the perhaps surprising omissions from the epidemiological work carried out so far in the UK is that none of the above ideas about the relationships between migration and the risk of developing MS have been tested with UK regional evidence. Scotland, for example, could represent an area of high MS risk and has been the origin of much migration to the rest of the UK in the recent past, most of which would represent a much lower risk area. For example, during much of the 1990s approximately 50,000 people a year left Scotland for elsewhere in the UK (Regional Trends on line, various editions). Now, if these people carried with them the Scottish MS prevalence rate of approximately 200/100,000 it would suggest that during this decade as many as 100 people a year left Scotland with the immanent probability of developing MS. But, how many developed the illness and how that may have related to their age of migration is not yet known?

5.7.4 Stayers

The above analyses have already shown that a large number of PwMS remain resident in a particular region not only in the short term, but also over a much longer period. In Leeds, for example, from April 1996, 90 per cent of PwMS remained in the region for the next 42 months (Ford et al. 2002). In South Cambridgeshire, 81 per cent of PwMS in 1990 were still resident in the same area 3 years later (Robertson et al. 1996b). For the same length of time in South Glamorgan from 1985 the proportion was 84 per cent (Hennessy et al. 1989) with 40 per cent surviving in the region for 262 months (Hirst et al. 2009). It has also been shown that of these 3 areas, Leeds recorded the lowest proportional loss of PwMS through death at 7 per cent compared with 8 per cent for South Cambridgeshire and 9 per cent for South Glamorgan. But, why Leeds should appear to be so favourably placed regarding surviving with MS is unclear.

Even from this variable evidence two deductions may be drawn. First, that 'stayers' and their apparently increasing longevity have made an important contribution to the recent increase in MS regional prevalences through time, most notably in north Northern Ireland and South Glamorgan. Second, and as was shown in the last chapter, the cohort of PwMS in a region was slowly becoming an aging one. And, for an increasing subset of this group of PwMS they will be accompanied by a full range of MS symptoms and age-related co-morbidities. It also adds support to the development of a life-course approach for the understanding and modelling of the development of MS in individuals and groups. The necessary information on the natural history of regional groups of PwMS, however, is just not available to take such ideas much further.

5.8 Conclusion

This chapter began by reviewing attempts to estimate the number of PwMS in the UK and came to the conclusion that the estimate of 100,000 by Thomas et al. (2009) adopted by the MS Society was likely to be an underestimate by approximately 10,000 for the end of the first decade of the twenty-first century; the estimate of 127,000 by Mackenzie et al. (2014) therefore probably an overestimate by a similar amount. The chapter then progressed to review recent regional MS prevalence work that for the countries of Scotland, Wales and Northern Ireland failed to concur with the results of Mackenzie et al. (2014). This may be because the data sources used were fundamentally irreconcilable. It is also important to observe that recent regional evidence on the numbers of PwMS was sparse. In fact, for England, Wales and Northern Ireland only one empirical study of this nature had been carried out in each country since the year 2000. The conclusions that could be drawn therefore were weak and poor indicators of what might happen in the future.

Nevertheless, this prevalence research revealed two important trends. The first trend was an increase in prevalence through time; the numbers of PwMS had been increasing. The second trend was an increase in prevalence with latitude such that the highest rates were to be found in Northern Ireland and especially in Scotland. The mapping of hospital admissions evidence for Scotland and England separately added support to this geographical pattern along with a suggestion that large urban areas for whatever reason tended to record relatively low MS prevalence rates.

A 'components of change' system to help account for the changing regional frequencies of PwMS was introduced but a lack of available evidence prevented the scheme being taken very far. Nevertheless, the discussion of the categories used in this system resulted in some important conclusions. The first conclusion was that incident cases of MS, especially among women, had been increasing through time although a note of caution was introduced. This was because in some cases incident cases may not be exclusively through the newly diagnosed but also through the in-migration of PwMS into an area. On the deaths of PwMS three important points should be made. First, the available evidence although weak suggested that in the UK PwMS tended to die at an earlier age than members of the general public. Second, on suicide, that although some PwMS do take their own lives, there was no convincing evidence that their suicide rate was any higher than among the British public generally. Finally, that in terms of the proximate causes of the deaths of PwMS, infectious and respiratory diseases appeared to be disproportionately high.

6
The Impact of MS

6.1 Introduction

This chapter is concerned with the ways in which Multiple Sclerosis (MS) impacts on peoples' lives and in essence will follow the World Health Organisation's (WHO's) International Classification of Functioning, Disability and Health by beginning with impairments, or the primary symptoms of MS as Burgess (2002, 76) called them, and move through activity impacts to consider limitations on participation in social and economic activities. The primary symptoms of MS such as bladder dysfunction and muscle weakness are those caused directly by the disease processes of demyelination, axonal damage and loss. This chapter reviews the range of symptoms experienced by people with MS, their prevalence and how over time they begin to affect people with MS (PwMS) not as individual symptoms but more likely collectively as bundles of symptoms either intermittently or indefinitely. The text proceeds to consider three particular symptom groups in detail: physical disablement emphasising walking and falling, fatigue and psychological distress.

Primary symptoms and the problems associated with their management may result in secondary medical problems or symptoms such as urinary tract infections, injuries from falls and pressure ulcers. For example, in an audit of medical services used by PwMS in Oxfordshire during the first 10 months of 1996, 15 PwMS reported injuries from falls that needed formal medical attention (Wade and Green 2001, 29). These secondary symptoms will not be considered in any systematic way in this chapter. However, it must be emphasised that the distinction between these two groups of symptoms is not always clear cut. For example, fatigue, depression and pain may all occur as both primary and secondary symptoms in MS. It also should be borne in mind that these secondary symptoms can have a direct and very serious impact on someone's life and may even be life threatening. For example, it was noted in Chapter 5 that deaths from infections would appear to be higher in PwMS than in the United Kingdom (UK) population generally.

In this chapter a distinction is made between symptoms and their impacts on the lives of PwMS. This separation is important because people differ in their abilities, aspirations and personal circumstances and especially in their coping skills. Thus, the impact of any one symptom or group of symptoms will vary between individuals. For example, a person may be able to adapt with some ease to a degree of walking disability if their lives, work and hobbies were relatively sedentary. This would be very different for parents of young children whose jobs and past-times required them to be on their feet for much of the day. But, it also means that someone with significant physical disability and limitations on activities of daily living could regard themselves as having a high and positive quality of life if they were still able to do the things that mattered most to them. Unfortunately, it also means the opposite is possible too. As Ford et al. (2001a, 520) observed, 'there is not a straightforward exchange between health status and quality of life.' However, the impact of MS on a person's life is not just in terms of their levels of activity and social participation, it is also in terms of their cognition and mood that in a reciprocal way may affect their ability to cope with their illness too. Furthermore, many of the symptoms of MS are of themselves subjective in nature such as sensory changes and fatigue and often transitory, difficult to pin down in time and bodily location. Two important points follow directly from these observations. The first point must be that measures of disease impact do not neatly correlate with measures of life satisfaction or subjective wellbeing. The second important point is that to try to capture the impact of MS may have on a person's life is a complicated and multidimensional task. This, of course, has not stopped people trying. Indeed, there is now a burgeoning literature on health status and quality of life measures both of a generic and of an MS-disease specific nature, including those assessed by clinicians and those by patients themselves (see Gruenewald et al. 2004; Zajicek et al. 2007, 44–65). However, it is not the intention of this review to consider them all, only those most relevant to this book's evolving argument. These will include, for example, the most widely used measure of physical disability the Expanded Disability Status Scale (EDSS), the generic measure of health-related quality of life EQ-5D and the disease-specific instruments the MS Impact Scale (MSIS-29) (Hobart et al. 2001) and the Leeds MS Quality of Life Scale (LMSQoLS) (Ford et al. 2001b).[1]

MS does not just affect the sufferer. It has impacts too on their spouses, partners, close family members and friends. These will also be considered where appropriate in this chapter with the specific issues facing the carers of PwMS, who are often close family members, considered in the following chapter on the care of people with MS. It is also worth remembering at this point that MS only reduces life expectancy by a few years and therefore someone with the disease will most likely suffer many years of increasing disability and, while there may be a plethora of ways of measuring disease impacts for particular points in time, much less has been done to look at change through time. Furthermore, there seems to be little research evidence on how people's coping strategies change with the symptoms thrust upon them especially given their almost certain prospect of more to come.

In their influential attempt to construct a patient-based outcome measure for MS, Hobart and colleagues (2001) concluded that all the possible health impact descriptors could be usefully summarised in terms of physical impacts and psychological impacts. This is one of the reasons why this review gives special attention to a symptom from each of these groups, physical disability emphasising walking and psychological impacts. The first of these symptoms was chosen because it is probably the most overt physical impact of the illness often requiring a major piece of technology to overcome, such as a wheelchair; the now iconic symbol of physical disablement. By contrast, the impact of MS on a person's mind, thoughts and mood has been included because it is a clear invisible symptom of MS that in its most extreme case depression can have profound impacts on a person's life. In addition, the symptom of fatigue will also be reviewed for four reasons. The first reason is because in impacts and possible aetiology it probably has both physical and psychological aspects. The second reason is because it has been one of the most common symptoms experienced by PwMS. The third is because it was the first symptom chosen by the membership of the UK Research Network of the MS Society for attention under that Society's Symptom Relief Initiative and, the final reason is because in a research priority setting exercise in partnership with the James Lind Alliance in 2013 the members of the MS Society and their health-care professionals identified 'which treatments are effective for fatigue in MS?' as the third most important unanswered research question (MS Society 2013).

Given the types of symptoms MS can generate and the time of life these symptoms materialise, this illness has the potential to exert major impacts on the lives of people with the disease and on their families. One way in which this has been usefully conceptualised in the academic literature that will be discussed in what follows is through 'biographical disruption' (Green et al. 2007). Under this umbrella concept the impact of MS on relationships, employment / careers, costs, standard of living and quality of life can be explored; consequences that are often a direct result of the way in which a society is organised and consequences that are often a heavy blight on the quality of life of PwMS. This latter group of MS effects, however, are not the result of an immutable symptomatic natural history of MS; rather they are the result of decisions made by individuals and groups of people. As a result they will be subject to change through time as the values of society and of the individuals within that society change through time. Thus, the social and economic consequences of having MS in a particular place at a particular time may not necessarily be repeated in the same place at another time or in a different place at the same time.

In the last section of this chapter a much more eclectic view of quality of life is advocated to assess PwMS in which the more recent political buzz-word of 'happiness' is introduced to the analysis. Here the emphasis is on what PwMS do in their lives and how that may change as their disease develops. The chapter then concludes on two of the major constraints MS may impose on peoples' lives, its economic impact and its impact on human relationships.

6.2 The primary symptoms of MS

In their document on 'Managing MS in Primary and Secondary Care' NICE (2003, 26) made the important observation that in MS the 'range of potential symptoms is vast.' They went on to list 16 specific impairments:

1. Fatigue
2. Bladder problems
3. Bowel problems
4. Muscular weakness
5. Spasticity and spasms
6. Ataxia and tremor
7. Sensory loss
8. Visual problems

9. Pain
10. Cognitive loss
11. Emotionalism
12. Depression
13. Anxiety
14. Swallowing difficulties
15. Speech difficulties
16. Sexual dysfunction

It is a list not too dissimilar from the one of 12 commonly experienced symptoms offered in the Media Planet MS Times Supplement of 2008 noted in the Introduction to this book:

- Fatigue, an overwhelming sense of tiredness making physical or mental activity difficult, and for some impossible.
- Balance problems and vertigo, walking difficulties, problems with coordination.
- Visual problems, blurred or double vision, temporary loss of sight in one eye or both.
- Numbness or tingling, commonly in the hands or feet.
- Pain, sometimes mild, sometimes severe.
- Loss of muscle strength and dexterity.
- Stiffness and spasms, tightening or rigidity in particular muscle groups.
- Sexual dysfunction.
- Anxiety, depression or mood swings.
- Cognitive problems, difficulty with memory and concentration.
- Speech problems, slurring, slowing of speech, or changes in pitch or tone.
- Incontinence, a lack of control of bladder or bowel functions.

Unfortunately, there is a definite lack of consistent evidence on the number of people who experience specific MS-related symptoms, along with the severity and duration of their suffering. All that can be said is that the frequency and rate of suffering would both appear to be high for most identifiable symptoms. Burgess (2002) for example, suggested that most people with MS will suffer motor and optic disturbance during the course of their illness, 80 per cent will have continence problems, up to 90 per cent sexual dysfunction, more than 50 per cent pain at some time and approximately half will experience a major episode of depression. Further evidence of symptom prevalence, that refreshingly notes its lack of general application, comes from the 223 usable responses to a symptom management survey of MS Society members (MS Society, undated). Here the most active problems experienced over the last two years before the survey were, fatigue 86 per cent, balance 73 per cent, muscle weakness 69 per cent, continence 66 per cent, numbness and tingling 64 per cent, muscle stiffness 64 per cent, pain 54 per cent and muscle spasm 51 per cent. Very similar findings were obtained from those PwMS who agreed between 2004 and 2008 to participate in the South West Impact of MS Project (SWIMS) project in Cornwall and Devon, with the top three symptoms reported at the time of joining being fatigue (80%), poor balance (75%) and pain (70%) (Zajicek et al. 2010, 10:88 table 4). By contrast, Ford et al. (2001a) from focus group work in Leeds suggested that cognitive and swallowing problems had a particularly strong impact on quality of life.

For those in the early years of relapsing remitting MS (RRMS), their symptoms will probably be temporary events, lasting only a few days or weeks, but for those with a progressive form of the condition there may be little prospect of relief without medical intervention. What is worse they may not be individual impairments but form one of a suite of concurrent symptoms that collectively are miserable to experience and difficult to treat effectively with a seriously negative impact on a person's quality of life. For example, in their investigation of the health-related quality of life of 929 PwMS frequenting 7 neurology treatment centres in various parts of England, Forbes et al. (2006b, 71) discovered that 16 per cent suffered seriously from the dreadful combination of the 'invisible' symptoms of pain, fatigue and depression as a result of their MS. Two further examples demonstrate this phenomenon more generally and just how varied the symptom combinations may be. First, in an audit of PwMS in Oxfordshire in the 10 months from January 1996, Wade and Green (2001, 29–32) detailed the symptoms that occurred throughout the period for 150 MS patients in which the control of legs, balance and fatigue were the principal permanent symptoms. What is more, the particular problems that required specific medical attention during this audit included 39 PwMS with urinary problems (18 more than once), 58 with mobility issues (3 more than once), 12 with emotional problems (1 more than once), 6 with fatigue (1 more than once) and 2 with cognitive problems (both more than once).

The second example of MS suffering comes from the work of Higginson and Hart (2006) on people with severe MS where one would expect the symptom burden to be at a maximum. In this case 51 PwMS with little or no mobility but still able to communicate, were referred to a palliative care initiative in south east London by local health and social care professionals. These individuals had a mean of nine separate identifiable symptoms, with a range of one to seventeen, three of which on average were regarded as severe or overwhelming, three moderate and three mild (Higginson and Hart 2006, 161). Lower limb and bladder disability were the most common afflictions with visual and swallowing difficulties the least prevalent. What may be surprising to discover though is that the mean age of this group of PwMS was only 53 years, with a range of 33 to 75 years, with 72 per cent female and 95 per cent of white ethnic origin that makes them very similar to the national survey results of members of UK MS societies observed in Chapter 4. This group of severely disabled PwMS therefore were not substantially older than the average regional or national cohort of PwMS. Clearly and tragically some PwMS have a very difficult time indeed with their illness from a relatively young age.

From this evidence it should be of no surprise to discover that in their document on managing MS, NICE (2003, 26) was able to point out that 'in most people there will be several if not many symptoms,' from which it directly followed that the symptomatic relief for most PwMS during their lifetimes and for existing PwMS who have already entered a progressive phase of the illness will not just be about relieving one symptom it will be about relieving many. In other words, most PwMS require many different forms of simultaneous medical intervention (Wade and Green 2001). But, it must be emphasised that any one of the symptoms of MS has the ability to cause concern for individuals with the condition and when added to even minimal physical disablement could have serious negative impacts on their quality of life. Physical disability, tremor and incontinence are not the comfortable bed-fellows of successful employment and social interaction!

So far only general descriptive categories have been used to group together the primary symptoms of MS. However, as shown later, to move on to treating these conditions further definition is required. For example, MS fatigue may have many different forms including general lassitude, short-circuiting fatigue and heat sensitivity (MS Society 2014a, Schwid et al. 2002) that may suggest both different aetiologies and modes of treatment. Unfortunately, uncertainty over the causes and remedies for many MS symptoms seems a common feature of the state of medical knowledge at the moment. Testament to this sorry state of affairs can be found in the NICE (2003) document on managing MS. The vast majority of symptom treatment recommendations came from very low-grade evidence. Indeed, of the 138 evidential references in the managing specific impairments section, only 25 (18%) were awarded the highest 'A' category, with 104 (75%) receiving a low 'D' authority.

The symptom burden generated by MS not only varies from person to person, making the experience of each person with MS unique, but also vary through a person's life. Figure 6.1 represents a hypothetical example of the symptomatic experience of a person with MS who, perhaps optimistically, lived for 80 years. During this time they experienced four primary symptoms concerned with the control of their walking, bladder and sight along with pain. It is, of course, most likely that people with MS who lived for four decades or more with the disease will experience rather more symptoms than this. Nevertheless, during their first 25 years of life this individual had no clinical indication that they were suffering from a serious chronic illness at all. After this point they experienced a series of distinct relapses with respect to their eyesight (3), ability to walk (3) along with three episodes of trigeminal neuralgia later in life. In most cases they recovered virtually all of their former competence after theses relapses. However, in sight and pain a modest deficit remained through the remainder of their life. Their ability to walk followed a different course by getting progressively worse from their late 30s onwards such that they needed a walking stick at age 42 years and a wheelchair at

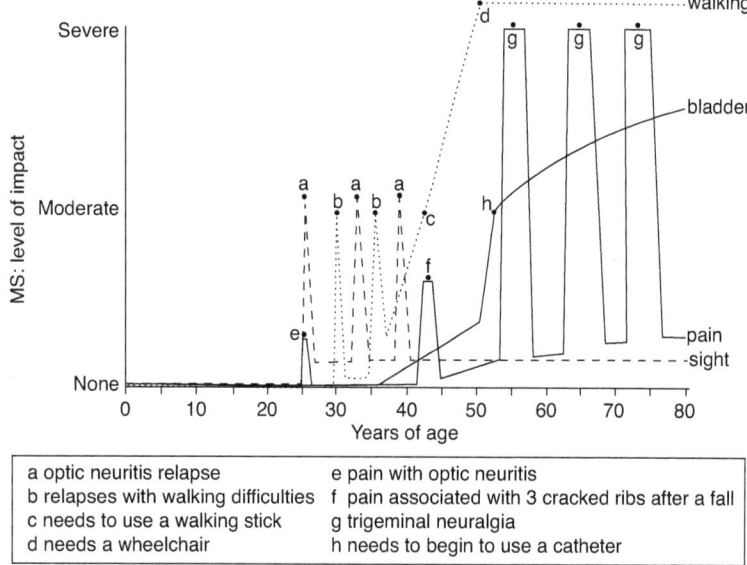

Figure 6.1 Hypothetical impact of MS on a person's life

age 50 years. Their ability to control their bladder showed no remission from the point it became problematic at age 35 years and became rapidly worse during the person's 50th year. Thus, in their mid-50s this individual with MS experienced a combination of walking and bladder failure with a period of serious facial pain. What impacts such medical problems may have had on their familial relationships or employment is not known. At the very least they would have been challenging. It would not be unreasonable to suggest therefore that this person with MS may have also experienced psychological distress at this time.

Unfortunately, severe evidence limitations prevent any formal calculation of the symptom burden of PwMS and the suffering that ensues. As a result there remains a need for the collection of more consistent evidence on this attribute of the disease. Perhaps the establishment of MS Registers in various parts of the world noted in Chapter 3 may ultimately provide suitable evidence on this issue.

6.3 Specific symptom groups

6.3.1 Disability, walking and falling

The EDSS detailed in Table 6.1 (Zajicek et al. 2007, 46–7) is a useful starting point for this discussion because, although it is a compound measure of neurological status, it is dominated by ambulation (Burgess 2002, 52–3). For example, EDSS 3.5 to 8.0 all include assessments of walking ability with EDSS 6.0, needing to use a stick for walking, regarded as a major disability milestone. In addition, it has often been used broadly to categorise PwMS as either mildly, moderately or severely disabled by their MS. For example, both Freeman and Thompson (2000) and MacLurg et al. (2005, 383) regarded EDSS 0 to 4.5 as mildly affected, or as having minimal disability and getting on with their lives, EDSS 5.0 to 6.5 as moderately disabled, or as 'working hard to stay on their feet' but starting to fall (sic) out of employment and EDSS 7.0 to 9.5 as severely disabled, those who have become dependent on their family and social services. By contrast, while Craig et al. (2003, 1227) agreed with the severe category, they regarded the slightly broader range of 4.0 to 6.5 as moderately disabled.

The EDSS scale with 20 distinct phases needs to be discussed because it has been so widely used in MS research. It may well be what Thompson and Hobart (1998) have termed the tarnished gold standard of measures of disability in MS research, but it is the one that has been used and 'published information on people with MS at different levels of functional disability is scarce' (Kobelt et al. 2006a, S96).

Table 6.1 Kurtzke's Expanded Disability Status Scale

0.0	Normal neurological examination
1.0	No disability, minimal signs in one FS*
1.5	No disability, minimal signs in more than one FS*
2.0	Minimal disability in one FS*
2.5	Mild disability in one FS* or minimal disability in two FS*
3.0	Moderate disability in one FS*, or mild disability in three or four FS*. Fully ambulatory
3.5	Fully ambulatory but with moderate disability in one FS* and more than minimal disability in several others
4.0	Fully ambulatory without aid, self-sufficient, up and about some 12 hours a day despite relatively severe disability; able to walk without aid or rest some 500 metres
4.5	Fully ambulatory without aid, up and about much of the day, able to work a full day, may otherwise have some limitation of full activity or require minimal assistance; characterised by relatively severe disability; able to walk without aid or rest some 300 metres
5.0	Ambulatory without aid or rest for about 200 metres; disability severe enough to impair full daily activities (work a full day without special provisions)
5.5	Ambulatory without aid or rest for about 100 metres; disability severe enough to preclude full daily activities
6.0	Intermittent or unilateral constant assistance (cane, crutch, brace) required to walk about 100 metres with or without resting
6.5	Constant bilateral assistance (canes, crutches, braces) required to walk about 20 metres without resting
7.0	Unable to walk beyond approximately five metres even with aid, essentially restricted to wheelchair; wheels self in standard wheelchair and transfers alone; up and about in wheelchair some 12 hours a day
7.5	Unable to make more than a few steps; restricted to wheelchair, may need aid in transfer; wheels self but cannot carry on in standard wheelchair a full day; may require motorised wheelchair
8.0	Essentially restricted to bed or chair or perambulated in wheelchair, but may be out of bed itself much of the day; retains many self-care functions; generally has effective use of arms
8.5	Essentially restricted to bed much of the day; has some effective use of arms; retains some self-care functions
9.0	Confined to bed; can still communicate and eat
9.5	Totally helpless bed patient; unable to communicate effectively or eat/swallow
10.0	Death due to MS

Source: Abstracted from the MS Trust information, education, research and support pages at www.mstrust.org.uk/atoz/edss.jsp. See also Kurtzke (1983) and Zajicek et al. (2007, 46–7).

* FS – Functional System of which there are 8: pyramidal, cerebellar, brainstem, sensory, bowel and bladder, visual, cerebral and mental, 'other'.

To understand EDSS evidence properly a number of its characteristics must be borne in mind. First, and fundamentally it must be realised that this data is ordinal in nature referring to specific categories of disability that are each designated by a number from 0 to 10. As such there is no sense in which the distance between any two adjacent categories can be measured or assumed to be the same. Similarly, there is no way of knowing what the distance between EDSS 3.5 and EDSS 5.5 may be or whether it is the same as the distance between EDSS 5.5 and 7.5. There is no EDSS 'interval' scale of measurement. Thus, a mean EDSS score is an arithmetic nonsense; it merely indicates a broad tendency and nothing more. This point becomes more important when it is realised that the frequency distribution, or histogram, of EDSS scores may not be 'normally' distributed, and certainly has not been for the few studies that have presented appropriate information.

The regional distributions of EDSS scores from different parts of the world and for different points in time display substantial unanimity, tending to be bimodal in form with a major maxima at EDSS 6.0 and subsidiary peaks near the lower end of the scale near EDSS 2.0. For example for the 1,099 PwMS surveyed in London Ontario between 1972 and 1984, EDSS maxima occurred across EDSS 6.0 and 7.0 and also between EDSS 1.0 and 3.0 such that 47 per cent of the sample possessed an EDSS score of 6.0 or above with 11 per cent at EDSS 8.0 or above (Weinshenker et al. 1989). For the UK as a whole the only available EDSS evidence comes from a postal questionnaire survey by Orme et al. (2007, 57) from which information on the self-rated Adapted Patient Determined Disease Steps scale was converted into EDSS equivalents for the 2,048 members of the MS Trust who responded. The frequency distribution of this attribute was bimodal with a major peak at EDSS 6.0, the modal group, and a minor peak at EDSS 2.0. There were few recordings for EDSS 0, 3.0 and 9.0.

The regional EDSS evidence in the UK shows remarkably similar results too for three very disparate regions, north Northern Ireland, South Glamorgan and the combined areas of Aberdeen City, Orkney and Shetland. In the former in 1996 for the 259 individuals with definite or probable MS, and for whom an EDSS score had been calculated, the median was 5.0 and the mode 6.0 with an important outlier at EDSS 2.0 or minimal disability in one functional system (McDonnell and Hawkins 1998, 425–6). For the same region 8 years later in 2004, the 370 definite or probable cases of MS recorded a median and a mode of 6.0 but now the subsidiary peak was lower at 0.5 and 1.0 (Gray et al. 2008, 883–4). For the three areas in North East Scotland in 2009, the individuals with probable or definite MS the recorded median EDSS was 5.0 (Visser et al. 2012, 721). Interestingly, in this latter study, men recorded a much higher median EDSS of 6.0 than women at 3.5 (Visser et al. 2012, supplementary table S2). But, no explanation for this difference was offered. In South Glamorgan between 1985 and 2005, the percentage distributions of EDSS scores given in the text strongly suggest that the principal measures of central tendency were in the range of 5.5 to 6.5 with more than 20 per cent, more than 120 people, in 2005 at EDSS 8 or worse, that is 'essentially restricted to bed or chair'. What is more, even when just considering people with RRMS, disability distributions displayed a bi-modal form. For example, for 182 patients with this form of MS in South East Wales between 1999 and 2006 whose disability levels were established before and after relapses both showed maxima at EDSS 6.0 and 6.5 with the pre-relapse distributions displaying major subsidiary peaks at 3.5 to 4.5 (Hirst et al. 2008c, 282).

Collectively what this disability evidence tends to suggest is that half of all people with MS, one million worldwide and 50,000 in the UK, have some form of walking difficulty ranging from minor limitation to not being able to walk at all. As a direct consequence the development of physiotherapy techniques and drugs such as Fampyra, that help PwMS remain ambulatory for as long as possible become extremely important to maintaining their quality of life.

Given the importance of being able to stand and walk to the ways in which most people live, some of the most important questions both MS patients and their clinicians face are how long will it take to reach EDSS 6.0, and more generally how quickly will my disability progress? Evidence on disability progression in the UK is certainly hard to find, a point emphasised by Richards et al. (2002, 27) in their discussion on modelling the natural history of MS. A modest degree of empirical material is available from South Glamorgan between 1985 and 2005. Here for the 149 PwMS who were alive at both points in time their mean EDSS score increased from 5.15 to 8.01 (Hirst et al. 2008b) which meant this group had moved from an average score for all PwMS in the region in 1985 to the upper quartile of the whole group's range by 2005, that is displaying significant disability and certainly being unable to walk. In addition, there have been a number of pessimistic views expressed by neurologists from their clinic-based cohorts that were, of course, going to be dominated by the most severe cases. For example, Young (2008, 15) stated that 'About half of people with MS will reach EDSS 6 (need assistance of a stick to walk 100 metres) within 15 years of onset'. Coles (2008, 20) offered a slightly less gloomy prospect that a woman diagnosed in her early 30s will need a stick by 53 years. But, this is very weak material that fails to answer the earlier questions; a problem likely to persist for many years until an appropriate register of PwMS in the UK is developed.

MS register evidence, however, from other parts of the world has begun to answer these disability progression questions. Disappointingly though, the first important point that must be emphasised from this research is that individual outcomes were so variable that any positive prognostic factor could only serve as a rough guide to long-term disability outcomes (Degenhardt et al. 2009, 681). Nevertheless, as far as the time it may take from disease onset to reach the important disability milestone of EDSS 6.0, when the use of a stick to aid walking may be required, there appeared to be some common ground. Specifically, the median time to this disability level from Newcastle Australia was 27.0 years, for Olmsted County in the United States (US) 28.6 years, British Columbia 27.9 years, Lyon 23 years and London Ontario much lower at 15 years (Hurwitz 2011b). In addition, early clinical features such as relapse rate in the first two years of the disease and the time interval between the first two relapses were shown to be directly related to the time to EDSS states 6.0, 8.0 and 10.0. But, once patients had reached the progressive phase of the disease, relapse activity had no association with higher EDSS scores. It has also been observed that better outcomes may be associated with the following characteristics: female gender, younger age at outset, RRMS at onset, optic neuritis as the first symptom and degree of recovery from the first symptom (Confavreux et al. 2003, Scalfari et al. 2010, Hurwitz 2011a and 2011b). Furthermore, a good example of the way in which disability in people with primary progressive MS (PPMS) may progress faster than in people with RRMS can be found in the work of Confavreux and colleagues (2000, 1433) from the EDMUS data base in Lyon. Here the time for patients to reach EDSS 4.0, 6.0 and 7.00 from onset for the 1,562 patients with RRMS were 11.4, 23.1 and 33.1 years respectively, whereas for the 282 patients with PPMS it was 0.0, 7.1 and 13.4 years.

Mobility, especially in terms of being able to walk, climb stairs and cross uneven ground is of fundamental importance to a person's independence, to their ability to have a job and earn a living, to live successfully in their own home and to take part in social and communal events. Its loss or diminution therefore can have a significant impact on a person's life. But, very little is known about the actual walking ability of PwMS or their need for walking aid equipment. Some limited evidence is available from, for example, the CAMS randomised placebo-controlled clinical trial on the use of cannabinoids in the relief of MS symptoms (Zajicek et al. 2003) that demonstrated the many different aspects of walking inadequacy. In this study 666 people with clinically definite or laboratory-supported MS, who in the opinion of their doctor had had stable disease for the last 6 months but with problematic spasticity completed the Rivermead Mobility Index that included 7 questions about walking and climbing stairs. Of these individuals, 67 per cent could not manage a flight of stairs without help, 87 per cent could not manage to go up and down 4 steps with no rail (but using an aid if necessary), 46 per cent could not walk 10 metres with an aid if necessary (but with no standby help), 66 per cent could not walk around outside on pavements without help, 86 per cent could not walk 10 metres inside with no calliper, splint or aid, and no standby help, 86 per cent could not walk over uneven ground (grass, gravel, dirt, snow, ice) without help, and 99 per cent could not run, or quickly walk, 10 metres without limping in 4 seconds (Hobart and Cano 2009, 37).

What is known about walking is that it is a complicated motor activity involving the integration of a number of different components and for which a number of different measures exist both of a generic and of an impact-orientated nature (Hobart et al. 2003). What is also clear is that the inability to walk competently in terms of loss of balance and falling is an important issue for a substantial number of PwMS such that both the MS Trust (2008) in 'Falls' and the MS Society in Essentials 26 'Balance and MS' have felt it necessary to publish guidance on possible causes and how to avoid such events. For example, 'Falls' noted both health and environmental reasons for falls that included the fear of falling itself, along with the problems of mobility and balance (of actually being able to get the legs to move appropriately), vision, coordination (of sensory inputs and motor response), continence, concentration, medication, footwear and unfamiliar surroundings. Like many other MS symptoms mobility is seen as a multifactorial one, with no simple one-fix solution.

According to the MS Trust's 'Falls' booklet (2008, 4), falling was the commonest cause of accidental injury in the UK with more than 2.7 million people affected each year. In addition, the Able Community Care Newsletter in November 2008 stated that approximately 60,000 people break their hip from a fall every year with 14,000 people dying. This has led to Falls Clinics being widely available in the UK offering advice on medication, balance and vision checks, home aids and exercise suggestions. It is also known that many PwMS have falls with serious consequences. For example, Bazelier and colleagues (2011) demonstrated with evidence on 5,565 incident cases of MS from the GPRD linked to the National Hospital Registry for the period from 1997 to 2008 each matched to 6 controls who did not have MS (by year of birth, sex and GP practice) that PwMS had a 1.2 increased risk of all fractures. However, for hip fractures (neck of femur) the risk increased threefold and for osteoporotic fractures by 1.4. Furthermore, fracture risks were higher for those who had been prescribed steroids and antidepressants during the previous six months and increased with age. Such findings received additional support for England from Ramagopalan et al. (2012) with the aid of the complete English National Hospital Episode Statistics 1999–2010 covering approximately 50 million people. In this case it was shown that PwMS had a particularly elevated risk of fractures of the neck of the femur (hip), other femur (thigh) fractures, tibia and ankle, in that of the 87,873 admissions to hospital of PwMS, 4,414 had fractures of which 1,579 with fractures of the neck of the femur. Unfortunately, the role of disability in these events could not be interrogated for lack of suitable evidence. However, disability is known to be one of a set of inter-related factors involved. Others, commonly related to MS would include low bone mineral density, osteoporosis, low vitamin D levels, low mobility and smoking and alcohol usage (Dobson et al. 2012).

Research findings from the US would support and extend such a view. Peterson et al. (2008, 1031), for example, have suggested that approximately 50 per cent of middle-aged and older PwMS had fallen in the past 6 months. And, from a telephone survey of 354 self-selecting members of NARCOMS aged 55 years and above that included 177 fall-related injuries needing medical attention (80 fractures), 2 further important observations were made. The first observation was that receiving medical attention from recent falls was associated significantly with osteoporosis and the fear of falling, but not with balance and mobility problems, concentration and forgetfulness or greater fall frequency. Thus, it was primarily an age-related medical issue and a psychological problem. These were the factors that helped most to explain the statistical variation in injurious falls in this group of PwMS. Second, that the fear of falling and actually falling can become a circular self-fulfilling prophecy through the former leading to reduced activities that lead to reduced fitness (muscle strength and bone density) that in turn increased the risk of falling and then the fear of falling once again (Peterson et al. 2007).

Mobility is an important, taken for granted part of most people's lives. It is directly related to their ability to work, socialise and their success at achieving most functions of daily living. When this ability is impaired therefore through, for example the impact of MS, that denies them the control and movement of their legs to a lesser or greater extent it can have a serious negative impact on nearly every aspect of their lives. This is especially so when the world in which many PwMS have to live is predicated on the needs and capacities of the able bodied. For example, a limited ability to walk, or the need to use a wheelchair, may challenge a person to find work, impede their ability to travel to a place of work and limit their ability to move around such a place of work safely, all of which will almost certainly lead to a reduction in income. Similarly, in social terms immobility may limit the opportunities of a PwMS to socialise and meet friends, increase their chances of social as well as physical isolation with possible negative psychological impacts.

For a large minority of PwMS a time will come when they need to use a wheelchair; some temporarily when their legs tire, others permanently when they cease to be able to walk. For many this is a moment in their lives that is strenuously resisted, and usually against medical advice, because it represents psychologically a serious defeat in their battle against their MS (Robinson et al. 1996, 29). Some disabled people, however, begin to view their wheelchair as a 'liberator', not as a symbol of failure, simply as a means of mobility (Sapey et al. 2005, 496–7). But, others view their wheelchair as a symbol of societal oppression because they are forced to use it in an inappropriate built environment. As the UK MP Anne Begg exclaimed, there are 'still too many physical barriers making life for us in wheelchairs unnecessarily difficult' (Sapey et al. 2005, 496). But, no matter how they view their new situation, all begin to enter the frustrating and discriminatory world of life in a wheelchair.

There are many social implications of having to use a wheelchair. At worst there is the hate crime that some disabled people have had to endure. But, despite laws against disability discrimination, as Kingston (2010, 59) emphasises 'minor nastiness goes on all the time'. This can range from name calling to bullying in the workplace where, for example, perks and outings are arranged in places inaccessible to wheelchairs or where there are no accessible toilets. It can also include acts of selfishness and carelessness such as parking on footpaths and across drop curbs, taxis refusing to stop and the use of spaces reserved for the disabled for other activities such as 'disabled toilets' as stationary cupboards. Indeed, such pointed indifference to the problems people in wheelchairs face may lead to some of them believing they are 'invisible'. Despite taking up a relatively large area of floor space, they are regularly ignored on footpaths and in queues, bumped into and overlooked, making it increasingly difficult to get about and be served. And, when they have someone accompanying them the situation may be even worse because their companion is recognised and not them. It is assumed that because they are unable to walk, they must be incapable of all other physical and intellectual activities too; the 'do they take sugar?' phenomenon (Kingston 2010, 49).

Surprisingly though, the effect of mobility change on the lives of PwMS has rarely been the subject of academic research except in vocational terms reviewed in the following chapter. One of the few exceptions was carried out by Dyck (1995) on the changing 'lifeworlds' of unemployed women with MS in Greater Vancouver at the end of the twentieth century. In this case the 24 women investigated in detail experienced shrinking geographical and social worlds as their contacts with people declined and their access to public spaces became more difficult such that their lives became increasingly hidden from view.

These women lost their jobs mainly because of the challenging symptomology of their MS including visual disturbances, loss of fine motor skills and incontinence, but mainly because of fatigue and mobility losses that made it difficult for them to get to their places of work and once there operate successfully within the working environment. To compensate for their mobility problems many of these women had moved home or were considering doing so in order to improve accessibility both into and out of their homes and to valued external resources such as shops. This was only possible though when financial resources permitted, an issue that was becoming increasingly problematic since many were without paid employment. At the same time some attempts were made to reorganise the internal spaces of their homes too to include ramps, stair lifts, wider door frames, grab rails and changing furniture positions. This went hand-in-hand with the reorganisation and where possible the delegation to others of household tasks that included for the person with MS the pacing and spacing of jobs to make them less physically demanding and if possible the hiring in of help such as cleaners. Mobility problems in conjunction with fatigue and fear of falling limited their use of space outside the home by these women too so their ability to undertake many activities of daily living such as shopping and socialising with friends declined. Issues of this nature will almost certainly have equal resonance in many other parts of the world. But, it must be remembered that this Canadian research was undertaken in the pre-Internet era when propinquity was necessary for much more social and economic interaction than it is today during the second decade of the twenty-first century. For PwMS in recent times the Internet can in part form an important, and some would argue crucial, element of social interaction and psychological adjustment to having MS. Through the

Internet PwMS can join virtual communities to discuss their symptoms and possible remedial action, collect evidence that may help challenge standard medical opinion, or at least converse more authoritatively with their doctors, but perhaps most importantly simply socialise (Parr 2002). Furthermore, these contacts need not be confined to their local area or even their own nation but can be truly global in reach. However, the sorts of PwMS who use the Internet and those who are denied access to it have not been investigated. Nor is it understood how its use may vary by gender, race, age and health. Yet these are important questions to answer to help improve the lives of PwMS.

6.3.2 Psychological impacts

PwMS face a series of challenges because of their illness of both a physical and a psychological nature. These include unpleasant and unpredictable symptoms such as physical disability, fatigue and pain; difficult treatment options with often uncomfortable and serious consequences; often serious disruption of employment, income, activities of daily living and relationships; significant disruption to life's expected trajectory and identity; a need to confront one's own mortality at a relatively early age. These issues in turn can lead to substantial psychological impacts such as increased anxiety and distress, low mood, elevated risk of depression and feelings of worthlessness, hopelessness, reductions in subjective quality of life and emotional wellbeing.

It has already been shown that psychological issues are of serious concern in the lives of PwMS. It is possible that 50 per cent of PwMS will experience a bout of serious depression at some time during their lives and in particular during periods of relapse (Moore et al. 2012). It is also possible that at any one time 10 per cent of PwMS, that is more than 200,000 people worldwide, will be suffering psychological distress because of their disease. But, are these impacts any higher than for the public in general or for individuals with other chronic diseases? More generally it is clear that the psychological reactions to having MS vary hugely between people; some cope well whereas many succumb to low mood, perhaps clinical depression and in a few rare cases even suicide. What factors might explain such behaviours? These are crucial questions too from a therapeutic perspective because if the important explanatory factors are modifiable in nature then appropriate interventions may be possible. In the more popular MS press it has been suggested that a certain kind of personality leads to successful adjustment to MS (Cook 2008) such that people who are stoic, hard-working, submissive, compliant, eager to please and good at putting up with things will do best. There is no supportive credible research evidence for such a view. However, there is weak support for the cognitive quality of self-efficacy, a belief that one can cope competently with any challenging situation along with having a high degree of control over one's lives may be associated with positive health status outcomes of both a physical and a psychological nature (Riazi et al. 2004). This was assessed as part of a much wider investigation of health outcome measures such as MSIS-29 and MSWS-12 already noted above on two different samples of people with MS who attended the National Hospital for Neurology and Neurosurgery (NHNN), one for rehabilitation (43 PwMS) and the other for steroid treatment following a relapse (46 PwMS). Interestingly, their measure of self-efficacy was better at statistically predicting the health outcomes for the steroid group, with people who were the less disabled, younger, more likely to be in employment and more likely to have RRMS, than for the rehabilitation group. This might appear counter-intuitive in that it may have been expected that the rehabilitation group would have had more experience of MS and therefore exhibit higher levels of self-efficacy and control. However, in this case both groups had the same mean time since diagnosis of 12 years (Riazi et al. 2004, 63).

In an attempt to discover what factors might assist a positive psychological adjustment to MS, Dennison et al. (2009) undertook a systematic review of the 72 relevant studies in English from around the world, concluding with a useful working model of adjustment to MS. It began with a set of MS Critical Events such as symptoms, the diagnosis, relapses and progression that disrupted emotional equilibrium and current quality of life. It then went on to list two sets of factors that had been found empirically to be related to successful and to unsuccessful adjustment to the disease, listed in Table 6.2.

On coping strategies two relationships seemed particularly clear. First, and most destructively, the adoption of certain emotion-focussed strategies were strongly related to negative adjustment outcomes. These included wishful thinking (e.g., hoping a miracle might happen) and escape/avoidance (e.g., trying to forget the whole thing). By contrast, problem focussed coping and seeking social support (e.g., talking to someone to find out more about the situation) and the more adaptive emotion-focussed strategy of positive reappraisal (e.g., rediscovering what was important in life) tended to be related to more positive adjustment (Dennison et al. 2009, 4). But, what stands out in particular from this table is the number of mentions of social support for positive adjustment. Indeed, one of the conclusions of Dennison et al. (2009, 5) was that

Table 6.2 Factors aiding successful and unsuccessful adjustment to MS

SUCCESSFUL ADJUSTMENT
Helpful factors.
Cognitive Factors.
- **Coping by using positive re-appraisal**
- Perceived control over generic life situation
- Self-efficacy regarding MS management
- Optimism
- Hope
- Benefit finding
- Self-efficacy regarding generic life situation
- Acceptance of illness
- Spirituality

Behavioural Factors
- **Coping by using problem-focussed strategies or seeking social support**
- Health behaviours

Social/environmental factors
- **High perceived social support**
- Positive relationships/interactions with family/spouse

ADJUSTMENT DIFFICULTIES
Unhelpful factors
Cognitive Factors
- **High perceive stress**
- **Coping through wishful thinking or avoidance**
- **Uncertainty about illness**
- Appraisal of MS as threatening
- Dysfunctional cognitions/cognitive errors and biases
- Helplessness
- Perceives barriers to health behaviours
- Unhelpful illness/symptom representations
- Unhelpful beliefs about pain

Behavioural factors
- **Coping through avoidance**
- Unhelpful responses to symptoms (avoidance/resting)

Note: Bold text indicates strong evidence in that many studies have been conducted and literature consistently supports the role of this factor.

'having satisfactory social support and positive interactions with significant others are associated with better adjustment.' Unfortunately, little detail on specific aspects of positive social support was given other than generic scores. Was it the support from specific groups of people such as partners, family, friends, medical professionals or work colleagues that was particularly important in securing a favourable outcome to coping with MS? Or, could it be the type of support such as instrumental, physical, companionship that was crucial? Or, was it a combination of the two? Finally, could it be that the dominant force in these relationships was the negative one of lack of support; when no social support of any kind was available, or when social contacts were reproachful and negative, that poor psychological adjustment to MS took place? It is crucial that these issues are sorted out by clear in-depth research because they have profound implications for positive interventions to help PwMS adjust to their situation successfully and to assist them in developing their own support networks. Furthermore, could it be that the same psychological qualities that help PwMS adjust successfully to their illness in its early years (Dennison et al. 2010) need to persist through time as their illness progresses? Certainly there is evidence to support their importance relating to the adaptation of some older individuals with MS (Dilorenzo et al. 2008). And, do they apply also to the adjustment of their partners, family, friends and work colleagues? These are important areas of concern too not only for the creation of social contacts for PwMS but also for them to develop successful support networks as their disease progresses. Some research already exists on the relationships between PwMS and their partners, families, carers and medical professionals. Partners and family members are considered later in this chapter with the other two groups discussed in Chapter 7 on caring.

6.3.3 Fatigue

There can be no doubt from the literature reviewed so far that fatigue is a serious issue for many PwMS and for some may be one of the most debilitating in terms of affecting their normal daily lives. Indeed, Kingston (2010, 86) claims it can happen at any time without warning and regularly effectively shortens her day. More generally the problem of fatigue was emphasised by focus group work of the Research Network members of the MS Society of GB and Northern Ireland who prioritised this symptom above all others for attention. However, after a poor response from the research community for projects in this field an International Working Group on MS fatigue chaired by Sir Michael Peckham was established in 2005 that included research scientists, clinicians, therapists and PwMS. Their unpublished report succeeded in confirming the ambiguous and intangible nature of the fatigue issue complaining there were too many perspectives expressed to permit unanimity. And, Thompson et al. (2010, 1190) would go much further in this counsel of despair by suggesting that for MS: 'Fatigue is a complex symptom that defies definition and measurement.' What remains therefore is great uncertainty as to how MS fatigue should be understood, described and treated other than an acceptance that it exists and that it may have many different causes. Some of these causes may be related to the MS disease directly such as damage to the CNS and immune activity, while others may be related to secondary aspects of MS such as nocturia, muscle deconditioning, pain and stress. In addition, it needs to be understood to what extent MS fatigue is an extreme version of the lassitude and exhaustion people without MS may experience after concerted physical and cerebral activities?

Nevertheless, what this discussion of fatigue implies is that although the notion of any pure MS fatigue may be a theoretical chimera, from a practical perspective it strongly suggests that PwMS may have to confront simultaneously more than one form of fatigue and consider more than one form of therapy. It should also come as no surprise given the above that attempts at overcoming the fatigue PwMS experience have so far led to few positive results. For example, Lee et al. (2008) in a systematic review of the English literature of both pharmacological and psychosocial treatments up to and including 2006 made the following conclusions. For pharmacological therapies: 'There is no reason...for concluding that either any one drug (or drug interventions as a whole) lead to reliable clinical symptom decrease in fatigue in individuals with MS' (Lee et al. 2008, 83). For psychosocial therapies that included CBT, energy conservation strategies and pulsed electro-magnetic therapy, they concluded: 'no single treatment approach merits recommendation' (p.90). Finally, they concluded with the depressing comment that 'there is little evidence-based advice that can be offered to people with MS to help manage their fatigue' (p. 90).

Such desultory success in finding effective therapies was confirmed by a Cochrane systematic review of pharmacological interventions for fatigue in advanced disease that included MS (Peuckmann-Post et al. 2010) although it has to be emphasised that this was often due to a profound lack of any reliable evidence. Nevertheless, it has been suggested by Dennison and Moss-Morris (2010) that certain psychological interventions more often used for combating depression along with the development of coping skills may be of help in alleviating fatigue in MS. Indeed, these authors have presented a plausible cognitive-behavioural model of the fatigue symptom that describes how a patient's beliefs and thoughts could exacerbate this problem. Such thoughts would include feeling helpless, feeling they have no control over their illness, 'catastrophizing' about their symptoms and being embarrassed about their symptoms. This has led to the testing of psychological interventions such as CBT and the promotion of helpful thinking styles in MS fatigue for which there has already been one controlled trial and a web-based intervention that have shown modest positive results (Dennison and Moss-Morris 2010).

6.4 Disability, health status and quality of life

The idea of health-related quality of life has been accepted enthusiastically into MS research practice in the recent past such that at one time the production of new measurement instruments and their testing reached almost industrial production-line proportions. For example, at the end of the 1990s, Rothwell (1998, 933) observed that a hundred or so papers linking quality of life to MS had been noted by MEDLINE between 1966 and 1998, 80 per cent of which had been published since 1991. Nearly 5 years later, Nortvedt and Riise (2003) were able to classify 83 quality of life studies in MS into 3 different groups: evaluating questionnaires and clinical scales, quality of life comparisons between different groups of PwMS and outcome measures as prognostic factors. And the following year, Gruenewald and colleagues (2004) published an extensive review of quality of life measures for PwMS and their carers printed in English that encompassed 16 generic measures and 19 disease-specific ones. Specifically, for PwMS they reviewed 16 studies that used focus groups and interviews to collect their evidence and 51 studies that used questionnaires (Gruenewald et al. 2004, 697). They also identified from this research evidence a comprehensive list of 15 different quality of life domains as shown in Table 6.3, where the emphasis seemed to be more on what PwMS could not do rather than what they actually could do.

Table 6.3 Domains of care for people with MS as identified by Gruenewald et al. (2004)

Mood/mental health
Role limitations
Family life
Impaired social function
Intimacy
MS symptoms
Disease course
Physical function
Control/autonomy
Support from others
Loss of dignity
Desire to remain at home
Accommodation/acceptance
Meaningful daytime activity/leisure
Unmet needs/access to care

Source: Gruenewald et al. (2004, 698).

For this discussion two different types of health-related quality of life assessment are of importance, but see Zajicek et al. (2007, 44–65) for the ones most commonly used in practice. The first type includes those of a generic nature such as the EQ-5D that allow the difficulties of living with MS to be compared formally with other medical conditions. Thus, some form of comparative context can be given to living with MS. In addition, such measures have been used to compare the quality of life of PwMS with different demographic, life-style and disease characteristics. The second important group of quality of life measure used in MS research has been disease specific ones such as the MSIS-29 and the LMSQoLS. Unfortunately, this did not result in the listing, or even the ranking, of the elements of the lives of PwMS that they themselves believed to be important in defining their quality of life. What occurred was the listing of the principal problems PwMS faced in their lives with no mention of the elements that gave them most pleasure and contentment; an emphasis on incapacity not capacity. Thus, these measures are biased towards the inadequacies and unworthiness of PwMS, not their strengths and by no means offer a balanced assessment of their quality of life; they are not so much measures of well-being as measures of 'bad-being'.[2]

Nevertheless, one of the defining characteristics of much of this quality of life research was the substantial effort and care expended on the development of its constructs. For example, the MSIS-29 development methodology had three distinct stages. First, a 129-item questionnaire was generated on the main issues and concerns PwMS faced in their lives from 30 patient interviews, expert opinion and literature review. Second, this was then sent for assessment to 1,530 randomly selected members of the MS Society of Great Britain and Northern Ireland. After screening for redundant items and item-grouping using factor analysis, the list was eventually reduced to 29 items (Table 6.4). And, third, the psychometric properties of this scale (i.e., data quality, scaling assumptions, acceptability, reliability and validity) were evaluated in a further independent random sample survey of 1,250 members of the MS Society (Hobart et al. 2001, 963). The original MSIS-29 questionnaire asked a respondent to assess each statement on a 5-point scale from 1 representing 'not at all', 2 'a little', 3 'moderately', 4 'quite a bit' and 5 'extremely'. After a detailed Rasch analysis, this scale was altered to 4 points in which 1 represented 'not at all', 2 'a little', 3 'moderately' and 4 'extremely' to produce an MSIS-29 version 2 (MSIS-29v2) (Hobart and Cano 2009, 63–96 and 173–4).[3]

The LMSQoLS was also developed through an extensive three-stage process. First, from 2 focus group sessions involving 30 PwMS a list of

Table 6.4 The MS Impact Scale (MSIS-29)

In the past two weeks how much has your MS limited your ability to:
1. Do physically demanding tasks?
2. Grip things tightly (e.g., turning on taps)?
3. Carry things?

In the past two weeks how much have you been bothered by
4. Problems with your balance?
5. Difficulties moving about indoors?
6. Being clumsy?
7. Stiffness?
8. Heavy arms and/or legs?
9. Tremor of your arms or legs?
10. Spasms in your limbs?
11. Your body not doing what you want it to do?
12. Having to depend on others to do things for you?
13. Limitations in your social and leisure activities at home?
14. Being stuck at home more than you would like to be?
15. Difficulties using your hands in everyday tasks?
16. Having to cut down the amount of time you spent on work or other daily activities?
17. Problems using transport (e.g., car, bus, train, taxi, etc.)?
18. Taking longer to do things?
19. Difficulties doing things spontaneously (e.g., going out on the spur of the moment)?
20. Needing to go to the toilet urgently?
21. Feeling unwell?
22. Problems sleeping?
23. Feeling mentally fatigued?
24. Worries related to your MS?
25. Feeling anxious or tense?
26. Feeling irritable, impatient or short tempered?
27. Problems concentrating?
28. Lack of confidence?
29. Feeling depressed?

Source: Hobart et al. (2001).

25 areas of concern was developed (Table 6.5). Second, to test different aspects of the construct further including its psychometrics it was sent to three different random samples of PwMS who lived outside the Leeds study area. Finally, a reduced 16-item scale was evaluated through a random sample of 199 PwMS from within the Leeds population prevalence register. From these final results, it was decided that the overall construct could be accurately and efficiently represented by just eight elements shown in bold in Table 6.5, what they (Ford et al. 2001b, 256) believed to be 'those aspects of the disease that impact most on the

Table 6.5 Original areas of importance identified by the LMSQoLS

1. I have joined in family activities
2. **My health has affected my relationships with my family**
3. We have taken family holidays
4. I have contributed to the family finances
5. I have enjoyed the same hobbies and interests
6. I have taken part in sports or other outdoor activities
7. I have been out with friends
8. **I have spent evenings out with my partner**
9. I have looked after the house (cleaning/repair)
10. My health causes problems with my job
11. I feel secure in my present job
12. **I feel lonely**
13. **I feel good about my appearance**
14. I am interested in sex
15. **I worry about my health**
16. **I worry about other peoples' attitudes towards me**
17. **I feel tired**
18. **I have as much energy as usual**
19. **I feel happy about the future**
20. I can make plans for the future
21. I can walk without help
22. I can control my bladder
23. I am sexually active
24. My doctors have helped me understand my illness
25. I have learned about my illness from other sources

Source: Ford et al. (2001b, 252).

well-being of the person with multiple sclerosis.' This is a very different set of criteria from the MSIS-29 scale with only three elements referring directly to health, two of which effectively relate to the same symptom of fatigue in terms of energy and tiredness. But, the objective of the LMSQoLS was never comprehensively to describe the MS experience, but the complete opposite of brevity and may be thought of as encapsulating the extent of adjustment of a person to their MS.

Each of the eight items of the LMSQoL was to be assessed on a scale of 0 to 3 where '0' represents 'very much', 1 'quite a lot', 2 'a little' and 3 'not at all', giving the construct a range from 0 to 24 with higher values indicating a better quality of life.

Initial findings from the above research in Leeds in which the median LMSQoL was 14.00 demonstrated statistically significant differences in the LMSQoL between early RRMS and progressive forms of MS, in which early was defined as below the median disease duration of 12 years. However, after this time no significant difference was to be found between the different disease types. This was interpreted as showing a separation of quality of life from disability (Ford et al. 2001b, 255).

This lack of close association between disability and subjective quality of life was explored further by Ford et al. (2001a). They began by making clear the major differences in disability between those with RRMS and benign MS on the one hand and those with progressive forms of the disease on the other hand. To take just one example of the comparison, 95.7 per cent of the latter group reported some difficulty walking outside of their home, whereas only 41.6 per cent of the relapsing group reported such a problem (Ford et al. 2001a, 518). However, there was no significant difference in the LMSQoL between these two groups. Ford and her colleagues suggested the reasons for this lack of congruence between disability and quality of life were complex that related to both health status and demographic factors. For example, the stage of a person's MS career appeared to have a strong impact with those near to diagnosis recording particularly poor quality of life results in contrast to those with a longer disease duration who tended to report relatively favourable results; a finding that may suggest a 'learning to live with it' phenomenon. Indeed, in terms of the variables that were the most useful predictors of quality of life in a step-wise multiple regression analysis, older age and longer disease duration were associated with a more positive quality of life along with absence of cognitive and swallowing difficulties, higher physical functioning and using a wheelchair. Curiously perhaps, being 'in work' and having a current sexual partner did not score well (Ford et al. 2001a, 520).

Interestingly, in a much later project with a small sample of only 90 members of the Northern Ireland branch of the MS Society who took part in a clinical study of the use of TENS (transcutaneous electrical nerve stimulation) for the treatment of lower back pain (Nicholl et al. 2005), only modest differences in the LMSQoL measure were observed between three different disease states and three different ambulation abilities (Table 6.6). In this case the differences between the different disease types and walking states were not statistically significant; unsurprising given the small number of cases that must have been involved. But, the scores do trend in the expected direction such that being able to walk scored higher than using a wheelchair and RRMS higher than PPMS. What is unexpected in these results though must be the range of scores in each of the six categories, from the relatively high to the relatively low that must in a modest way give support to the idea that quality of life for PwMS can be independent of both level of disability and type of MS. In other words, it is possible for a good quality of life to

Table 6.6 LMSQoL scores by disease state and ambulation status

	Mean LMSQoL*	LMSQoL* range
Disease state:		
RRMS	13.7	7.0–22.0
SPMS	11.7	4.0–23.0
PPMS	11.6	3.0–19.0
Ambulation status:		
Walking independently	12.9	6.0–23.0
Walking with an aid	12.3	3.0–22.0
Wheelchair use	10.9	4.0–17.0

Source: Nicholl et al. (2005, 709).

* Possible range from 0.0 to 24.0 in which the higher the score the better the level of wellbeing.

be achieved by many if not all PwMS. Sadly the opposite of this may also be true too. But, why there should be such a difference between these different states of disability and disease type has yet to be explored.

The LMSQoL has been used to demonstrate an increase in quality of life over a 3-year period for 56 people taking a range of DMDs in the Leeds area that was independent of baseline age, disease duration, disability or number of prior relapses (Lily et al. 2006). In this case it was those with the worst self-assessed quality of life at the start of their treatment phase that tended to record the most favourable increase in subjective quality of life. However, there was no control group involved in this study to eliminate placebo effects.

These measures of health-related quality of life take into account a set of attributes for a particular person at a particular point in time or over a short period of time. For example, the MSIS-29 scale asks for impacts over the last two weeks and the LMSQoLS over the preceding month. But, rapid change in health and functionality over very short periods from one hour to the next, and most certainly from one day to the next are characteristic of MS too. To capture these sorts of events an MS Impact Diary was developed by Greenhaigh et al. (2004) with an earlier version used in a cost and quality of life appraisal of the use of interferon β by Parkin et al. (2000, 145). However, its use has been questioned by Beaumont (2004) on the possible adverse psychological impacts on respondents being reminded on a daily basis of the problems they and their families face because of MS.

One of the curious manifestations of this type of research, however, must be the degree to which the medical research community has accepted such 'social science' constructs into their own work. They seem not to have baulked with any strength at the use of perhaps less-rigorous forms of measurement of such terms as quality of life and wellbeing. Perhaps they have at last begun to accept that their own methods and measurement scales, especially in neurology, can also be 'woolly' and vague. As the neurologist Rothwell (1998, 433) observed to 'put our faith in our own measurements, or those of our machines, than in the apparently subjective assessment made by our patients... is not only arrogant, it is also deluded.' However, much of this early research has been understandably absorbed in defining and testing measures of quality of life epitomised by the seminal work of Hobart and Cano (2009) rather than actually describing the quality of the lives of PwMS. Thus, the evidence in this area for the PwMS is surprisingly thin. Neurologists may also have reluctantly begun to realise that health is but one component of a measure of quality of life and that their expertise is only relevant to part of the answer to a contented life. And, this must be especially so for an illness such as MS that the medical world cannot yet cure or with any certainty stop progressing and one in which observable damage to the CNS seems not to correlate well to bodily disability and malfunction. The unwary cynic at this point might argue that measures of quality of life are becoming acceptable to the medical community because they will almost certainly show a positive increase with the application of any new medical procedure as a result of the placebo effect if nothing else. Defining a matching control group may, of course, help to obviate such a problem. However, at least in terms of the pioneering crop of DMDs for MS the initial impact for many patients was a series of uncomfortable 'flu-like' side effects. This was not the context in which a positive quality of life measure could be expected. But, in the longer term, after these initial symptoms had subsided, a positive increase in quality of life may take place irrespective of any clinical impact of the DMD. Thus, research on the quality of life impacts of MS medications and its interpretation must be viewed as challenging.

When completing the original MSIS-29 questionnaire each element was scored from 1 to 5, that is, from 'not at all' to 'extremely', and then summed to produce a grand total. For the scale as a whole or for the physical (20) or psychological (9) groups separately these results can be presented in a range from '0' to '100', where the former would indicate the highest possible health-related quality of life and the latter the worst. For the sample of members of the MS Society undertaken by Hobart et al. (2001), the results for specific subgroups suggested the anticipated results that for both the physical and psychological groupings those in employment had a better quality of life than those who retired because of their MS (Table 6.7). Similarly, those who had no mobility problems had a better quality of life than those confined to bed, with these two groups recording both the worst and best scores in their analysis. Those who were better educated also tended to record relatively favourable quality of life scores. However, the difference between the sexes was not so clear cut. While admittedly the differences between these two groups were small, males tended to record a poorer quality of life on the physical scale and women a poorer result psychologically. The reasons for such findings were not forthcoming. Differences in quality of life using the MSIS-29 were also observed between rehabilitation and steroid treatment groups at the NHNN in London with not unexpectedly the latter reporting the more favourable results. This was because although the two groups had very similar average ages of 44.7 years for the rehabilitation group and 42.6 years for the steroid group, far more of the latter had a relapsing remitting form of MS at 80.4 per cent (i.e., they were in a relatively early stage of their MS) and therefore a greater propensity for employment, at 63 per cent, compared to the rehabilitation group with only 23.3 per cent having RRMS and 28 per cent in employment. Thus, the steroid group reported an MSIS-29 score of 52.1 for the physical component of the index and 33.5 for the psychological element

Table 6.7 Average group scores for the physical and psychological components of the MSIS-29

Group	Number	Physical	Psychological
Employment:			
Employed	107	30.6	31.1
Retired due to MS	390	64.3	49.9
Mobility:			
No problems	61	17.5	27.7
Confined to bed	70	82.6	51.4
Gender:			
Female	489	55.0	46.1
Male	197	58.1	43.5
Degree/prof' qualification:			
Yes	183	53.2	41.6
No	411	56.7	46.8
Range:			
Max' score		100 – poor quality of life	100 – poor quality of life
Min' score		0	0

Source: Hobart et al. (2001, 969).

compared to the rehabilitation group where the results were higher and therefore worse at 67.7 and 45.6 respectively (Riazi et al. 2004, 63).

One of the regularly used generic health-related quality of life measures in MS research has been the European Quality of Life Scale, EuroQoL or EQ-5D. This consists of five domains: mobility, self-care, usual activities, pain/discomfort, anxiety/depression. For each domain a respondent is asked to rate their experience on a scale of 1 to 3, where 1 is no problem, 2 some problem and 3 major problems. Thus, each individual may be represented by a 5-digit code made up of 5 numbers from 1 to 3, of which there are 243 possibilities. For example, 11223 would mean the individual had no problems walking about, no problems with self-care, some problems with performing usual activities, some pain and discomfort and severe anxiety or depression.

However, to be a useful descriptive device such codes need to be able to be transcribed into a single index value, or 'utility' score as it is often rather disparagingly called (Orme et al. 2007). This was achieved in a much earlier study by Dolan et al. (1995) in which the results of a representative survey of 3,395 non-institutionalised people in England, Wales and Scotland in 1993 were asked to state how long they would be willing to spend in full health to make it equivalent to one year spent in any of a range of given alternative health states. Such a time trade-off analysis allowed a utility value to be calculated for each of the possible health states in which 1 = full health and 0 = death, but in which negative values were also possible indicating health states that were regarded as worse than death. However, and notwithstanding theological life after death, the experiential possibility of negative values for the EQ-5D when experience ends with death may cause some problems of comprehension even if permitted theoretically.

The McCrone et al. (2008) investigation on MS health costs and quality of life not only provided mean EQ-5D scores for specific groups of PwMS it also provided response frequencies in its five separate health domains. From this evidence it would appear that members of the MS Society with MS (MwMS) performed best in self-care where 41.1 per cent had no problems and worst in 'usual activities' in which 67.1 per cent had some problems and 23.8 per cent had major problems (McCrone et al. 2008, 851). It should be noted, however, that this domain is a very broad category indeed that includes 'work, study, housework, family and leisure activities' (Dolan et al. 1995, 2) and is essentially about what people do with their lives. It must be a domain therefore in which getting a poor score is relatively easy. This investigation also suggests that except in self-care most MwMS had some problems in all 5 quality of life domains, especially in mobility where 11.6 per cent had severe mobility difficulties and only 8.5 per cent claimed they had no problems, a much lower proportion than would have been expected from earlier EDSS evidence.

The McCrone et al. (2008) research provided some disquieting evidence too on the way in which MwMS viewed their affliction in that 339, or 17.6 per cent, of them regarded their quality of life as worse than death. Indeed, 9 individuals (0.5%) recorded the lowest EQ-5D score possible in this research of –0.59. At the other extreme 49 people (2.5%) recorded the best possible score of 1.00 indicating no problems at all in all 5 domains. It is important to note, however, that this frequency distribution of EQ-5D scores is skewed towards the lower end of the scale because of a large number of relatively low scores with a median of 0.52 and a mean of 0.41 (McCrone et al. 2008, 851). This must raise concerns about the relevance of this measure of quality of life to the MS case and perhaps more importantly counsel prudence when comparing EQ-5D scores for MS with other conditions.

When comparing health-related quality of life with the demographic and functional ability of MwMS, it was discovered that EQ-5D tended to be higher for the employed, those who had retired because of age not disability and as the number of children aged under 18 years of age increased. By contrast, it tended to be lower for the unemployed, for those who were divorced, separated or widowed and for those with a progressive form of MS. And, in terms of relationships across all the MwMS, quality of life was strongly associated inversely with disability, duration of illness and disease costs (McCrone 2008, 855). It is also worth observing that the research on costs and quality of life in patients with MS in three neurological centres in England (Leeds, Birmingham and Newcastle-upon-Tyne,) by Kobelt et al. (2000, 27) demonstrated an inverse relationship between quality of life and disability too. Here, for the 597 patients involved mean EQ-5D increased from 0.277 for those patients with an EDSS level of more than 6.0 to 0.574 for those with EDSS 3.5 to 6.0 and to 0.698 for the least disabled cohort of all with an EDSS of 3.0 or less.

The survey of MS Trust members by Orme et al. (2007) produced a mean EQ-5D score of 0.49, higher than the McCrone (2008) analysis, along with additional evidence of very poor EQ-5D scores for people with serious disability. Using the pre-existing weights given from the earlier research from York University, they suggested that living with the most severe EDSS states 8 and 9 was worse than death; that is a negative EQ-5D score. What is more, a strong inverse correlation between disability and this measure of quality of life was observed. However, it must be emphasised that the authors (Orme et al. 2007, 59) admit to bias entering the results at the higher end of the EDSS distribution, 8 to 8.5, because of the involvement of carers in completing the questionnaire who tend to report significantly worse utilities than the people with MS to whom they provide care.

One of the potential advantages of using a generic measure of health-related quality of life such as the EQ-5D is that it facilitates direct comparisons with different diseases and conditions including a control sample of people who have no illness. In the McCrone et al. (2008, 856) research a population norm for the EQ-5D in the UK of 0.86 is suggested, much higher than the averages so far noted for MS. It is also true that MS has tended to report lower EQ-5D scores than a number of other serious chronic conditions. For example, Brazier et al. (2004) recorded mean (and median) EQ-5D scores for seven different conditions and populations: Chronic Obstructive Airways disease 0.54 (0.62), Osteoarthritis 0.44 (0.59), Irritable Bowel syndrome 0.66 (0.73), lower back pain 0.64 (0.69), leg ulcers 0.55 (0.62), post-menopausal women 0.73 (0.80) and elderly people 0.61 (0.69). This is indeed depressing news for PwMS because all these values were higher than the mean and median values for MS reported earlier. Does this suggest that PwMS have a lower health-related quality of life than people with many other chronic diseases? The evidence presented by Orme and colleagues (2007, 59) on the recent EQ-5D results for 20 other conditions all of which except Rheumatoid Arthritis were higher than MS would suggest this was so.

Furthermore, similar comparative research from other countries also supported relatively low subjective quality of life assessments for MS. For example, in Cleveland Ohio in the early 1990s, Rudick et al. (1992) demonstrated for admittedly relatively small numbers of subjects that people with MS had a lower quality of life than people with either Inflammatory Bowel disease or Rheumatoid Arthritis and with evidence from a number of sites across the US, Hermann et al. (1996) demonstrated that PwMS had a lower quality of life in physical and emotional dimensions but not in terms of pain compared to individuals with Epilepsy and Diabetes. What is more, in a secondary analysis of a multidimensional measure of health-related quality of life from existing data sets in the Netherlands, 1993–6, that included more than 15,000 patients Sprangers et al. (2000) observed the most favourable outcomes were to be found in urogenital conditions, hearing impairments, psychiatric disorders and dermatological conditions. Meanwhile conditions with an intermediate impact included cardiovascular conditions, cancer, endocrinologic conditions, visual impairments and chronic respiratory diseases, whereas the most adverse consequences were found to occur in gastrointestinal conditions, cerebrovascular/neurologic conditions (including MS), renal disease and musculoskeletal conditions. Once again the impact of having MS appeared to be unrelentingly bleak. Furthermore, this view would appear to be a pan-European one because in comparative research across France, Germany, Italy, Spain and the UK, using admittedly very small sample sizes, similar disease EQ-5D values were discovered by Karampampa et al. (2012, 12).

Nevertheless, there are three possible ways this apparently bitter pill may be sweetened, at least as far as the British evidence is concerned. First of all it must be asked whether in these comparisons like was being compared with like? The MS figures in the McCrone et al. (2008) came from a survey of members of the UK MS Society and were therefore likely to be older and more disabled than the wider MS community, both of which would tend to depress the EQ-5D figure. A similar concern would apply to the evidence from the research of Orme et al. (2007) too because it came from a sample of members of the MS Trust. But, much more serious was that this latter sample was self-selected and therefore likely to be biased towards the educated aggrieved. A lower EQ-5D score than for all PwMS should therefore have been expected from this cohort.

The second point of mitigation concerns the stability of estimates of quality of life over time. Should one expect social tariffs for disease states estimated in the early to mid-1990s to have equivalent relevance in the 2010s? Even in MS as individuals become more familiar with their disease and the ways of ameliorating its impacts the illness perhaps may be becoming less frightening. And, this may be true of society too with respect to many conditions including cancer and disability generally. But, whether this is quite so true for neurological illnesses may be more of a moot point. Nevertheless, the concern must remain that quality of life estimates in the mid-1990s could be poorer than for equivalent states in the 2010s.

The final point of concern regarding an EQ-5D measure for PwMS must be that it fails to take account of impacts that are of direct importance to PwMS such as fatigue (see Hemmett et al. 2004) that have no place in its calculation. In addition, how should the impact of MS on the family of a person with the illness be taken into account? It may be therefore that a range of different health states particular to MS need to be researched to estimate a new type of disease-specific EQ-5D for MS? Whether this would increase the score for MS though may be open to doubt.

McDonnell and Hawkins (2001) took their analysis of the disabled of north Northern Ireland a step further by calculating the Incapacity Status

Scale (ISS) and the Environmental Status Scale (ESS) for 248 PwMS out of the 259 for whom they already had an EDSS score. They were concerned that at that time the enthusiasm for the new DMDs that were only of use for the relatively recently diagnosed might lead to people with more established disease being overlooked and to emphasise their plight they needed to demonstrate just how impaired they were. Their analysis does not make for happy reading demonstrating that the majority of PwMS in north Northern Ireland at that time were significantly troubled by their illness. Three quarters of their patients were unable to climb a flight of stairs without assistance, 50 per cent were unable to walk 50 yards without help, 48 per cent needed help with toilet, bed or chair transfers and two thirds needed help with bathing (McDonnell and Hawkins 2001, 112-3). In fact only 29 per cent were fully independent with activities of daily living (McDonnell and Hawkins 2001, 114). In terms of the direct symptoms, 73 per cent had bladder problems, 46 per cent abnormal bowel functions and the overwhelming majority, 84 per cent, were affected to a lesser or greater degree by fatigue. Indeed, one third of patients required significant help with personal care and a similar proportion had to move home or become institutionalised because of their MS. It perhaps should not be unexpected to discover therefore that 30 per cent of PwMS in this part of Northern Ireland were unable to work and that 79 per cent were in receipt of some form of external financial support, while it might be refreshingly surprising to note that as many as a quarter were in full time employment (McDonnell and Hawkins 2001, 114).

The evidence reviewed so far clearly indicates that MS directly affects bodily functioning and the activities of daily living people with the illness can undertake independently. But, how did this change the lives of PwMS? Did it stop them carrying out the activities they wished to do, or did it just make them more difficult to achieve? Unfortunately, there is very little longitudinal evidence on the way in which MS changes the lives of PwMS in terms of what they actually do with their time. Conceptually Green and colleagues (2007) have attempted to capture such change by the phrase 'biographical disruption'; a short-hand for the alteration in life's trajectory caused by a chronic illness such as MS. Although originally intended by Bury (1982) to tackle the ways in which chronic illness could affect a person's identity and 'taken for granted' worlds of experience and expectation, it is relatively easy to envision the idea being stretched to include more structural elements of a person's life such as employment, income and relationships. Furthermore, Green et al. (2007) attempted to operationalise the concept for the UK through a large survey of MwMS. Now, although there were some serious methodological issues with this research already discussed in Chapter 3, if it is interpreted with caution, it may offer some useful evidence on the self-reported impact of MS on people with the illness and on their households. This can be achieved by first presenting evidence on how MS has affected the functioning of PwMS and second through a comparison of selected social and economic characteristics of MwMS with their equivalents from the 2001/2 British General Household Survey (GHS). It is important to note this was not a longitudinal study of the way in which MS changed the behaviour of an individual and their family over time, but a cross-sectional comparison at a particular point in time. It therefore told us nothing about how MS changed what people did with their lives.

For the Green et al. (2007) sample of MwMS living in GB, it was clear that MS had a major impact on their lives and on the lives of other members of their households. In terms of functional disability, use of the legs seemed to dominate with 75.1 per cent having problems walking for more than 10 minutes and 63.6 per cent having difficulty climbing stairs. Of course, the degree of difficulty is not shown in these figures, but at the very least MS was causing some serious irritation to most of the respondents to this survey and in some cases its effects were much more serious. For example, in only 13.3 per cent of the 900 cases was MS deemed to have no effect on their lives, whereas 8.7 per cent of respondents needed someone to look after them all the time with a further 9.1 per cent needing assistance if they wanted to do anything. Clearly almost 20 per cent of this sample was in serious physical difficulty because of their MS. And, it is likely this proportion could have been higher because the most seriously disabled PwMS may not have been able physically or cognitively to answer the questionnaire.

These difficulties led to impacts, and we must assume for the most part negative ones, on the lives of PwMS in the realms of social life in 79.9 per cent of cases, standard of living (55.9%), employment (76.2%) and relationships (46.0%) and in 27 per cent of cases on the employment status of others in their households too (Green et al. 2007, 529). What this latter observation exactly means is unclear but it could include a partner cutting back on their hours of work, or even giving up work altogether, to care for a loved one with MS.

When the sample of MwMS were compared with people in the GHS, it was found that a higher proportion of both men and women with MS were owner occupiers, less likely to be in the lowest annual income categories, less likely to be in paid employment, more likely to be in receipt of state financial benefits, have a lower proportion living in single-person households, and for women with MS more likely to be divorced (Green et al. 2007, 529).

On employment issues specifically, Green et al. (2007) made a number of important observations not only from their empirical evidence but also from the accompanying qualitative remarks by their survey respondents. The first of these observations must be that the chances of unemployment were highly positively correlated with disability. This supports the view that a large number of PwMS lose their jobs or retire early because of the disability caused directly by their illness that could include mobility problems with getting to work and coping with the work environment, cognitive impairment, fatigue and visual difficulties. One such individual was Meg Kingston (2010, 127) who exclaimed in her autobiography: 'I never made the decision to stop working, my body and my MonSter made it for me'. However, Green et al. (2007, 533) go on to make the following telling observation: 'people with MS whose disability is less severe and who are able to live without assistance are still significantly less likely to be in employment compared to the general population'. The reasons for such a depressing state of affairs were not considered. Could it be that MS provided a suitable reason for firing someone, not employing them in the first place, or a reason to leave or retire early for those already in employment with MS? Given the importance of employment not only to financial wellbeing but also to psychological wellbeing, this area demands further research, understanding and policy prescription.

Green et al. (2007, 533) continued their analysis by attempting to match GHS and MS cases through a propensity grouping technique in which scores were derived via logit regression. Given the problems with the representativeness of this sample of PwMS stemming from the way in which the newly diagnosed, young and minimally disabled groups were included, understanding what exactly may be going on in this elegant analysis becomes challenging. Nevertheless, even though this research may flatter to deceive it does make potentially two further important points regarding income and marital status. On income Green and colleagues (2007) observed the impact of MS was heavily associated with disability level for both men and women. While there was no significant difference between MwMS who were able to live independently and members of the British public across both genders, this was not the case for those with MS who needed assistance. Here the differences in income between the significantly disabled with MS and people generally were profound. On marital status Green et al. (2007, 533) observed that differences between the MS and GHS groups were observed for women in the initial analysis, but that 'this difference becomes non-significant when demographic variables are controlled for in the matched analysis'. Thus, people with MS 'whether dependent on others or able to live independently, are no more likely to be divorced than people in the general population. Any apparent increase in divorce rates for MS populations...would appear to be attributable to confounding factors such as age'. However, it is not explained how age may confound this relationship and in what direction. Of course, this does not mean MS has no impact on marital relationships. Its impact is likely to be serious especially as disability and sexual dysfunction both increase along with potential financial difficulties. Some substantial readjustments are almost inevitable. But, it does not mean that marital relationships will inevitably fail.

This analysis was extended both quantitatively and qualitatively by Green and Todd (2008). For the former they were able to show statistically how as disability increased so too did the impact of MS on their lives differentially in the eight domains of household composition, household modification, children, own employment, employment of others, standard of living, intimate relationships and social life. For example, for those with minimal disability MS had very little impact on household composition and household modifications with only 6.7 per cent and 5.9 per cent respectively reporting such effects. Yet in employment and social life terms for the minimally disabled 56.7 per cent and 41.4 per cent respectively noted an impact. By the time major disability had set in substantial changes occurred across most domains of life with now impacts on employment and social life being reported by 91.9 per cent and 93.8 per cent respectively, yet still only 16.3 per cent noted an impact on household composition (Green and Todd 2008, 166); a result that may suggest that one of the few elements of relative stability in the life of a person with MS may be the family unit to which they belong.

From the written comments made on their respondents' questionnaire replies, Green and Todd (2008) were able to characterise the impact of MS on the lives of people as 'restricting choices' and 'limiting independence', suggesting that in the early phases of the illness the impacts were borne mainly by the individual with MS but, as the illness developed with increasing disability its reach stretched across more members and activities of the household and family to which the person with MS belonged. In particular, Green and Todd (2008, 170) argued that MS had a powerful impact on 'the interaction with others in public places outside the household' especially on social and leisure activities.

6.5 Quality of life and happiness

Quality of life is about more than levels of personal disability and functionality, it is much more about being able to participate in a range of chosen activities, varying from person to person, that can ultimately lead to personal happiness and contentment. Indeed, the detailed interview research of Somerset et al. (2002) of admittedly only 16 purposely sampled PwMS came to the conclusion that achieving an acceptable quality of life was dependent first on being reasonably happy and second on being as socially active as desired, irrespective of disability level. It was further admitted that these qualities were influenced by two broad factors. The first factor over which they probably had very little control was the trajectory of their illness, while the second over which they wished as much control or autonomy as possible, was what they did in their life including the care they received. These observations emphasise three important points in any quality of life analysis. First, that quality of life, happiness and contentment are relative, subjective qualities that individuals may achieve in many different ways and under many different sets of circumstances. Second that improving a person's sense of being in charge of their own destiny is a fundamental element of this issue and, third that while poor health may be an important constraint on achieving an acceptable quality of life it does not preclude it.

Such a view on the quality of life may be usefully developed through the work of Smith (1977) on a welfare approach to human geography that advocated an eclectic normative view on this concept to provide people with the basic necessities of life and allowed them to become involved in as broad a spectrum of activities as possible; that is taking as full and as active a part as they wished in the society to which they belonged. This should involve them being able to secure the following elements:

1. An income, usually in terms of having a job, being self-employed or receiving state financial benefits. For many disabled people, depending on the state and charitable organisations for their income may replace having a job.
2. Shelter or housing, having somewhere to live. This can be extremely challenging for some disabled people especially for those using wheelchairs.
3. Health and a good diet. Having access to appropriate physical and mental health services if and when required. This is explored in the next chapter on caring for PwMS.

4. Education, at an appropriate level throughout life.
5. Transport, being mobile. This, of course, is a very significant issue for the physically disabled.
6. Recreation, being able to participate in normal leisure past-times and have holidays.
7. Justice; access to the legal system if required; free from crime and threats to social disorder.
8. Participation in society's democratic institutions. This is not just about being able to vote but also about being able to hold public office. Disabled people should not be excluded from society's decision-making institutions.
9. Social belonging, that is free from alienation, either from a family, community or from a wider society; an individual must have the opportunity to feel they belong to a larger group of people.

Many of the all-too-common consequences of having MS discussed above and especially physical disability may limit a person's ability to take part in some of the elements on this list; that is they act as constraints on a person's ability to participate fully in the society to which they belong. Furthermore, many of the elements on the above list are inter-related. Thus, a person with a low income (perhaps unemployed) may have limited access to good housing, live in an area with high rates of crime and family disintegration, have a poor diet, limited opportunities for recreation and as a result be in poor health. Indeed, they could be so significantly excluded from normal societal behaviour that they must be regarded as being in relative poverty, socially excluded or multiply deprived. This may well depict an extreme case but, it has been clearly shown by Ackroyd (2003) and the Strategy Unit (2005) that disabled people generally in the UK at least and most probably elsewhere too tend to have relatively poor housing, employment, health and education prospects; their disablement becoming a direct route into social exclusion. Although there is no specific evidence on this issue for PwMS, it is not unreasonable to suspect this may also be true for some of them too, especially when they begin to suffer many of the attendant depressing symptoms of their condition. Worse, it is possible that over time such individuals may become so seriously ruptured from normal social behaviour they could struggle to find a way back.

Following the WHO's quality of life prescription a set of international MS experts under the aegis of the Multiple Sclerosis International Federation (MSIF) attempted to define a set of principles to promote the wellbeing of PwMS, that is a move from a generic measure to a disease specific one (MSIF undated). The former WHO formula included the five domains of physical health, psychological health, level of independence, social relations and the environment (very broadly defined), while the MSIF group postulated ten principles they believed that focussed on the following issues most commonly faced by PwMS.

1. Independence and empowerment.
2. Medical care.
3. Continuing (long-term or social) care.
4. Health promotion and disease prevention.
5. Support for family members.
6. Transportation.
7. Employment and volunteer activities.
8. Disability benefits and cash assistance.
9. Education.
10. Housing and accessibility of buildings in the community.

As one might have expected for a disease-specific construct three of these principles, 2 to 4 inclusive, were concerned with medical matters. However, the other seven were not, emphasising once more that a good quality of life with MS is concerned with much more than just health. Indeed, what is remarkable is the degree to which these principles promote the social aspects of a person's life such as support for family members (principle 5), education (9), employment and volunteering (7), access to the community (10) and especially the first principle of independence and empowerment that emphasises participation in a full range of community activities. It is also interesting to note how closely these principles match the quality of life construct of Smith (1977) proposed 30 years earlier and now how closely they match the UK government's thinking on the definition of wellbeing. For example, in 2006 the Whitehall Wellbeing Working Group agreed the following statement of common understanding on wellbeing for policy makers:

Wellbeing is a positive social and mental state; it is not just the absence of pain, discomfort and incapacity. It arises not only from the action of individuals, but from a host of collective goods and relationships with other people. It requires that basic needs are met, that individuals have a sense of purpose, and that they feel able to achieve important personal goals and participate in society. It is enhanced by conditions that include supportive personal relationships, involvement in empowered communities, good health, financial security, rewarding employment and a healthy and attractive environment. (Skelton 2009, 6)

It may be reasonable to assume that in theory the above list of possible quality of life components could be used to describe a person with a high standard of wellbeing such as having a nicely appointed home in a beautiful area with a loving family, a rewarding job and a set of reliable friends, and by inference the opposite of low wellbeing. It does not help though to define which elements of this list stand the greatest chance of making a person happy or happiest. Is it a good family life, a respected job, high income, good friends, good health or something else? This issue has been investigated recently using evidence from the British Household Panel Survey for the years from 1992 to 1995. In these exercises respondents were asked questions about the major events in their lives and their families over the previous 12 months and on their level of happiness (Ballas and Dorling 2007). The latter referred simply to the question: 'Have you recently been feeling reasonably happy, all things considered?' for which there were four possible answers: more than usual, same, less so and much less so. The major events were coded according to the person to whom they referred (self, spouse, child, etc.) and were divided into 7 categories: health-related events, education, employment, leisure, births and deaths, relationships, finance and others. This in turn produced 34 subject-event combinations each accounting for more than 1 per cent of all recorded events. The vast majority of respondents, 94,911 or 66.1 per cent, reported no major events over the previous year. It is also important to observe that the importance of life events varied markedly between age groups with the old prioritising health and the young education. An ordinary least-squares regression equation of subjective happiness against major live events was then calculated adjusted for age, gender and education attainment to indicate which events were related to greatest happiness. The top and bottom ten event/subject combinations are given in Table 6.8 for which it should be noted that the death of a child does not feature because it did not reach the inclusion criterion of 1 per cent or more of all events.

These results, no matter how provisional, raise some important issues for PwMS and their families. The first must be how important relationships appear to be for generating personal happiness and sadness when they fail. Second, the significance of health and its stalking partner, death (of relatives and friends), in making people feel unhappy. Thus, while poor health because of a chronic illness such as MS may be only one element of achieving a poor quality of life, it is a crucially important one. If to this in midlife employment and relationship losses also take place, then it is little wonder many PwMS succumb to low mood and depression because they are all in the top six events likely to make

Table 6.8 The ten subject-event combinations producing most and least subjective happiness

Most happiness:
1. Relationship starting, mine
2. Employment job gain
3. Finance (house)
4. Pregnancy/birth, mine
5. Pregnancy/birth, child's
6. Education, mine
7. Leisure
8. Employment job change
9. Relationship, child's starting
10. Pregnancy/birth, family

Least happiness (sadness)
1. Relationship ending, mine
2. Death, parent
3. Health, parent
4. Death, other
5. Employment job loss
6. Health, mine
7. Death, family
8. Health, partner
9. Health, child
10. Health, other

Source: Ballas and Dorling (2007, 1249).

people in the UK feel most unhappy! Third, that leisure activity may not be as successful at making people happy as successful relationships, employment or family events. Finally, it may not be 'living states', such as being married, having a steady job, that make people feel most happy but events, that is a positive change, such as starting a new relationship, taking on a new job, that generates most happiness. Unfortunately, the converse may also understandably apply, that change for the worse such as losing a job or a partner may make people least happy; a prophetic observation for PwMS whose health can only be expected at best to stabilise and most probably get worse.

6.6 The economic burden of MS

Economic evidence has been used in the UK to establish the direct cost of MS in the country as a whole (Holmes et al. 1995, McCrone et al. 2008, Kobelt et al. 2000 and 2006a, Tyas et al. 2007), in England and Wales (Blumhardt and Wood 1996) and the cost in the UK compared to a selection of other European countries (Murphy et al. 1998, Kobelt et al. 2006b, Karampampa et al. 2012). This has been achieved with varying degrees of success using survey material from the MS Society membership (Holmes et al. 1995, McCrone et al. 2008), MS Trust members (Tyas et al. 2007, Kobelt et al. 2006a) and clinic-based cohorts from London and Liverpool (Murphy et al. 1998), from Newcastle upon Tyne, Leeds and Birmingham (Kobelt et al. 2000) and from a set of unspecified treatment centres (Karampampa et al. 2012). Such analyses provided evidence on the economic burden of MS but they gave no indication of how resources might best be used to treat PwMS. For this task some form of cost-effectiveness or cost-utility analysis is required. In such work it has to be remembered that any medication or treatment for PwMS uses scarce resources that could be employed to treat other conditions and therefore to be acceptable it must satisfy a given cost threshold. In the UK this has been established by NICE expressed in terms of cost per quality-adjusted life year (QALY) gained of between £20,000 to £30,000/QALY (Sharac et al. 2010, 1685). Unfortunately, so far few of the economic assessments of the utility of recent DMDs in the UK have fallen below this range (Sharac et al. 2010); an issue that caused great consternation in the MS community along with an innovative method of overcoming the problem. This issue is considered in Chapter 7 on providing care for PwMS.

From the results of a survey of 1,942 members of the MS Society, McCrone et al. (2008) offered an estimate of the mean annual service cost for a PwMS in the UK as £16,794 in 2006/7 prices of which £16,144 (87.3%) was for direct MS-related care. The main components of these cost estimates can be seen in Table 6.9 in which the profound importance of informal care that provided without payment by family and

Table 6.9 Mean annual costs per PwMS by category (£s in 2006/7)

Inpatient use and contacts with professionals	890
Tests and investigations	74
Medication	764
Aids and adaptations	444
Informal care	12,038
Total service costs	16,794
Lost employment	8,480
Total costs	25,310

Source: Adapted from McCrone et al. (2008, 854).

Note: Not all categories were available for all participants and therefore numbers cannot be added.

friends at 71.7 per cent of service costs and 47.6 per cent of total costs is clear. The lost employment at 33.5 per cent of total costs was a further significant element of this cost structure, as emphasised in the methodological arcane work of Tyas et al. (2007). It represented a summation of the income lost due to early retirement, days off work due to illness and reduced working hours as a result of having MS. To some extent such losses could be mollified in the UK by state benefit payments such as Incapacity Benefit (Employment and Support allowance since 2011), but no account has been taken in any study of productivity losses due to the possible premature death of people with MS.

What is also important to note is that this cost structure for a person with MS in the UK was not repeated in other European countries. As Kobelt et al. (2006b, 923) observed, 'The profile of MS resource provision in the United Kingdom is unique, with this country frequently appearing at the top or bottom of a list of resources ranked by utilisation.' In particular the UK had relatively high indirect and informal care costs and relatively low costs for DMDs because take up rates were low.

Kobelt et al. (2000) estimated mean annual direct costs in the UK per person with MS to be £12,050, 72 per cent of the McCrone figure with the main reason for the difference probably to be found in the use of informal care. Fewer people in the Kobelt study made use of this resource, 56 per cent compared with 76 per cent in the McCrone et al. (2008) research, and with the unit costs being lower. By contrast, Kobelt et al. (2000) estimated indirect costs to be 31 per cent more at £10,278 compared with £8,480 by McCrone et al. (2008).

In a later report by the Kobelt group (2006a), mean annual service costs per person with MS of £20,035 were estimated from a survey of members of the MS Trust that was 19 per cent higher than the McCrone et al. (2008) study and 66 per cent more than the original Kobelt et al. (2000) research. This may be due to rises in medication and medical professional unit charges. It may also be due to an older and more disabled sample. Nevertheless, from the review of Trisolini et al. (2010, 26) annual costs per PwMS in the UK in 2007 (€39,742) were the third highest nation state in Europe after Norway (€42,706) and Sweden (€42,687) and only slightly lower than in the US (€39,742). Given these mean annual cost figures per person with MS, it became possible to calculate an estimate for the total cost burden of MS in the UK on the assumption of 100,000 sufferers. This produced a figure of between £2.2 billion (Kobelt) and £2.5 billion (McCrone) for direct costs, with lost earnings (indirect costs) additionally amounting to between £845 million and £1.03 billion respectively at 2006/7 prices. Thus, the total annual cost of MS in the UK exceeded £3 billion whichever approach was adopted, the highest of all European countries according to Trisolini et al. (2010, 27).

The fact that a heavy burden of the costs of having MS are borne by the individual with MS and their family was demonstrated by the research of Holmes et al. (1995, 187) in a survey of members of the UK MS Society but with a very different accounting system to that adopted by McCrone et al. (2008) or Kobelt et al. (2000).[4] In this case within an overall annual national cost of MS of £1.2 billion, lost employment by both PwMS and their carers accounted for 33.0 per cent of this total with private expenses a further 11.7 per cent. The work of McCrone and Kobelt also demonstrated this. However, none of them gave an indication of the private costs to PwMS for home adaptations or medication. Much of this is often borne by the state through the NHS or local social services, but not all. For many PwMS in the UK, prescription charges may apply and often means-tested contributions are applied to home adaptations. Only Tyas et al. (2007, 389) offered an estimate of mean annual medical and non-medical out-of-pocket expenditure at between £1,100 and £2,600 per PwMS. This may appear a relatively small proportion of total service costs, say 10 per cent at most, but this has to be borne by the person with MS and their families on an annual basis at a time when earnings would most likely be declining. This, therefore, could have a very serious effect on quality of life and the sorts of things PwMS and their families can afford to do; an issue that needs thoroughly researching in the future.

Some of the above economic assessments of the impact of MS went on to relate the costs of MS to levels of disability and quality of life, all not unexpectedly supporting an increase of costs with the former and a negative relationship with the latter. With respect to disability both Holmes et al. (1995, 188) and Kobelt et al. (2000, 27) divided their responses into three levels of disability, modest, moderate and severe. Then, in the case of the Holmes study, if the annual cost per person with a low level of disability was equal to 100, moderate disability was 294 and severe disability 477. For the Kobelt et al. (2000) study the equivalent figures were 100, 177 and 367. Thus, the mean cost of a person who was severely disabled because of MS was substantially more than a person of modest disability, a phenomenon shown to have international resonance by Naci et al. (2010, 373).

Intangible costs of MS, that is the costs due to pain, grief, anxiety and social handicap according to Kobelt et al. (2000, 15) have often been ignored in the costs of the illness. They, however, following research on quality adjusted life years suggest a value of £5,170 per person at 1999 prices (Kobelt et al. 2000, 28) or £6,902 in 2006/7 prices. This could add more than 30 per cent to the cost burden of MS in the UK.

Finally, the research by Parkin et al. (1998, 28) on a cost-utility analysis of Interferon β offered an estimate of the cost of an MS relapse by comparing the mean direct costs over a six month period of two groups of patients with MS attending the neurological service at Newcastle-upon-Tyne towards the end of the 1990s: 60 patients in remission with 40 who had had a relapse within the last 6 months. The former group consumed resources at a mean cost of £529 and the relapse group at a mean cost of £2,644, resulting in a cost per relapse of £2,115, more than half of which was due to additional inpatient care. But, these are, of course, direct costs to the health-care provider, not to the individual with MS and their family.

6.7 Relationships

In the discussion on the psychological adjustment of a person with MS to their disease the importance of social relationships appeared regularly as a positive attribute. The number and form of relationships between PwMS and others are extremely varied in quantity, type and quality and include those within their family (both immediate and extended), work, through activities of daily living such as shopping, recreation and through acts of worship. Some of these interactions may be ephemeral and trivial, others may be indefinite (at least intended to be) and serious, but all are of importance in maintaining a person's contact with the society to which they belong. After a diagnosis of MS many of these relationships may change in magnitude and form. The most immediate impacts, and almost certainly the most significant, will be with the family members of the person with MS, with their partner/spouse, children and parents. As Courts et al. (2005, 20) from research in America evocatively described it: 'the effects of MS ripple through the family, with each person's reaction affecting other family members.' There would appear to be no research what-so-ever on the psychological and relationship impacts on parents who have progeny with MS unless they themselves have the illness, while there is a growing international literature on other groups such as spouses/partners (Courts et al. 2005, Bogosian et al. 2009, Dennison et al. 2010) and children (Blackford 1999, Cross and Rintell 1999, Bogosian et al. 2010 and 2011). It is also likely these relationships may vary according to the stage of disablement experienced by the PwMS as family members become care-givers and progress to formal carers and then perhaps ultimately to long-term visitors if permanent residential care is necessary. Thus, there have been separate analyses of early stage MS (Bogosian et al. 2009, Dennison et al. 2010) and late stage MS (Bowen et al. 2010, Bowen and MacLehose 2009, Edmonds et al. 2007a) on close familial relationships.

The most extreme response to the stresses MS may place on a marriage, namely divorce, has already been discussed where it was explained there was no convincing evidence for the UK case that people with MS were any more likely to be divorced than members of the general public but, that this may not be true in other countries. What is more, even for the most severely disabled people with MS where one might imagine the pressure for divorce could be at its greatest, marriage may still dominate adult relations. For example, in the modest survey of Edmonds et al. (2007a, 103) of 32 PwMS of EDSS 8 and above, 7 people lived with a wife or female partner, 7 with a husband and, although the accounting system was not exactly clear, it would appear that 1 more male in residential care during the week went home to his wife at weekends and 2 additional females in hospital would be going home to live with their husbands.

From a semi-structured telephone interview survey of just 15 partners of people with relatively early stage MS, Bogosian et al. (2009) distilled a number of key themes in their responses to the illness entering their lives and the ways they tried to cope. For most the initial diagnosis phase was difficult, long and frustrating with poor communication skills exhibited by the senior medical staff involved. The diagnosis for some came as a shock because initial symptoms did not appear serious to the lay observer while to others it was a relief in that it did not lead to a much more life-threatening conclusion like a brain tumour. The impact of MS on the life of the partner of the person with MS was then discussed under five major themes: loss of control, constant worry, lifestyle changes, relationship changes and attempts to adjust. It was also stressed that often the person with MS had difficulties in accepting their diagnosis and new identity especially during periods of relapse and symptom deterioration. These often led to the person with MS being reluctant to disclose their illness to others and to go out to socialise, both of which in turn led to a diminution in the support and understanding from their existing social contacts and a reduction in their social circle. This was a lifestyle change that was difficult to accept by both parties.

Attempts to adjust to the arrival of MS by partners were varied. They included seeking out relevant information, making practical changes such as house adaptations, sharing their worries by talking to friends, accepting their new situation with the need simply to deal with each new problem as it materialised, encouraging their partner's independence and engaging in hobbies away from their home to distract their mind. It was certainly true that many of these sorts of adjustments were faced by the partners and families of PwMS during a particularly bad relapse or for progressive disease but this analysis may not necessarily be confined to early stage MS because the mean age of the 13 partners for whom quotations were included in the text was 49 years; the mean age of most regional cohorts of PwMS so far studied in the UK and not the mean age of diagnosis (see Chapters 4 and 5). This was usually in the early thirties. So unless PwMS in the Southampton area were systematically choosing partners over 10 years older than themselves, this information may not be indicative of the partners of people with early-stage MS merely of partners of PwMS.

One issue that does confront people with early-stage MS and their partners, however, is whether to start a family. In fact until recently there was anecdotal evidence that some medical practitioners as late as the 1980s had been regularly advising women with MS not to get pregnant at all and if they were to consider seriously having a termination. For example, a pregnant Poppy Hasted only 18 months after being diagnosed with MS was asked when she wanted an abortion on the grounds that her doctor did not believe she would be able to cope with a child and her almost certain future disability (reported in MS Matters 2009, Issue 87, 12–13, 'Just say no – I dare you'). This issue, and its relevant decision-making processes, has been tackled in research in Australia (Prunty et al. 2008) and the US (Smeltzer 2002) but not yet in the UK. The British context for such work though would be one of delayed pregnancies generally due mainly to economic reasons than any others with, for example, over the last 40 years in England and Wales the mean age of mothers giving birth rising from 25 years of age in 1970 to what is believed will be 30 years of age in 2010 (Dorling 2010, 193 and 197).

When the disablement caused by MS becomes severe it may be necessary for individuals with the illness to be placed in indefinite residential care. Bowen and colleagues (2010) presented a model of the experiences of family members of this phenomenon; 'a life-changing experience for all the family' (Bowen et al. 2010, 12). Their analysis came from a set of 25 detailed structured interviews of the relatives of

PwMS who had either recently entered respite care (7 cases) or who had recently entered (or were just about to enter) permanent residential care (18 cases). This information produced four over-arching themes:

Information, communication and understanding
Family relationships, rules and responsibilities
Emotions, coping and support
Life outlook and reflection

What was particularly surprising in this case was that some family members, and especially the children of PwMS, still had many unanswered questions about MS even though it had been a long standing part of their family. This was explained by a culture of not talking about this 'difficult' subject. But, that resulted in family members often being unprepared for deterioration, cognitive change and the eventual necessity in some cases of residential care for their close relative with MS. What was important to observe in these cases though was that the provision of information, or even its collection by the family concerned, did not necessarily lead to understanding or acceptance.

Significant changes in relationships took place not only because the person with MS needed help with activities of daily living but also because of their change in behaviour, outlook and beliefs that led them to becoming far more self-focussed. In some cases the need to look after the person with MS can bring families closer together, but it can also fracture them apart if insufficient time is devoted to the other members. There is also a distinct worry on the part of the children of PwMS, whether justified or not, of becoming involved in the care of their parent with MS, especially in terms of more intimate tasks and in limiting the time they can spend with their peers.

The impact of MS was felt by every member of the family with many difficult emotions experienced such as guilt, frustration, despair and relief. They often expressed sadness as friends started to drift away because of lack of contact but, at the same time some families chose to keep their difficult situation private. In a similar way some family members failed to prioritise their own needs and, while accepting they probably needed support, would at the same time have found it difficult to accept that support. Finally, the experience of living with a person with MS who eventually needed to go into residential care led, or so the authors claimed, to a set of profound reflections on how caring impacts on family life, and especially on how it had changed their outlook on an uncertain future.

The adjustment of children to having a parent with MS was considered in a review essay of 16 studies in English by Bogosian et al. (2011) and researched in practice for adolescents by Bogosian and colleagues (2010) through a set of 15 face-to-face interviews. Three of the papers reviewed in the former analysis found no impact of parental MS on the children's adjustment whereas the other 13 demonstrated that the children faced a number of psychological problems that led to stress, anxiety and in the worst cases depression and behavioural difficulties. However, it was also suggested from this work that a set of five factors might help positively to moderate this behaviour. These were parental responses, illness characteristics, family environment, gender and child factors. Thus, child adjustment to parental MS would be most favourable if their parents coped well (i.e., minimal anxiety, tension and depression), where the severity of the illness was least and progression slowest, where the family environment was most supportive (limited dysfunction, positive support from the well parent, responsibilities at a minimum), female gender in that girls coped better than boys and healthy mother and daughter coped better than healthy dad and son, the higher the levels of social support not only from within the family but from friends too and opportunities for recreation outside the home. Finally, it seemed to be the case that the older the child the greater the chances of maladjustment. Adolescents in particular were worried about their futures and their continuing familial responsibilities and obligations. Thus, analytically it would seem appropriate to separate this older group of young people from other children as indeed Bogosian et al. (2010) decided to do in their study of adolescents.

The response of adolescents to having a parent with MS was found to vary greatly. Some adolescents responded positively saying the experience made them feel more independent, thoughtful and grown up, with the benefits of carers regularly coming into the house to do the chores and their ability to queue jump when their disabled parent was with them. Others were overwhelmed by their new responsibilities and resented the way it limited their social activities especially in terms of transport options. What appeared to be general in all responses, although of course has no wider application given the small number of observations in this research, was that the response of the adolescent to parental MS mirrored the family's attitude towards it. Where the parent with MS seemed to be coping and support was available from the well parent and other relatives (and friends) then adjustment was more assured.

However, where the parent with MS did not accept their illness, refused outside help and took their frustration out on those around them; when the family was more dysfunctional and especially when the well parent left, then adolescent adjustment was less successful. Nevertheless, in conclusion Bogosian et al. (2010, 800) observed that 'Having a parent with MS does not necessarily mean that adolescents have to face adjustment difficulties. In some instances it can mean that adolescents can develop the self, become more independent and more thoughtful and understanding of other people.' Indeed, as Blackford (1999) poignantly made clear from her own experience in Canada, that one should not assume that home caring activities for children were necessarily negative if it resulted in increased feelings of self-worth, self-reliance and a healthy sense of altruism.

It has already been pointed out in the previous chapter that PwMS may often lose their employment as their symptoms develop and as a consequence lose the social relationships that went along with it. Of course, it is perfectly possible that some of the friendships developed during a working life will endure beyond retirement. It is also likely that some may wither with time. Such trends may be true for hobbies and past-times too although, perhaps, the prospects will be more positive for philately than fell walking. Finally, as a direct consequence of having MS, new social relations will most certainly develop; some whether the person with MS likes it or not and others out of choice. The former will include contact with members of the medical and social services communities, while the latter may include MS-support organisations including the virtual community via the web. These are discussed in the next chapter on 'Care'. But, what is important for the person with MS is that they are all opportunities for social contacts, vital for their positive adjustment to their changing situation.

One of the recent areas of growing research interest in the lives of PwMS has been concerned with gender issues especially through the pioneering work of Coyle (2005) and colleagues (Jobin et al. 2010). These not only consider the decisions about family formation and women's health during pregnancy and child rearing, but also the possible differences between the sexes in coping with MS and caring for PwMS. For example, it has been suggested from focus group research in the US that men tended to try to protect their wives with MS by intervening to do things for them, whereas wives attempted to promote the independence of their husbands with MS by encouraging them to do things for themselves (Courts et al. 2005). But, it should not be forgotten that while the well spouses and partners may be expected to give support to their respective spouses and partners with MS, they themselves may need support too, to help them cope with their own self-care and possible changes of role, career, social contacts and financial security.

6.8 Conclusion

In reviewing the impact of MS on people's lives this chapter began by describing the wide range of symptoms the illness may produce from physical disablement to cognitive impairment, fatigue to incontinence. Unfortunately, though, lack of suitable evidence prevented any precise calculation of the person years of suffering from any particular symptom. In addition, it was shown that for people with a progressive form of MS, symptoms will rarely be experienced individually more as collections that steadily get worse through time.

In this discussion special attention was given to three specific symptom groups: physical disablement, fatigue and psychological problems. In the former, it was suggested that up to half of all PwMS may have some form of walking problem from limping and foot dragging to not being able to move their legs at all. For fatigue the problems of description and definition were emphasised, whereas for a successful psychological adjustment to the illness the importance of positive social relationships were highlighted.

The analysis progressed to consider a number of measures of the quality of life from which one observation dominated; although at the population level disability and quality of life were inversely related, for any disability group or type of MS, there was a very wide range of associations such that it was possible to have a high quality of life with significant disability. The opposite was possible too with some people with only limited disability regarding their quality of life as very poor. Indeed, some PwMS regarded their life as so dreadful they recorded it as worse than death. When some generic measures of quality of life were employed such as the EQ-5D, that almost by definition missed much of the essence of having MS, yet allowed comparisons with other medical conditions, MS did not fare well at all, being regarded as one of the worst illnesses possible to endure.

When trying to understand how MS impacts of people's lives two problems emerged. The first problem was the lack of published research in this area, while the second problem was that what research had been undertaken often suffered from serious methodological flaws compromising their findings. It was therefore not at all clear how people generally were affected by having MS or how they spent their lives after they received an MS diagnosis. Nevertheless, with these points in mind the available evidence did point towards five main conclusions:

1. Increased disability was associated with financial disadvantage especially among the most disabled.
2. PwMS were less likely to be in employment than members of the public generally irrespective of disability. This finding needs careful further research to discover why this should be the case.
3. Notwithstanding the two previous findings, PwMS in the UK appeared to live in better off households than people generally in the UK.
4. There was no convincing evidence that PwMS in the UK were any more likely to be divorced than people without MS.
5. A person's MS may be seen as developing through time such that their choices and independence become increasingly restricted and its impact extending increasingly from the individual with MS to their entire family.

Further understanding of the plight of many PwMS may face was revealed when the concept of happiness entered the analysis. Here it was shown that taking part in new relationships and securing new employment opportunities were powerful generators of happiness with their losses generators of sadness. It should, therefore, be of no surprise that in early middle age as many PwMS face the prospects of job loss and the contraction of their social contacts as their disability and symptoms develop that their quality of life declines too.

Two aspects of the quality of life of a PwMS were considered in detail: the costs of having MS and the disease's impact on relationships. Although, again there were methodological issues with the analyses, the mean annual cost per PwMS was approximately £25,000 in the UK of which almost half was in terms of informal care and 30 per cent in terms of lost employment. Finally, on relationships the limited small scale qualitative research that had been undertaken suggested that successful adjustment to MS encroaching into their lives of either a child, spouse, parent or friend seemed most closely related to the way in which the person with MS accepted their new situation. Where the response was one of rejection, anger and frustration with outside help refused then relationships of all types were likely to be dysfunctional.

7
The Care of People with MS

7.1 Introduction

This review of research on the care of people with Multiple Sclerosis (PwMS) begins by detailing the services they use and then proceed to assess the adequacy of their provision relating to the United Kingdom (UK) through comparisons with published standards of care by the MS Society, National Institute for Health and Care Excellence (NICE) and the Department of Health. The chapter considers in detail four care-related issues of particular concern to PwMS in most places: informal carers, the use of disease modifying drugs (DMDs), the use of complementary and alternative medicine (CAM) and vocational rehabilitation. Other general MS-care concerns such as the delivery of the diagnosis, the role of MS nurses, rehabilitation, respite care, palliative/end-of-life care and the success of self-help programmes are then discussed briefly in an MS care-research miscellany.

However, before reviewing research evidence on the provision of care for PwMS it is worth making a number of important points about the disease and the social contexts in which that care is offered. First, and most fundamentally, it must be remembered that as currently understood MS is a chronic illness that the sufferer will have for life; it will not resolve itself spontaneously and cannot be cured. Thus, once diagnosed a PwMS will be in need of some form of care to a greater or lesser degree for the rest of their life and that that care will not be concerned with trying to return them to full health, but in stopping their health getting worse or trying to mitigate the presenting symptoms and their consequences. What is more, the nature and intensity of the care required will vary hugely throughout their life time and between different people with the condition.

The second important point to observe is that before the end of the twentieth century there were no treatments available for PwMS that could actually affect the course of their disease and very little research interest in MS symptom-relief research either. As Parkin et al. (1998, 1) observed, 'Until recently, no specific therapy was available for MS, and patient management consisted of symptom control, provision of physiotherapy and disability aids, and psychiatric and social support.' And, to demonstrate what a new phenomenon medical care for PwMS really has been, Alan Thompson, a key player in setting standards of care for PwMS and establishing neurological rehabilitation as an intellectual research activity and practical reality, made the following remark about the 1980s. 'MS was regarded as a hopeless, depressing condition, and of relatively low interest in neurological research. Neurologists thought that they could do nothing for patients with MS and generally just wanted them to go away' (Mayor 2009, 230). In addition, although there may now be a growing number of DMDs on offer to PwMS, or at least those in the early stages of the condition, symptom-relief therapies are still poorly developed. This is not just a problem for MS. It is a general medical phenomenon as Wall (2000, 164) remarked in his exposition on pain: 'Symptom control was historically not worthy of the attention of serious men. So this task was assigned to the denizens of the depths of the hierarchy.' But, it is certainly a serious issue in MS as Thompson, once again, and colleagues (2010, 1195) made clear: 'For most treatments, however, the supporting evidence is weak and often relies on evidence provided by other disciplines...This restricted evidence base is attributable not only to the paucity of trials done so far and their methodological limitations, but also to the difficulty in measuring the effect of treatments in a chronic condition such as MS in which impaired functions often interact (impaired cognition, mood disturbance, and fatigue).' And, it is a point that has been reiterated by (Zajicek et al. 2010, 2): '[T]here are relatively few effective symptomatic treatments, and many clinical trials of symptomatic treatments have been disappointingly negative.' What is worse, even when a therapy has been developed and received regulatory approval some health organisations will not allow its use. For example, Sativex, the cannabis-based mouth spray for treating spasticity in MS, that was finally given a licence for use in Britain by the Medicines and Healthcare Products Regulatory Agency in June 2010, was not being prescribed in some Primary Care Trusts (PCTs) in Scotland and England, including parts of London, the West Midlands, Yorkshire, East Midlands, Suffolk and the South West (*New Pathways* 69, Sept/Oct 2011). Thus, in the areas where it was not directly available through their General Practitioner (GP), patients with MS needed a neurologist to make an individual funding approval request or the individual needed to pay privately approximately £176 per month to buy the drug. Through these mechanisms therefore Sativex was directly and indirectly being rationed geographically and financially.

It should be of no surprise to discover that as a consequence of the above, PwMS and their families have a long history of trying to find solutions to their problems for themselves, of trying to manage their own care, long before the current vogue of active patient participation. To begin with this was out of necessity because health-care professionals had little to offer them. It has also been a regular element of the pre-diagnosis period in which many patients who ultimately were diagnosed with MS questioned the opinions of their doctors that they did not have MS (Robinson 1988, 47). Unfortunately, what we do not know to judge the significance of such mild belligerence is the proportion of these patients who did not go on to be diagnosed with MS. Nevertheless, the self-care approach has received a degree of legitimacy from recent self-help Expert Patient Programmes. However, the extent to which PwMS are truly able to take on this role needs careful consideration. But, one of the drivers for such an initiative may be a phenomenon that is affecting all fields of health-care provision in many parts of the world in the early twenty-first century, financial restraint that is leading directly to the questioning of the provision of specialist neurological services for MS such as their nurses, physiotherapists and expensive DMDs compared to other health-care demands. Furthermore, it raises the much wider issue about which elements of care should be funded and provided by the state and what should be the responsibility of the individual and their family, or the voluntary and private sectors? But, a discussion on the sort of national health-care system that may be most favourable for PwMS is beyond the scope of this book.

The evidence on the provision of neurological services in the UK generally and for MS in particular is both partial and challenging to interpret. At the international level within Europe, UK neurology may be thought of as a Cinderella service, under-resourced and of unrecognised worth. For example, in 2006 there was just 1 neurologist per 15,000 people, less than a third of the European average and, while excellent support may be found in regional neuroscience centres, inadequate provision existed at local and district hospitals (Lancet Neurology Editorial 2011a, 671). And, such a situation does not bode well for the growth or even maintenance of this specialism and the care of PwMS in the future when it will be under severe pressure from three different sources:

1. Financial restraint and budgetary cutbacks when the costs of new drugs and treatments are growing.
2. An increasing demand for their expertise as the population ages and more people begin to suffer from age-related brain conditions such as dementia, Alzheimer's and stroke.
3. A major internal reorganisation of the National Health Service (NHS) that has rested commissioning more with consortia led by GPs (Department of Health 2010). It is these groups that in the future must be convinced that expenditure on neurological and MS-specific care is a worthwhile exercise compared to all other competing demands.

However, in terms of the actual expenditure on neurology and its share of the NHS budget this specialism appears to have been doing relatively well recently. For example, between 2006–7 and 2009–10 total spending on neurological services increased from £3.2billion to £4.1billion at an average annual percentage change of 9 per cent and with the neurology proportion of the NHS budget increasing from 3.6 to 4.0 per cent (National Audit Office 2011, 19). Nevertheless, as will be shown the delivery of care to PwMS has often been poor. Perhaps this rise in expenditure has not been able to keep pace with the rise in demand for neurological services. It certainly does not seem to have been capable of delivering care of an acceptable quality for many PwMS. But, what is particularly frustrating for any attempt to evaluate the neurology service provided by the NHS is that, as the National Audit Office (2011) pointed out, it has no way of showing the benefits of any increase in the neurology budget, no way of knowing whether it has been value for money, because appropriate evidence has not been routinely collected.

7.2 Care-services used by PwMS

Evidence on the services used and contacts made by PwMS reveal a number of common patterns. First, PwMS require many different services and types of medical support to help them cope with their condition. Indeed, Wade and Green (2001, 19) from their audit of services used in Oxfordshire from January 1996 for 10 months discovered that for their 226 PwMS, 284 new problems arose needing 31 different professional groups and 15 different hospital specialisms where they never formed the sole or main focus of the service. They concluded that 'The totality of services that someone with MS might need is little different from the totality of services the population might need'.[1] Meanwhile of the 1,000 or so PwMS in Devon and Cornwall who joined the South West Impact of MS Project (SWIMS) project by 2010, 16 different types of specialist were contacted during their previous 12 months of which neurologists, MS specialist nurses, GPs, Ophthalmologists, Continence advisors, Physiotherapists and Occupational Therapists (OTs) were dominant (Zajicek et al. 2010). Similar results were also obtained by Ford and colleagues (2000, 24) from interviews with 30 randomly selected PwMS in the Leeds conurbation, from a questionnaire survey of 318 PwMS selected through their GP practices in England and Scotland (Somerset et al. 2001), a set of PwMS from a supposed representative sample of 30 GP practices in Northern Ireland (MacLurg et al. 2005) and from a set of 150 patients consecutively attending the National Hospital for Neurology and Neurosurgery (NHNN) at the very end of the twentieth century (Freeman and Thompson 2000).

The second general observation to come from this suite of research was that the three services that dominated the contacts PwMS made to secure the care they needed were their GP, hospital neurology departments and physiotherapists. For example, in the Northern Ireland study 99 per cent of PwMS had visited their GP during the previous 12 months, 55 per cent had visited their GP 4 or more times, and half had had contact with their neurologist, with 13 per cent having contact with physiotherapy (MacLurg et al. 2005, 381). Furthermore, in the Somerset et al. (2001) research, 78 per cent of respondents had made contact with their GP during the previous 12 months, 50 per cent with a hospital consultant and 38 per cent with a physiotherapist.

Two further important points about the provision of care services to PwMS emerge from this research. The first concerns the fragmented nature in both time and location of many of the health-care services required by PwMS, such that attending all appointments at different locations and on different time-cycles could prove expensive and most certainly time-consuming especially by public transport. A new geography of effort may therefore be required to understand how attending all their medical appointments fitted into the lives of PwMS, especially when employment and familial responsibilities were involved too. The second important observation is that while many PwMS were accessing a range of care services to help them cope with their condition, some were not. For example, in the NHNN based study 45 per cent of these individuals were currently receiving no community services at all other than their GP including 12 per cent of the severely disabled (Freeman and Thompson 2000, 730). In addition, they observed that 'Wide and unacceptable variations in the provision of outpatient and community services remain a fundamental problem for people with multiple sclerosis.' And, the services a person with MS may be able to access becomes 'just a matter of chance' (Freeman and Thompson 2000, 732).

However, this research referred principally to the services contacted and not to those services that were in demand and could not be contacted either because they were unavailable or because access was rationed in some way, by for example restriction or cost. One way of approaching this issue would be to compare actual provision with agreed basic standards of care PwMS should expect to receive from their health and social care services.

7.3 Standards of care for PwMS

The UK case offers a good example of the setting of standards of care for PwMS that have then been audited against actual experience. The setting of these benchmarks began in earnest in 1997 with the collaborative publication of 'Standards of Health Care for People with MS' between the MS Society and the NHNN. These standards were significant for three main reasons. First of all they led to the Measuring Success Awards Scheme through which the MS Society could recognise formally excellence in service provision. Second, they led to an assessment of the degree to which the basic needs of PwMS were being met by the NHS published by the MS Society in 2002 in the document 'Are we being served: health care experiences of people with MS'. Now, although this research had a number of serious methodological problems, detailed in Chapter 3, that prevented any general inferences being drawn, it did indicate that many PwMS in the UK had received a poor and uncoordinated service from the NHS. In particular this survey (MS Society 2002, 5) highlighted the following impacts:

1. The process of diagnosis was poorly managed, with little or no information about MS given out, and little on-going support offered.
2. Following diagnosis, people with MS and their families received almost no information and support from health professionals.
3. In the course of their illness people with MS had great difficulty accessing the services they needed, at the time they were needed.
4. There was almost no involvement of people with MS in the planning and management of their services to do with MS.

The third, and most important impact of the original standards of care document, however, was the development of a set of new evidence-based recommendations for MS services by the MS Society and the MS professional Network (Freemen et al. 2002) that included a complementary workbook for service providers and a Charter for MS Services for service users; a prescient reminder perhaps for NICE who at that time were preparing their own set of guidelines for the care of PwMS. This 2002 report began with the telling observation from Thompson that it 'describes the strength of evidence available for current practice and perhaps more importantly the many areas in which evidence is sorely lacking' (p.4).

For practical purposes the recommendations were divided into four phases of the condition for which the key issues were highlighted, in what may be regarded as a rehabilitation approach, an evolving and on-going process of the promotion of physical, psychological and social adaptation to a patient's particular circumstances to maximise their quality of life (Zajicek et al. 2007, 174). These four phases were

7.3.1 Diagnostic phase

Key issues:

1. Certain and clear diagnosis
2. Appropriate support at diagnosis
3. Access to information
4. Continuing education

7.3.2 Minimal impairment phase

Key issues:

1. Continuity in service provision
2. Access to support and informed advice
3. Access to appropriate treatment and self-management
4. Access to treatment for conditions unrelated to MS

7.3.3 Moderate disability phase

Key issues:

1. Responsiveness of services
2. Access and location
3. Expertise
4. Communication and co-ordination
5. Self-management

7.3.4 Severe disability phase

Key issues:

1. Access to information
2. Expertise
3. Communication and co-ordination
4. Adequate community care services
5. Community mobility
6. Provision of respite care
7. Appropriate long-term facilities, including palliative care

Despite the observation that the bulk of supporting evidence was of low grade (Freeman et al. 2002, 6), the report concluded optimistically that the recommendations 'provide people with realistic expectations of their entitlements' (2002, 28); perhaps intimating what a person with MS in the UK ought to expect from their nation's health and care services. Unfortunately, for many PwMS this has not materialised.

The guidelines published by NICE (2003) specifically on the 'Management of multiple sclerosis in primary and secondary care' began by identifying 6 key priorities for the implementation of their guidance and ways in which they may be audited, and went on to offer specific advice on diagnosis, the treatment of the disease process, relapses, rehabilitation and 19 specific impairments. The six specific key priorities for implementation (NICE 2003, 4) were specialised services, rapid diagnosis, seamless services, a responsive service, sensitive but thorough problem assessment and self-referral after discharge.

An attempt at an audit of these recommendations in England and Wales was undertaken by the Royal College of Physicians and the MS Trust (2008) that included a self-selected survey on the MS Trust website to represent service users (1,300 responses), along with questionnaires to 157 NHS Trusts as service providers (127 responses), 172 service commissioning (140 responses) and 13 organisations responsible for performance management (7 responses). From this evidence six key results emerged:

1. Access to specialist neurological services was generally good.
2. Access to neurological rehabilitation was unacceptably low, with very limited commissioning and only slightly less limited actual provision.
3. Time between initial referral and final diagnosis remained long.
4. Integration of care between health and social services was felt to be poor.

5. Patient involvement both in the planning of individual personal care and in service provision and development was very poor.
6. Assessments were perceived by PwMS generally to be carried out in a sensitive and thorough manner.

Thus, although some caution needs to be exercised with the self-selected nature of some of the evidence collated in this survey, it would nevertheless appear to be the case that for a large number of PwMS in England and Wales the majority of NICE guidelines on their care had not been implemented five years after their publication. It would seem that only one of the six key priorities (number 5) had been met along with part of the first key priority. And, in this priority, the principal deficit in care provision was to be found in access to neurological rehabilitation. As the RCP and MS Trust (2008, 7) commented: 'This is particularly important for people with a chronic disabling condition which is characterised by periods of relapse and by a wide range of neurological losses.' In an editorial in their *Way Ahead* magazine the MS Trust went on to emphasise that 'it is the inadequacy of symptom management that causes distress, and may worsen disability' (Editorial MS Trust, *Way Ahead* 2008 12(4), 1) and as a result of the failure to implement the NICE guidelines for the care of PwMS: 'The postcode lottery is now about basic services – continence, prevention of pressure sores, wheelchair assessments, pain relief.' But, what is not known is how many PwMS were suffering unnecessarily with their condition as direct victims of this form of state failure? What was even more depressing was that the RCP/MST report went on to suggest that the improvements that could be identified were probably more the result of the commitment of local clinical champions than of the adherence to national guidelines. Clearly at this time care services for PwMS in much of the UK had failed to live up to reasonable expectations.

Furthermore, according to the NICE (2003, 36) guidelines document a review process should have begun four years after its publication to be available within two years of the start of that review process, that is in 2009. Unfortunately, that process did not begin until 2012 and it would appear only after intense pressure from the MS charities with the revised guidelines not published until October 2014; another example of a health-care expectation failing to materialise for PwMS. This new document (NICE 2014) has not met with unanimous approval, being praised for recommending the application of multidisciplinary teams, a named single point of contact and annual reviews by an MS expert for the treating of MS, it has been criticised for undervaluing the role of MS

Nurses, not bringing together all elements of MS care into a single document of best practice and for not recommending the drugs Fampridine and Sativex for the relief of immobility and spasticity respectively ((MS Society 2014b, MS Trust 2015).

The third set of standards of care against which the provision for MS could be compared were provided by the National Service Framework (NSF) for long-term conditions published by the Department of Health in 2005 that emphasised neurological conditions, designed 'to put the individual at the heart of care and to provide a service that is efficient, supportive and appropriate to every stage from diagnosis to end of life' (Department of Health 2005, 5). This was to be achieved through the implementation of 11 Quality Requirements over the following 10 years that would transform the care of people with long-term conditions and enable joint working across health, social care and the voluntary sector.

The 11 Quality Requirements were as follows:

1. A person-centred service
2. Early recognition, prompt diagnosis and treatment
3. Emergency and acute management
4. Early and specialist rehabilitation
5. Community rehabilitation and support
6. Vocational rehabilitation
7. Providing equipment and accommodation
8. Providing personal care and support
9. Palliative care
10. Supporting family and carers
11. Caring for people with neurological conditions in hospital or other health and social care settings.

Unfortunately, it became clear in 2010, half way through this programme's so-called 'implementation period', that very little of this document's agenda had been achieved. This may have been the result of no additional funding being provided for its execution, but with a change of government in the UK in 2010, immanent health service reform and serious future funding constraints it would seem unlikely that they will be in the foreseeable future either. Nevertheless, a review of progress on the NSF implementation was undertaken in 2010 using an audit tool called 'Quality Neurology' that included interviews and focus group work with both service users and professionals in 11 PCTs and their related Local Authorities (Thomas et al. 2010).

Although this was far from a formally representative sample of PCTs from which generalities may have been deduced, the results revealed exceedingly poor results. Indeed, not one PCT had fully met a single NSF quality requirement (Thomas et al. 2010, 368). Furthermore, with respect to specific Quality requirements some of the general findings of this audit made for depressing reading. Patients with long-term neurological conditions were not receiving even the basic information they needed to manage their condition, and they often spent significant amounts of time trying to locate it. There were insufficient numbers of appropriately trained health and social care staff to manage their needs properly. Integration of social, primary and secondary medical care was not common place leading to problems of service delivery. There was a postcode lottery of service availability and frequently provided too late to have any affect. Access to rehabilitation and the timely supply of equipment was often a significant issue. There was not enough emergency out of hours care for neurological conditions. And, the commissioning of neurological services for conditions that progressed rapidly was extremely variable across the audit sites because of a lack of understanding (Thomas et al. 2010, 368). Essentially the same information can also be found in a document published by Neurological Commissioning Support (2010), a partnership of Parkinson's UK, the Motor Neurone Disease Association and the MS Society to act as a consultancy service to health and social care to promote effective commissioning of services for people with long-term neurological conditions. It is also repeated in the findings of the National Audit Office (2011, 7) of services for people with neurological conditions that the achievement of quality requirements within the framework has been poor with no major improvements in many aspects of service provision since 2006. Such observations do not rest easily with the view of Zajicek et al. (2007, 172) on MS that 'this life-long disease requires a continuing relationship to be developed wherein the person with MS needs to be able to access services in a timely manner, as their needs change.' But, with their conclusion that 'the reality of many people...of health and social care input is overwhelmingly one of crisis management wherein interventions are provided as a fragmented series of short term quick fixes.'

From this evidence therefore it is difficult not to conclude that many PwMS have been treated poorly by health and care services in many areas of the UK compared to what they should have been able to expect. The UK health and care services for PwMS fail their inspection!

7.4 Specific care concerns

There are many elements of the care of PwMS that have attracted research interest, too many to include in this discussion. Instead, what will be attempted here is first an in-depth analysis of four aspects of their care that are of particular significance to PwMS generally namely informal care-giving, DMDs, CAM and vocational rehabilitation and, second a brief overview of some of the important research findings from other aspects of their care in an MS-care research miscellany.

7.4.1 Informal care-giving

An informal care-giver in this context refers to a person who offers care and assistance to a person with MS but is not formally employed to do so by them or by a health/social care provider. In most cases such an individual will be a member of the family of the person with MS receiving care and usually a spouse or partner. For many such individuals the role of carer may creep upon them slowly, beginning simply as caring for their ill partner as would be expected in any intimate, loving relationship. However, as the latter becomes increasingly disabled by their MS the care demands upon them inevitably increase. The degree to which a partner takes on these tasks or seeks help from others including health and social care professionals will vary hugely between individuals and between families. Some may attempt to abdicate their familial responsibilities completely while others may devote themselves to caring for their loved-one; some far more willing to accept and identify more readily with their new role than others. For example, from 40 narrative interviews with a wide range of different carers Hughes et al. (2013) discovered that many objected to the 'miserable' term carer as they saw it because they saw their role simply as a normal part of a relationship that they took on willingly. However, not all these interviewees took such an altruistic view with at least one man resenting the effort and expense of looking after his wife, exclaiming 'why couldn't I have a normal life?' (Hughes et al. 2013, 80). Similarly, it should not automatically be assumed that family members of a person with MS will be sympathetic to their situation with, for example, Hepworth and Harrison (2004, 55) reporting PwMS suffering with fatigue being accused of laziness and malingering.

Two aspects of informal care givers to PwMS have already become clear in this book. First, in terms of the costs of MS, they incurred the greatest burden when a monetary value was ascribed to the time they spent on their caring tasks. According to the research of McCrone et al. (2008) in the UK for example, this was as high as 71.7 per cent of the service costs of looking after PwMS and 47.6 per cent of total costs. Furthermore, it has been suggested by the research of Kobelt et al. (2006b) that the costs of informal care for PwMS varied markedly between countries dependent on the services offered by the state and the degree to which women entered the workforce. Where the state offered substantial support to its disabled citizens as in Sweden and Austria, then the need for informal care was relatively low, with the opposite the case in Italy and the UK. Another good illustration of the importance of informal care came from the work of O'Hara et al. (2004) from a self-selecting questionnaire survey of PwMS in Greater London and its immediate hinterland. During the 24-hours before they filled out their forms family members dominated the number of care providing contacts by accounting for 76 per cent of personal care contacts, 79 per cent in the domain of mobility, 84 per cent for household tasks, 81 per cent for leisure and 79 per cent for employment (O'Hara et al. 2004, 1404). In a number of ways therefore the immediate family was an indispensable part of the care package for PwMS. Whether this is an acceptable situation at the start of the twenty-first century is an important issue for debate. It also raises the issue as to whether personal and family relationships should form the basis for care–giving? Unfortunately, neither of these important issues can be tackled at this juncture. However, such research findings emphasise that carers are almost certainly knowledgeable agents in the care of their 'loved-ones' and need to be regarded as such by health professionals; that is they are one of the important stakeholders in the care-making decisions for PwMS.

The second aspect of informal carers that can be inferred from what has already been described above is their demographic characteristics. It has already been shown that approximately 70 per cent of PwMS in the UK were female and of an average age of approximately 50 years. In addition, national surveys of MS Society members have suggested that the vast majority of PwMS were either married or living with a partner. Thus, one might reasonably have expected most carers of PwMS to be male and on average about 50 years of age. Of the few surveys of carers of PwMS in the UK that have been undertaken the work of Woodroffe et al. (undated) and Forbes et al. (2007) provided evidence in support of such a view. In the former, derived from a random survey of members of the MS Society with MS (MwMS) with 317 carer responses, 65 per cent were male with the median age group of between 51 and 65 years suggesting carers could be slightly older than the PwMS who received their care. This was similar to the result drawn from the self-selecting survey of 257 carers in England by Forbes et al. (2007) where 60 per cent were male, 91 per cent married and with a mean age of 52 years.

While it may be that the general case of the informal care-giver to PwMS in the UK is a middle-aged male, the population of carers is in fact an heterogeneous one including female partners and spouses, friends, neighbours, parents and children. Unfortunately, there is very little evidence available on the size and nature of these different cohorts of carers, the tasks they carry out individually or collectively and the impact of their caring activities on their own lives. There are few large surveys of carers of PwMS such as the one by Forbes et al. (2007), but what does exist are a number of detailed qualitative inquiries into specific small groups of carers such as by Mutch (2010) that help to reveal some of the issues these individuals have to confront daily.

The discussions on caring for PwMS are understandably replete with the negative aspects this activity may bring on the care-giver's lifestyle, quality of life and health both physical and emotional, issues that are often subsumed under the headings of 'carer strain' or the 'carer's burden', although some argue such expressions devalue the person receiving care (Hughes et al. 2013, 79). Nevertheless, these negative impacts come in many different forms that do not act individually but collectively and cumulatively on the carer. They include the following impacts:

1. The physical health of the carer related to their age, health and gender; the seriousness of the symptoms of the person receiving care; the instability of the symptoms; the length of time the carer has been caring; the quality and timeliness of support received informally from family and friends and formally from health and social services.
2. The emotional health of the carer related to worry about: continuing their caring duties indefinitely, relentlessly into the future; what the future may bring; their helplessness to affect change; their finances; their possible other roles as parent or employee; their need to plan everything; their feelings of loneliness, isolation (confined to their home perhaps) and being taken for granted, undervalued; of being overwhelmed by responsibilities.
3. The intrusiveness of the illness; its impact on finances; disrupting lifestyles and leisure time, in doing the things you value; the effort needed to secure help from health and social care services, the fighting for everything phenomenon; the changing of your identity into a 'carer' that in many respects is very different to your peers.

Chipchase and Lincoln (2001) from 51 responses to a self-selecting carer survey discovered that 46 per cent were, as they defined it, under a form of carer strain with their principal worries being that their partner had changed substantially for the worse from their former self, the financial impacts of the illness and the impacts on their personal plans and goals, but no noticeable difference was observed between male and female carers. By contrast, the results of a questionnaire survey of carers by Forbes et al. (2007) with 257 responses concluded that their main health concerns were anxiety, tiredness and depression with women reporting a greater burden than men. The research by Chesson (2003), however, from 60 carer interviews in Scotland made no comment on gender differences, instead emphasising the major life adjustments caring roles often demanded in their social activities, financial affairs and employment including rearranging their working times, decline in promotional prospects and resigning early to concentrate on caring.

A completely different perspective on caring for PwMS that adds important detail to the generalities already discussed was provided by the interview work of Mutch (2010) in her attempt to understand the carer's role, motivations and coping strategies. From just 8 interviews with 4 male carers and 4 female carers of between 50 and 74 years of age and married for between 28 and 54 years to the person for whom they carried out caring duties, 3 major themes emerged to describe their role: Worry, Planning and Frustration.

Worry included the individual issues of a genuine concern for their spouse; the unpredictability of MS; helplessness; concern for their own health; concern for their own future.

Planning indicated that their lives were consumed by constant planning on daily, weekly and long-term issues.

Frustration included the issues of lack of sleep; anger; financial matters; inability to communicate with their charge because of cognitive problems.

The carers employed a number of coping strategies summarised under the themes of the phases of MS, relaxation, holiday/respite, attitudes of self and partner and avoidance. The ability of the spouse to cope with their partner with MS depended on the degree to which MS was affecting them at that time, on the phase of the disease being experienced. Their ability to escape their caring role and relax, or do something to avoid it altogether, being vital to the carers' ability to persevere with their task. But, the major motivational factors in these relationships persisting were marriage longevity, commitment to their marriage vows and the attitude and outlook on life by both partners, their ability to continue to laugh and have fun together. What may be more in doubt though is the likely continuance of spouses being prepared to support their disabled partner with MS in the future if society becomes more selfish and increasingly values personal fulfilment and possessions over family and community cohesion.

With the exception of the analysis by Chipchase and Lincoln (2001), the carer-related research reported here has indicated a gender difference in the care-giving phenomenon in that women reported higher levels of carer stress than men and had different attitudes towards their caring tasks. This view argued that women have more difficulty in putting their own needs first than men, less able to distance themselves from their caring duties. Women therefore may often be engulfed or overwhelmed by their caring duties such that they are unable to balance their own interests with the person they are supporting and become too easily dominated in that relationship. Boeije and van Doorne-Huiskes (2003) perceptively argue that the reason for this gender difference may be a cultural one in that women grow up in a society in which their gender is expected to undertake the nurturing and caring duties. It is expected that wives will provide some aspects of personal care for their husbands, but women do not expect this of their husbands and feel guilty for what their husbands do provide. According to Boeije and van Doorne-Huiskes (2003, 240) 'when women give care, they act in line with social expectations. When men give care, they believe they are doing something special that deserves attention and reward'. Does this imply that men would feel less guilty than women in not providing care for an ill spouse? And, could a corollary of this be that men might gain greater satisfaction from successfully carrying out care-giving tasks than women?

Nevertheless, whichever spouse was delivering care to an ill partner with MS, it would be wrong to believe that the task was one of unrelenting hard work, stress and despair. There can be some positive elements too including personal growth, strengthened relationships, a change in life's priorities, a greater appreciation of life and a sense of accomplishment and pride in what they had achieved (Mutch 2010).

7.4.2 Disease modifying drugs (DMDs)

The beginning of the twenty-first century marked a new era in the treatment of MS with the availability of a series of drugs that it was claimed could alter the course of the disease for the better, could reduce the number of relapses and the number of central nervous system (CNS) lesions as seen on Magnetic Resonance Imaging (MRI) compared with what otherwise would have been expected and perhaps even slow disability progression in patients with relapsing remitting MS (RRMS), the DMDs. The first three of these were beta-interferon preparations, Betaferon, Avonex and Rebif followed soon after by Glatiramer acetate (Copaxone) (Zajicek et al. 2007, 127) that collectively became the 'first-line' treatments for RRMS, or 'platform therapies' (MSIF 2013). Since that time a number of other DMDs have been developed for varying degrees of relapsing-remitting activity such that by the end of 2014 NICE will have approved ten of them for use in England. These included Extavia to be added to the first-line group that are all delivered by injection, Tysabri (Natalizumab) and Lemtrada (Alemtuzumab) administered by infusion (via a drip) and three tablet regimens, Aubagio, Tecfidera and Gilenya (Fingolimod). Others such as Plegridy are still in development and some established treatments in other countries such as the tablet Cladribine have failed to secure UK approval (MS Matters Issue 95, Jan / Feb 2011, 22–5). However, the availability to patients with MS of these platform therapies through their national health systems varies hugely between countries; available in 96 per cent of the high income countries of the world that took part in the MSIF (2013) survey but not available at all in the poorest countries.

For the richest nations of the world the development of many different kinds of DMDs must appear very positive because it offers neurologists and their patients with RRMS a range of different drugs they can use to try to slow the disease's progress, such that if one does not appear to work or has unacceptable side effects another can be tried (Ward-Abel et al. 2014). However, a cursory reading of the relevant literature reveals a much more troubled and confusing DMD world. First of all it is important to notice that no DMD has yet been licensed for progressive forms of MS, although some compounds such as the Simvastatin have been shown to have positive results in a Phase II clinical trial (Chataway et al. 2014) and others are being actively researched. There had been high hopes for the supposed neuro-protection drug Lamotrigine but it failed to show any beneficial effects compared to placebo in a double-blind phase II trial over a two-year period (Kapoor et al. 2010). Collectively what this implies is that at least half of all PwMS have no DMD to help slow their disease's progress. In reality this proportion must be much higher because existing DMDs are only relevant for early stage RRMS and up to 35 per cent of those who are eligible to take them do not stay on them long term (Nicholas and Wilkie 2011).

The second important issue to broach with respect to these new DMDs is that they all have side effects, the impact of which varies hugely from person to person. Some of these effects such as irritation at injection sites may be mild whereas others can be life-threatening. But, in general the more recent the preparation the more toxic it is likely to be. For example, the first set of DMDs often caused flu like symptoms for the first few weeks of taking them and are usually described as 'well-tolerated', whereas the more recent Natalizumab can release the JC virus to cause the potentially fatal Progressive Multifocal Leukoencephalopathy (PML) infection. By contrast, one of the latest DMDs Fingolimod has the common side effects of headache, liver enzyme increases, influenza, diarrhoea, back pain and cough, plus the rarer possibilities of temporary changes in heart rate, blood pressure, shortages of breath, macular oedema (a swelling in the eye affecting vision) and serious herpes infections (Nicholas and Wilkie 2011). At the very least this all means that PwMS considering embarking on a course of DMDs that may have to be for many years must carry out a detailed and careful risk/benefit assessment with their consultant neurologist taking account of how these likely impacts will fit into the type of life they realistically can hope to live.

There are three other important contentious issues over the use of DMDs that need to be considered: when to start taking DMDs; whether the outcome measures used to assess their impact have any real value; whether under conditions of limited medical resources their use can be justified.

The view expressed so far in this discussion has been that, because damage to myelin and its underlying axons begins early in the MS disease process often at a subclinical level, and because it is the latter process that may lead to permanent disability, DMD therapy should begin as early as possible in individuals presenting with a demyelinating episode. In other words, it should begin when patients present with a Clinically Isolated Syndrome (CIS). As Zajicek et al. (2007, 129) suggest, 'if we want to use drugs acting on the immune system to treat MS, then we will need to intervene at a stage before significant disability has accumulated.' They therefore say it would be 'prudent' to begin at the first event, that is the CIS and thereby the time to any second demyelinating event will be extended, the formation of any new inflammatory plaques will be reduced and the development of definite MS postponed. CIS is seen in this context as a 'window of opportunity' to prevent irreversible CNS damage and disability.

However, by 2010 not all neurologists supported this view, and not even those who agreed that treating CIS patients with beta-interferon would delay a first relapse (Gilmore et al. 2010). This possibility arose because CIS is not synonymous with early MS and a large minority of individuals with such a presentation will either never relapse again or experience infrequent ones. For example, Gilmore et al. (2010, 756) reported on a set of PwMS seen at the NHNN in London in which 18 per cent of those with CIS and abnormal MRI imagery had not converted to confirmed clinical MS after 20 years of monitoring and of the patients with at least 10 brain lesions 35 per cent of whom had minimal disability. Would it have been right to give such individuals 20 years of DMD therapy with all the injections and discomfort involved in the knowledge that 30 per cent and more of them would have gone on to experience only minimal disability? Would it have been acceptable to have expected the state via the NHS to have paid up to £10,000/year for each patient to receive such therapy under conditions of limited financial resources? These are issues society and neurologists must confront, compounded by the knowledge that perhaps 50 per cent of their CIS patients will eventually struggle with future MS and a much smaller proportion will have an absolutely dreadful experience of the disease. But, at the start of the twenty-first century it is simply not possible to differentiate between those who will progress badly with MS without treatment and those who will not? Worse, if patients with CIS began DMD treatment and experienced few subsequent relapses and/or disability, then it would not be known whether this was the result of their therapy or simply the natural evolution of their particular disease. Finally, it could theoretically be possible to justify early DMD therapy if it was known to prevent long-term irreversible disability at a later time. Unfortunately, the evidence does not exist to demonstrate this either. But, there is some persuasive evidence from Canada to suggest it may not (Ebers et al. 2010, Shirani et al. 2012). As a result, it would seem that the remark made by Paty and Ebers in 1998 (p.516) that 'no known treatment for MS significantly alters the long-term outcome of the disease,' may still hold true.

The solution of Gilmore and colleagues to the 'when to treat' conundrum was predicated on the view that significant and permanent disability in MS was caused by the processes of disease progression or neuro-degeneration and not during relapses caused by inflammation and demyelination. Relapses may cause temporary disability but in most cases PwMS recover completely or virtually so from such events. It is the disability caused by the processes of progression that remain and appear to be beyond the body's capacity to repair with its own resources. Relapses therefore, although they may be distressing to experience are to all intents and purposes irrelevant to the acquisition of sustained disability and long-term outcomes. It follows directly therefore that delaying DMD therapy until the first relapse has no detrimental effect on long-term disability. The speed and character of this event, though, may give some insight into the form a person's MS may take and the appropriate DMD to administer. However, such a view raises the important issue of the significance of relapses. Many of the early DMDs were championed on the basis of reducing the number of expected relapses. But, if relapses have little impact on sustained disability does it matter whether DMDs are taken at all? Furthermore, does this imply that many of the early DMD trials were measuring almost irrelevant outcomes or even the wrong outcomes? On both these issues there is no unanimity.

One powerful view at this time would be that DMDs ameliorate relapses 'but have little or no proven effect on progression or long-term disability' (Bennetto et al. 2011, 2) supported by Ebers et al. (2010). Lublin et al. (2003) and Hirst et al. (2008c) would disagree, with Bennetto and colleagues (2011) also attempting a reconciliation based on the different measurement time periods, the way disability was measured, the areas of the CNS affected and the difference between impairment and immobility. But, although the argument continues in the academic literature (Hutchinson 2011), the cautionary view of Giovannoni and colleagues (2011, 335) may be the most prudent counsel at this time that: 'Although many studies have attempted to uncover the relationship between MRI measures, relapses and disability progression, the effect that these endpoints have on one another remains elusive.'

Regarding whether there is any real point in taking DMDs during the early years of MS there is some modest evidence of a benefit from the early two-year Prevention of Relapses and Disability by Interferon beta-1a Subcutaneously in Multiple Sclerosis (PRISMS) trial and its two-year extension study. In the former, those taking interferon did better than those on placebo in terms of the time to 'sustained' progression of one or more EDSS points for more than three months and in the latter those in the 'always-treated' group did best. Additional evidence from the recent clinical trial of Alemtuzumab in which disability actually declined may add weight to this view. In this case 51.6 per cent of patients taking the DMD recorded a decrease in disability over a six month period compared with only 27.2 per cent taking interferon (Coles et al. 2011).

The prime objective of any new DMD therapy must be to try to free a person of their MS, or more realistically expressed as to stop any MS disease activity and thereby prevent the development of disability. However, because MS, as understood so far, is a chronic condition any new therapy would need to work throughout a person's whole life time from diagnosis to death, perhaps over more than 40 years. The testing of such therapies in clinical trials is instantly faced with a number of daunting, if not intractable, challenges to do with their time length and their outcome measures.

Clinical trials are usually relatively short-term experiments of two to three years at the most, not over a life time. And, they can rarely be longer because people leave trials. These 'drop-outs' will include those who wish to start a family, those who find the side-effects too uncomfortable, those who realise they are not on the active therapy from well-known side-effect profiles (*de-facto unblinding*) and those who simply feel that whatever they are on is not doing them any good.

The second clinical trial problem concerns the characteristics of a person's MS that could be measured in the short term for which long-term outcomes are known. Are there any such surrogates? Indeed, the fact that it is not known yet whether any putative short-term measure of DMD performance can be extrapolated indefinitely forms the basis of much serious criticism of many of the early DMD clinical trials (Ebers et al. 2008).

In reality these issues should not have been of great concern because the majority of DMDs tested so far were only ever designed for RRMS during its inflammatory phase, that is, during the first few years of the disease. The idea of projecting their results too far into the future should not have been countenanced.

The outcome measures that have been used in DMD clinical trials fall into three distinct groups:

1. Radiological, based on MRI observation of the number, volume and rate of change of lesions in the CNS, plus measures of brain volume shrinkage or atrophy.
2. Clinical, concerned with the number and annual rate of relapses and the measurement of disability usually in terms of the EDSS.
3. Combined measures of the above.

According to Ebers et al. (2008, 624), the prevention of 'unremitting disability' is the key therapeutic target for DMDs in MS, defined in a similar way by Giovannoni and colleagues (2011, 335): 'to prevent the long-term accumulation of irreversible disability'. But, both these aspirational objectives beg the practical question of how long to wait before a change in disability for the worse may be regarded as long-term and irreversible? According to the first of these groups of authors it must be for at least a year because it is known that relapses may take up to a year to resolve and perhaps even longer. In addition, the decline in disability must be of at least one point on the EDSS because the variation between different researchers using this rubric can be as much as one point (Goodkin et al. 1992). This is a crucial issue because most of these large DMD trials have been international involving many neurology centres and researchers. For example, the Cladribine trial reported in Giovannoni et al. (2011, 332) involved 155 clinics in 32 countries.

In most of these clinical trials the success in terms of disability was not shown by virtue of a reduction in the EDSS score but by a slower rate of growth of the EDSS in the group of PwMS taking the DMD under investigation compared to either placebo or another therapy. The remarkable exception to this situation occurred in the trial of Alemtuzumab in which 'sustained reduction in disability' (SRD) was a defined outcome measure (Coles et al. 2011). In this case, an SRD of one or more EDSS points for six consecutive months (for patients with a baseline EDSS of 2 or more) was achieved in 51.6 per cent of patients taking Alemtuzumab compared to only 27.2 per cent taking an interferon (Coles et al. 2011, 338). Why this took place, however, is not understood.

Following the research of Havrdova et al. (2009) on Natalizumab in the 'AFFIRM' clinical trial, compound or multidimensional output measures have been applied to DMD research to try to show the degree to which they damp down or stop altogether measurable MS disease activity. In this case, absence of clinical disease was defined as no relapses or progression of disability over a given time period, absence of radiological disease activity as no new or enlarging CNS lesions and absence of disease activity as a combination of the two. However, as the number of dimensions of the outcome measure increased the possibility of achieving it reduced. In the material reported by Havrdova et al. (2009, 254), 64 per cent of patients taking Natalizumab were free of clinical disease activity after 2 years compared to 39 per cent on placebo, while 58 per cent were free of radiological evidence of disease activity compared to 14 per cent on placebo. But, in the compound measure only 37 per cent were free of disease activity compared to 7 per cent on placebo.

A similar low proportion of PwMS free from measurable disease activity was discovered from a reworking of the Cladribine trial (CLARITY) evidence involving 1,326 patients. In this case, a measure of 'freedom from disease activity' had three components: no relapses, no sustained increase in EDSS and no new MRI lesions over a given period. At 96 weeks, 44 per cent of PwMS on the low dose of Cladribine remained free from disease activity, 46 per cent on the higher Cladribine dose, but only 16 per cent on placebo (Giovannoni et al. 2011, 332). Thus, although PwMS on Cladribine appeared to be doing much better than those on placebo, the proportion remaining free of disease activity was still less than half at 24 months. Whether this can be regarded as a success remains a moot point.

What has not been considered so far in any of the DMD trials is the opinion of PwMS on what they believe to be the important outcome measures of any DMD clinical trial. It is after all the PwMS who will have to endure the therapies and their possible side effects and, it is they who will have to take the risks of taking part in DMD experimentation in the hope their MS disease activity will be switched off or significantly reduced. This in turn will depend on how they view the likely course of their condition, how quickly it might progress, how their disabilities will proceed and how catastrophic they fear their future may be without pharmacological intervention? It has already been argued that the number of relapses bears little relationship to revealed long-term disability and therefore they may not be a useful outcome measure to adopt. However, for some PwMS relapses may significantly upset their preferred life course and therefore the substantial discomfort and risks with the DMDs that may help to limit them may be acceptable. Other PwMS may be more concerned about approaching the tipping point into secondary progressive MS (SPMS) when any acquired disability is deemed unremitting. This important milestone in a person's MS career seems to have been singularly missing from DMD analyses so far presumably because studies have not been long enough. But, whatever the reason, there seems to have been a lack of concern for the patient's view on what DMD clinical trials should be attempting to achieve, be it in the short or the longer term, that may be construed as an example of expert arrogance in the conduct of therapeutic research. At the very least it runs counter to the aspirations of many current health services for increasing public and patient involvement in medical research and health-care delivery decisions (Petit-Zeman 2010).

There seems little doubt that DMDs in early RRMS can alter the course of the disease for the better or perhaps more accurately slow the disease down relative to what would have happened without it. For example, Bates (2011) states DMDs in RRMS can reduce the relapse rate by 30 per cent. What has been in doubt though is whether the output measures for the clinical trials of these drugs have had any meaning in the long term, whether any short-term gains from taking these drugs were maintained in the longer term or soon forgone and, crucially for the MS community, whether their health-care services will fund them?

Under conditions of limited financial resources health-providing organisations inevitably have to make choices on what treatments to purchase and which ones they will not purchase. In England and Wales

NICE is charged with making recommendations on such matters by focusing on the improvements in the length and quality of life gained by medical and other health-care interventions. This is achieved by calculating the Quality Adjusted Life Years (QALY) gained, the extra years of life gained at a reasonable quality, from new interventions. In addition, such calculations provide a way in which different treatments may be compared using a common standard that in theory at least may provide a fair way of deciding which therapies are best at maintaining and improving life. Then, when the cost of a therapy is known, its cost effectiveness can be calculated per QALY gained. This in turn allows decisions to be made on which treatments produce the greatest good per unit of expenditure. In reality in making such decisions NICE has tended to set a benchmark cost per QALY over which treatments would not be recommended for the NHS to purchase (McCabe et al. 2008). In 2010, for example, this threshold stood at £30,000 per QALY gained (NICE website) above which a therapy would not be regarded as cost effective and therefore under normal circumstances should not be purchased by the NHS.

It is important to remember that a QALY is the outcome of any intervention in terms of the quantity and quality of life it achieves, a measure of the extent of any health gain from a health-care intervention, and is the product of life expectancy and the quality of remaining life-years. Its calculation depends crucially therefore on being able to measure:

1. Life expectancy, the number of years of expected future life.
2. The quality of that life, or its health utility.

Issues of this nature appeared in the cost-effectiveness study of the early DMDs by Chilcott et al. (2003). This paper was an over-condensed description of a simulation of the clinical course, costs and utilities of MS that is best understood if read in conjunction with material on the UK Risk Sharing Scheme by Boggild et al. (2009) and McCabe et al. (2010). Nevertheless, it attempted a comparison between those PwMS taking DMDs and those not taking them that should permit an evaluation of DMD impact. Evidence on the progression of PwMS through the disability stages of the EDSS and their relapses for at least 20 years was obtained from research in Ontario Canada simply because no such relevant UK data existed or indeed still exists. This may raise the question as to whether the non-DMD care given to PwMS in Canada was similar to the equivalent care given in the UK at that time. It also indicated a fundamentally important gap in the UK MS research base that data from the UK Register project may eventually fill. More peculiarly this simulation exercise made the assumption that improvements on the EDSS score, that is disability reducing, were not possible. This may be an acceptable axiom for SPMS, but it seems wrong in this case given most of the drugs assessed were primarily intended for RRMS. And, the reason is a simple one, as its name clearly states the condition remits, spontaneously gets better. Now, the reason for making such an assumption may be a practical one in that to take possible improvements in the EDSS state into account may place an almost intractable additional evidential demand on the analysis, but not to do so ignored the very essence of the condition.

The quality of life evidence in terms of the EQ-5D instrument for the Chilcott et al. (2003) assessment was supplied by the MS Trust from 1,532 PwMS who had taken part in an earlier survey (Hemmett et al. 2004). As was noted in the previous chapter this work cannot be regarded as representative of PwMS in the UK because it was a self-selecting survey and almost certainly biased towards older people with MS, those with above average disability and perhaps the educated aggrieved, that is those unlikely to be taking DMDs for early RRMS. Some of the analysis was difficult to comprehend too because of data withheld from publication because of commercial confidentiality. Furthermore, it cannot be thought of as representative of people with RRMS either, the main target group of the treatments being assessed, for similar reasons. For example, the mean age of the 1,554 respondents to this survey was 51.6 years (Hemmett et al. 2004, 673) much higher than the median age of the eligible and treated people with RRMS under the Risk Sharing Scheme of 38 years (Boggild et al. 2009, 5). Now, mean and median may be two different measures of central tendency but in this case they are wide enough apart to suggest real differences in the populations from which they came.

In the previous chapter the usefulness of the EQ-5D measure was questioned as a device for the MS case not least because it failed to take into account disease impacts of direct concern to PwMS such as fatigue (Hemmett et al. 2004). It may not be at all clear what impacts these problematic issues may have had on the cost-effectiveness calculations for DMD use in MS, but at the very least they suggest that the published assessments so far may not be as robust as their authors and NICE would seem to believe, a problem that Manouchehrinia and Constantinescu (2012) demonstrate was common throughout the world. They may have been the best that could have been achieved at the time, but they were a long way from being good enough to make important health-resource allocation decisions.

The use of DMDs to treat MS produces definite benefits in the short term but such gains are infrequent and it is unclear to what degree they are sustained in the longer term. Thus, they produce small quality of life gains to begin with that may increase through time to be more substantial. The cost effectiveness of DMDs, therefore, will increase with the length of the time horizon of their use. Unfortunately, reliable knowledge on the impact of DMDs in the longer term now and certainly when the first cost-effectiveness studies were carried out was scarce. Perversely, therefore the nearer in time DMDs appeared to becoming cost-effective the less reliable the evidence on which to make such a judgement became.

The pivotal cost-effectiveness study by Chilcott et al. (2003) calculated the cost/QALY gained in the range of £42,000 to £98,000 over a 20-year time frame, with commercial estimates quoted in the text (p.425) in the range of £35,000 to £104,000/QALY gained. These results therefore tended to confirm the high costs of interferon beta offered in earlier studies by Parkin et al. (1998 and 2000, 148) of £74,500/QALY all under the most favourable of assumptions. It follows directly from these results that NICE was never able to recommend the use of the early DMDs for the treatment of MS in the NHS as witnessed by their formal appraisal (NICE 2002). The knowledge of this impending decision generated vigorous political lobbying and protests by MS patient groups in the belief that the DMDs actually worked but were considered too expensive. This resulted in a political compromise: the Risk Sharing Scheme. Under the terms of this agreement the drugs would be made available to NHS patients in the context of a 10-year monitoring exercise: 'coverage with evidence development'. If the observed benefit was less than predicted by the NICE model (Chilcott et al. 2003), or by the DMD manufacturers, then their price would be reduced to a target cost-effectiveness of £36,000/QALY gained (McCabe et al. 2010).

The monitoring exercise was designed in particular to try to resolve two major uncertainties in DMD analysis so far:

1. Whether results from clinical trials of two to three years in length could be reliably extrapolated over a longer period.
2. Whether patients who stopped treatment retained any benefits beyond that point, with the disease progressing in line with that expected of untreated patients, or whether there was a rebound effect after cessation of treatment.

Patients began to be recruited into the scheme in May 2002 in 70 neurology centres across the UK. By April 2005 they numbered 5,583, believed to be 80 per cent of all patients with MS starting treatment during that time (Boggild et al. 2009, 8). Unfortunately, the first review of the evidence produced by the Risk Sharing Scheme monitoring (Boggild et al. 2009) did not support the case for the use of the early phase DMDs for the treatment of MS; they were not cost effective. Indeed, disability increased by 113 per cent among the treated patients, at a faster rate than among the comparator cohort of patients who did not receive treatment. With the usual caveats about the possible unrepresentativeness of these results, they must suggest at the very least that the cost of DMDs to the NHS should be reduced. At worst it may question the use of these DMDs altogether, to ask whether they were another example of the over-zealous prescribing of extremely expensive and profitable drugs that have little value in improving the health of those who take them.[2]

The evidence collected in this research could also have permitted a view on which, if any, of the four DMDs included performed best. There have already been major inquiries into the different impacts of these compounds such as the REGARD (Rebif vs Galtiramir Acetate in Relapsing MS Disease) and BEYOND (Betaferon Efficacy Yielding Outcomes of a New Dose) trials, but all were found clinically to do the same thing. What is not known, though, is whether their cost effectiveness differs in the UK. Unfortunately, the research design of the Risk Sharing Scheme was not set up to test this issue. But, not to have done so was almost certainly a disservice to both PwMS and the principal funder of their care in the UK, the NHS, even if for clear commercial reasons it would have been naïve to have ever expected it to happen.

Despite these misgivings there have been at least two very positive outcomes of DMD therapy and the Risk Sharing Scheme. First, DMD therapy will have stopped many relapses from taking place that, even if of relatively short duration, can be disabling, uncomfortable, frightening and life-style threatening to experience. Second, it should also be remembered that the Risk Sharing Scheme through the need to help PwMS self-inject their medication encouraged the growth of an infrastructure of MS nurses and neurology centres that have benefitted all people with the condition. But, given the increasingly constrained budget of the NHS in the future there is a huge opportunity cost involved in continuing the scheme with the annual drugs bill alone estimated at £50 million (McCabe et al. 2010). What other conditions that could have produced relatively high QALY gains may have been denied funding because of this expenditure on PwMS? Of course, no one will ever know, but it is a sobering thought to ponder that there may have been some. This should not be a reason for despair, rather it should be a motivation to question a resource allocation system dependent on arbitrary benchmarks and inadequate evidence; a system that treats QALYs equally but not people; a system that lacks political legitimacy because of its elitist arcane procedures that produce invidious comparisons between different therapies. The QALY system adopted by NICE is not the only way of making decisions on allocating scarce medical resources. There are many others of worth that were usefully introduced by Persad et al. (2009) although a discussion of them is beyond the scope of this analysis.

One final point is also worth making. It must be particularly confusing for PwMS to discover that the same DMD can be assessed differently in different countries despite access to the same experimental evidence and all contributing to the same international clinical trials. For example, Fingolimod was approved as a front-line therapy for RRMS in the United States (US), Switzerland and Australia but in Canada and in much of Europe has only been approved for use in patients who have not responded to existing front-line DMDs and whose MS is highly active. By contrast, Cladribine received a licence to be a front-line DMD for MS in Australia and Russia but not in the US or in the European Union. And, in 2013 the US Food and Drug Administration rejected Alemtuzumab for use in RRMS yet it was approved in the European Union, Canada, Australia and Mexico (Coles and Compston 2014). In some cases the reasons for these inconsistencies of appraisal lie in differing assessments of the long-term safety of the latest DMDs for which there is as yet little evidence simply because their drug trials lasted no more than three years. For example, in the case of Cladribine the particular worry lay with cancers and therefore the Australian regulatory authority restricted its use to just a two-year period. But, it must be remembered that the potentially fatal infection PML released by Natalizumab only became apparent years after the drug had received widespread international approval. It is not surprising, therefore, that some regulatory authorities are more cautious than others about granting licenses to new DMDs for MS. However, in the case of Alemtuzumab the issue seems to lie in an argument over appropriate research methodology. How is it possible for a methodology to be acceptable in one part of the world but not in another? For a potentially important life changing drug such an issue should not have been allowed to develop.

Unfortunately, these international inconsistencies in drug licensing may have a number of serious consequences for the MS community. First, and most importantly PwMS may be unnecessarily denied access to drugs that may limit their disability status and progression. Including more PwMS in the risk/benefit calculations for these new compounds might help to overcome this issue. Second, it may help to reinforce an already uneven international geography of access to DMDs for MS. Finally, it may lead to pharmaceutical companies only developing those drugs for which regulatory approval will be easiest to secure. If not it may lead to the cost of the drugs that are approved rising to cover the development costs of those that are not (Lancet Neurology Editorial 2011b, 491). More generally perhaps all this evidence demonstrates a brutal reality about most DMD clinical trials to date and especially about the early ones; not enough was known about the disease processes at work to specify clinically meaningful outcome measures or effective surrogates. More generously, this may be viewed as a sign that much of this work is at the cutting edge of neuro-science, fundamentally exploratory and therefore inevitably to involve mistakes and disappointments.

7.4.3 Complementary and alternative medicine

Complementary and Alternative Medicine (CAM) is a wide-ranging topic that includes many different techniques and therapies: biological (e.g., diets, hyperbaric oxygen); mind-body (e.g., hypnosis, meditation); manipulative (e.g., reflexology, massage); alternative medical systems (e.g., homeopathy, Chinese medicine); energy techniques (e.g., magnets, therapeutic touch) (Bowling 2007, 7). The available evidence on the effectiveness of many of these techniques generally and for the treatment of MS in particular varies hugely in both quantity and quality. Nevertheless, they are used enthusiastically by many PwMS around the world and, although their mechanisms and reasons for working may be uncertain or even wholly unknown, it is clear that for many individuals they appear to have a positive effect in relieving suffering. Now, even if this effect is some form of placebo or a form of therapeutic alliance, the effect of being in the presence of a positive empathic individual, the formal medical profession appears increasingly to be willing to consider such interventions. Some advocates of CAM see them as a positive complement to conventional medicine in which both are undertaken, while others see CAM as a definite alternative to conventional therapy. The latter may be when conventional medicine has failed to ease their suffering or when a decision has been made to take a 'drug-free' approach to self-treatment (Graham 2010, 2).

According to Bowling (2007, 9) between 50 and 80 per cent of PwMS in the US regularly use CAM, with the proportion perhaps being as high as 90 per cent in Germany and 36 per cent in Italy, although the definitions of CAM and the time periods considered varied between countries (Esmonde and Long 2008, 177). For the UK there is no such general evidence with only two small-scale surveys giving some insight into this issue. The first of these by Esmonde and Long (2008) made use of a questionnaire distributed among attendees at the biennial meeting of the MS Trust in April 2006 from which 138 completed responses were received. These revealed that 84 per cent had made use of CAM within the last year, with the six most popular therapies being reflexology, massage, yoga, relaxation and meditation, acupuncture and aromatherapy (Esmonde and Long 2008, 178). Interestingly, although between 25 and 40 per cent of respondents rated each of the top six therapies as 'extremely helpful', acupuncture received the least favourable response with 18 per cent of those who had used the therapy regarding it as 'not at all helpful'. Unfortunately, there were no discernible differences between the people using the six top therapies to explain their responses. Nevertheless, there was general agreement across all six main therapies that the most common benefit from them was 'relaxation' with 'empowerment', the ability to be proactive and take control of your own health care, being an important secondary benefit noted in a follow-up workshop session.

The second UK survey on CAM and self-treatment concerned a questionnaire sent to 318 PwMS in a set of randomly selected GP practices by Somerset and colleagues (2001) in which it was shown that during the 12 months before being contacted nearly half of the sample had taken oil of primrose, 37 per cent multivitamins, 18 per cent had tried a special diet, 5 per cent hyperbaric oxygen, 5 per cent homeopathy, 3 per cent sunflower seed emulsion and the use of cannabis was acknowledged by 8.0 per cent (Somerset et al. 2001, 34). Meanwhile, in terms of therapists consulted, 7 per cent had made use of an aromatherapist, 7 per cent a reflexologist, 6 per cent a masseur, 3 per cent a hypnotherapist all of which in the majority of cases were deemed to be helpful (Somerset et al. 2001, 35). What is more, 27 per cent of the respondents said they would like more advice and information about CAM.

The taking of cannabis usually by smoking is often linked to MS for the relief of pain and spasticity although it is not known how common the practice may be; a situation that is likely to persist because of its questionable and variable legality. In addition, according to Ashfield (2005) there was little agreement among experts as to its efficacy or safety with worrying stories of cannabis use being linked to pulmonary disease and psychotic disorders. Again a situation that is unlikely to be resolved soon even with the research of Zajicek and colleagues (2003 and 2012) whose clinical trials have moved from initial disappointment to much more promising results, because of the many different forms in which cannabis can be prepared, purchased and consumed. What cannabis use by PwMS does present, however, is a series of worrying ethical and legal dilemmas for the medical staff responsible for their care.

What has been presented so far cannot be viewed as positive evidence for the significant use of CAM in the UK in the early twenty-first century. The Esmonde and Long (2008) analysis must suffer from a worrying degree of selection bias, in that people with positive views about CAM would have been much more likely to take part in their survey than those who did not. And, the evidence on CAM in the Somerset et al. (2001) research was a minor element of a much broader quality of life study. But, CAM may have been used much more frequently in the recent past because Elian and Dean (1983, 1093) for the early 1980s reported 'the widespread resort by multiple sclerosis patients to alternative medical practitioners.' Furthermore, although the precise importance of CAM to the health care of PwMS cannot be precisely quantified, the fact that it is important can be inferred from three different sources. First, and perhaps most importantly, from the 13,000 PwMS in the UK who have joined one of the 57 MS Therapy Centres in the UK and the Republic of Ireland according to their federation the MS National Therapy Centres. The second indication of importance comes from the recent growth of self-care books, the regular featuring of CAM in popular MS magazines such *as New Pathways* and the production of information publications on the subject by the MS Society, the MS Trust and the MSRC (now MS-UK). Meanwhile, the third significant indication of CAM's importance in the UK comes from its formal recognition in the NICE (2003, 28–9) guidelines for the management of MS in primary and secondary care where they were viewed as complementary to and definitely not as complete alternatives to conventional therapies.

Almost by definition CAM therapies are on the margins of acceptance by the medical establishment. Some do go on to be shown to be beneficial such as cannabis and vitamin D whereas others such as the Cari Loder treatment and hyperbaric oxygen do not. However, this is not to argue that PwMS have not and will not in the future benefit in other ways from some of even these impotent treatments. Although they may have next to no impact on the MS disease process or impact on some of its symptoms they may well have significantly positive psychological, social and community gains. As Bowling (2007, 13) perceptively comments quoting from a personal story of someone taking CAM to help cope with cancer: 'Uncertain hope was better than hopeless certainty'. Nevertheless, these therapies in the penumbra of formal medical acceptance are ripe for exploitation by deluded physicians, quacks and crooks to offer procedures and treatments to the MS community with the tantalising promise of symptom relief or even a cure. Unfortunately, some PwMS have been so concerned about their current health and future prospects that they have been prepared to pay large sums of money and travel huge distances to take a chance on these new 'wonder' treatments despite the potentially huge health risks involved. Two recent therapies for MS that in some instances may fall into this category are stem cell therapy and the Liberation treatment for CCSVI. These are now considered in more detail.

Stem cell therapy offers great promise for the future (Rice et al. 2013), but at the moment must be regarded as experimental with many of the basic elements of the approach such as the type of stem cells to use, at what dose and how to deliver them into the body still to be decided for any element of the MS disease process. Thus, it is outrageous for clinics and physicians to be able to offer such therapies in the early part of the twenty-first century to PwMS with confidence and safety.

PwMS will probably have heard of the ground-breaking research in Chicago and Sydney on people with very aggressive disease and poor prognoses who may have had their immune systems favourably re-engineered using their own bone marrow stem cells. They have also possibly heard that stem cells may be employed to repair damaged myelin; perhaps in the longer term even fix broken nerve fibres to return parts of their body to long-denied cerebral contact. PwMS will almost certainly have also seen on the TV stories of people apparently 'cured' of their affliction by stem cell injections in far-away clinics in Costa Rica, China and Russia, encouraging a new form of medical tourism (Barclay 2009), and perhaps experienced first-hand the sophisticated and persuasive marketing for such procedures. The media hyperbole for this kind of therapy has been strong and the coverage in the more popular press enthusiastic. Who could not have been impressed by the seemingly miraculous results claimed by Canon Andrew White in *New Pathways* (2009, Issue 54, 26–7) who said he felt different 'within a matter of hours' after his stem cell session in a clinic in Baghdad and then in the following issue (*New Pathways* 2009, 55, 17) reported on a man with MS who could now walk more than a 100 metres having not been able to do so at all for 10 years.[3] Another good example can be seen in the MS Matters Magazine for Jan/Feb 2009, Issue 83. Here it is reported on page five that the UK government backs the MS Society's warning over rogue stem cell therapies including one operating from the Seychelles, offering false hope and no supporting evidence. Interestingly on the same page the first positive results from a real stem cell therapy on 21 people with MS in Chicago is reported that involved taking bone marrow cells, freezing them and hitting them hard with drugs to destroy the immune cells that cause damage and then transplanting them back into the body. It is easy to see how the unwary might be able to conclude that 'there must be something in this stem cell stuff that may be worth a punt?'

Hopes are therefore high that stem cell therapies will solve some of the medical difficulties PwMS struggle with on a daily basis. But, what is the scientific reality behind this stem cell enthusiasm? Can stem cell therapy really begin to cure MS now or at any time in the not-too-distant future? Tragically in this case it would appear hype and hope have conspired to give a massively unrealistic picture.

Towards the end of the first decade of the twenty-first century the scientific community became very concerned about the growth of unregulated stem cell therapies for MS and the lack of understanding among themselves about the state of knowledge of such activity. As a result a 'Consensus' meeting took place in London on 19 May 2009 attended by 27 experts from 7 different countries along with a number of patient-group representatives. From this meeting two different publications were produced, one for the scientific community and another for PwMS (MS Society 2010b) better to understand stem cell therapy and its future prospects.

The first practical point to emphasise from this work is that at that time in mid-2009 there were no properly licensed stem cell therapies for MS anywhere in the world. Two completely contrasting approaches to therapy were, however, available. First, there was therapy development based on meticulous, but unfortunately slow, progress in a highly complex area of biological science in which clinical trials for some novel stem cell therapies were only just beginning. These were for small numbers of patients with very specific MS characteristics. If successful such therapies will then need to be approved by national licensing authorities before health services can agree to purchase them. All these processes take an agonisingly long time. It is therefore most likely that very few people should expect to be able to receive stem cell therapy for their MS as a routine procedure from their national health systems for a considerable period. This does not, however, deny the possibility of a few individuals being enlisted onto clinical trials, nor, if early clinical work proves stunningly successful, many more benefiting from 'off license' therapies or the fast-tracking of approval. In this regard the experience of Stella Thornley undergoing haematropic stem cell transplantation to try to treat her highly active RRMS, in the injections with unpleasant side-effects and the chemotherapy she had to endure to make the harvesting of her own stem cells possible and then their re-implantation after manipulation into her own body, is a salutary reminder of just how complex, dangerous and uncomfortable such therapy can be (*New Pathways* July/August 2011, Issue 68, 17–20; *New Pathways* September/October 2011, Issue 69, 14–5) especially since by the March/April Issue of *New Pathways* 2012 the article about her treatment was entitled 'Stop the ride- I want to get off!'

The second available approach to stem cell therapy for MS is through scientifically unproven methods. These are available from two different sources. First, there have been pills and potions purporting 'to maintain healthy stem cell physiology' and thereby encourage them to go and repair damaged tissue of many different kinds. These products will not be named here but they benefit from being often classified officially as foodstuffs not medicines and therefore can be sold without proof of their supposed efficacy. Then there are the unregulated and expensive clinics in various parts of the world offering unproven therapies that carry a high degree of personal risk. These establishments may not have actually killed anyone yet but it is probably only a matter of time before they do; they have certainly been responsible for tumours, serious infections and huge disappointment (ISSCR 2008, Barclay 2009, Scolding 2009). Refreshingly too, there now seems to be an increasing number of PwMS prepared to admit that after undergoing such practices no obvious benefit took place. For example, Vicci Chittenden from Maidstone spent £3,000 at a Rotterdam clinic for stem cell therapy that made no difference to her MS (Wark 2009). But, many people have claimed stem cell therapy has improved their condition. Why can their 'anecdotal' evidence not be accepted? There are many possible reasons why people may have claimed stem cell therapy worked for them:

1. Dishonesty, always a possibility when financial gain may be involved. For example, Dr Robert Trossel who practised in both London and Rotterdam was exposed as improperly offering stem cells not designed for human use to MS patients and banned from practising medicine in the UK (*New Pathways* Issue 61, May/June 2010, 8; MS Matters November/December 2010, Issue 94, 26–9).
2. People wanted to believe that the therapy would work, they convinced themselves it had.
3. Placebo effect. Doing something for a patient is nearly always better psychologically for them than doing nothing. Thus, any form of

therapy no matter how benign can often make people feel better in the short term. It does not mean it has altered the course of their disease in any way.
4. Spontaneous remission. This is always a possibility in early stage (relapsing remitting) MS and is a real problem in assessing the impact of any MS therapy. It is one of the reasons why carefully planned clinical trials must be carried out for all MS therapies.
5. An unknown effect.
6. Any combination of the above.

When stem cells are transplanted into a patient with MS it may take several weeks, if not months, for them to reach the damaged parts of the nervous system and then multiply into sufficient numbers either to begin the repair process or to start to remodel the immune system (ISSCR 2008, Scolding 2009). It is for this reason that the claims from some unlicensed clinics of the rapid success for their brand of stem cell therapy appear unreasonable, if not perverse. If the process was going to work therefore it would need much more time. In addition, if any of these clinics regularly recorded consistently positive and enduring results their therapies would be rapidly lauded around the world; the fact this has not happened demonstrates their results have been poor! These clinics peddle hope and despair not care and cure.

The 'Liberation' treatment for chronic cerebrospinal venous insufficiency

The chronic cerebrospinal venous insufficiency (CCSVI) hypothesis of MS causation by Zamboni and colleagues (2009) offers an unorthodox view on the possible cause of MS that leads directly to a very different remedial therapy (Rhodes 2011). The traditional view of an MS lesion has it centred on a small blood vessel through which the inflammatory cells enter the CNS to attack the myelin sheath depositing iron in the process. Zamboni et al. (2009) suggested alternatively that iron deposition could be caused by back-pressure in the venous system due to restricted outflow through the large veins from the brain and spinal cord. And, it was the iron that attracted the inflammation resulting in demyelination. If true the vascular problem could be overcome by surgically widening the veins leaving the brain and spinal cord by inserting a balloon or a stent. This process, that has become to be known evocatively as the 'Liberation' process, is not a trivial matter because it involves feeding a catheter from a vein in the groin through the heart to the veins in the neck or by direct surgery on the neck. The research that has been undertaken in this field so far certainly shows that some

PwMS, and it may be a large proportion, have a narrowing of the main veins in the neck and spine, and there was some evidence of abnormal blood flow in some of them, but it has been far from a consistent finding across all those investigated (del Pilar Cortes Nino et al. 2010, Filippi and Rocca 2011).

The reaction of the neurological establishment to this new theory of MS causation and therapy was unenthusiastic, nicely encapsulated in the somewhat despairing title of a review paper on the subject by Qiu (2010) in the *Lancet Neurology*: 'Venous abnormalities and multiple sclerosis: another breakthrough claim?' and directly equating it with the exaggerated assertions for hyperbaric oxygen therapy in the 1980s. They pointed out that the narrowing of the blood vessels in the neck was a common phenomenon in people both with and without a neurological disease and that the head and neck had a surfeit of blood vessels such that a restriction in one of them need not constitute a problem at all. It has also been suggested that even if a positive and consistent association between CCSVI and MS was discovered it would not at all be clear in which way causation may lie. Did CCSVI cause MS or could CCSVI be a consequence of having MS? Finally, the practical problems of keeping stents in place for the long term in a very flexible part of the body have been raised, especially given Stanford stopped carrying out the procedure after a stent moved to the heart of one patient necessitating open heart surgery and another haemorrhaged to death.[4] At the very least it was argued that these issues needed to be resolved through careful research before any therapeutic actions could be recommended. It is now clear, however, that CCSVI is neither specific to MS nor has a causative role (Friedmann and Wattjes 2013).

The response of many PwMS around the world was very different. Powered often through electronic social media Liberation lobby groups were established in many western countries demanding that both their support charities and national governments fund CCSVI research, with some success. For example, the National MS Society in the US and the MS Society in Canada jointly sponsored a $2.4 million investment in seven research projects on the relationship between CCSVI and MS to report in 2012 (MS Trust website). In the UK the response was less vigorous with a petition to Downing Street, an international conference, 'CCSVI – the Way Forward', in Glasgow in October 2010 and a review meeting at the MS Society's UK HQ in May 2010. What this generated was a willingness to fund promising research projects into the hypothesis accompanied by a warning that until the idea was demonstrated to be true and remedial surgery safe the NHS would most certainly not fund either the investigatory procedure or the surgery if CCSVI was shown to be present. Nevertheless, because of the refusal of national health services around the world to recognise the veracity of the CCSVI procedures and the demand for any possible new remedial therapies by relatively well-off PwMS in the west, a private market for CCSVI testing and treatment developed such that in 2010 clinics were offering the procedures in the UK, Republic of Ireland, Poland, Italy, Bulgaria, Costa Rica, Australia, Jordan, India, Slovenia, Greece, Germany, Belgium, the US and Canada (Cook 2010) to which was added Malta and Kuwait in 2012. In addition, according to the *New Pathways* Magazine (Issue 72, March/April 2012, 17) more than 300 liberation procedures had been performed through the Essential Health Clinic in Glasgow by the end of 2011.

7.4.4 Vocational rehabilitation

In the discerning review essay by Simmons (2010) on 'life issues in MS' the benefits of work and employment in general and for PwMS in particular were clearly set out. Work establishes identity, creates a sense of self-worth and offers an opportunity for social interaction. What is more, as has been shown from a longitudinal study of members of the British household panel study between 1991 and 2001, if it is carried out in a healthy environment work reduces the chances of people becoming ill (Bartley et al. 2004). By contrast, if people lack work or have to carry it out in an unpleasant environment, then work can increase the risks of both physical and especially mental ill-health. Finally, paid work may bestow financial independence, reducing the need for any support from the state and the intrusion of its institutions into peoples' lives through, for example the claiming of means-tested benefits. Yet, a clear finding from many countries around the world is that PwMS experience higher rates of unemployment than the general populations of which they are part (Sweetland et al. 2012). Why should this be so given the clear benefits of work? What are the factors that lead to PwMS apparently leaving employment relatively early in life or what inhibits them from maintaining their employment? And, what are the barriers that reduce their chances of re-entering the labour force once they have left?

According to the extensive systematic review by Sweetland et al. (2012) of mainly small-scale qualitative research projects two sets of important factors appear to interact to disadvantage PwMS in the workplace:

1. The way MS affects the individual, or disease factors.

2. The social and workplace environments in which PwMS must attempt to function.

For example, from interviews with 100 PwMS between 18 and 65 years of age selected consecutively when attending the NHNN who all were in employment or education when diagnosed, the issues that had most impact on their ability to work were their handwriting or fine motor skills (26%), fatigue (28%), balance (40%) and walking difficulties (45%) (O'Connor et al. 2005, 894). In addition, there were two important environmental barriers to carrying out their employment in terms of the physical access to their work (39%) and their journey to and from work (48%). Furthermore, despite the clear benefits of employment only one fifth of these PwMS had received any formal vocational advice on work retention or return. Finally, it is important to observe that this was an urban-based cohort of people who could attend a large hospital in central London, and although we are not given any evidence on the sorts of jobs these people undertook they would most likely have been white collar ones dependent on sitting down for long periods of time. In more rural locations where more manual occupations are to be found and the ability to walk much more important MS would probably have had a much greater impact of job security.

But, for those PwMS who left work because of the effects of their MS, what factors or developments would have allowed them to stay on? According to a major international study by MSIF (2010) with more than 7,500 responses from 125 countries the main elements would have been

1. Flexible working.
2. Scheduled work breaks with a place to rest.
3. Improved awareness of MS among colleagues.
4. Increased support from both employers and colleagues.

This review while stating that fatigue (85%) and mobility problems (72%) were the two most important issues that prevented PwMS staying in work, it also listed the following principal factors that enabled the employment of PwMS.

1. Stable MS.
2. Medication for symptom treatment.
3. Seated work.
4. Flexible working hours.

Thus, the employment chances of people with progressive forms of MS would appear to be most severely compromised. This report goes on to emphasise that in general there were a number of other conditions too that enabled PwMS to retain and return to paid employment, most importantly the support of the people around them, their family, employers and fellow employees. Without their understanding, work becomes permanently stressful and wholly unrewarding as an opportunity for social interaction.

Sweetland and colleagues (2007) attempted to take the employment of PwMS further by trying to define an appropriate vocational rehabilitation service for them through 4 focus groups with 24 ambulant people with RRMS. These individuals emphasised two key needs, managing performance and managing expectations. The former would involve attempting to affect changes that would enable them to maintain their employment by treating their symptoms, changing their working environment and altering the demands of their jobs. The latter, by contrast, involved trying to moderate the expectations of both themselves and especially their employers that realistically would lead to fewer hours worked and a diminished or different output. However, the latter is crucially dependent on the PwMS disclosing their condition to their employers and work colleagues, and as soon as possible, so that plans can be put in place to cope with the almost inevitable changes MS will bring. This in turn raises the issue of possible discrimination, direct or indirect, bullying and even pressure to leave. Disclosure therefore could be viewed as a high risk strategy in a society and employment environment that is often unsupportive. In these areas the PwMS felt they needed help in developing advocacy skills and a much better knowledge of their legal position. But, according to Townsend (2008) from research with occupational therapists, it is in attempting to maintain the employment of PwMS already in work that is crucial, because this is a great deal easier than trying to help PwMS back into employment once they have left. From a practical perspective what is also needed is the testing of the different forms of delivering vocational rehabilitation to discover which is most efficacious.

7.4.5 An MS-care research miscellany

The Diagnosis. Receiving a diagnosis of MS has been associated with four significant concerns. First, the insensitive way in which it is too often been given, in a rushed clinic, by phone or letter, by a junior doctor, with the once common practice of telling a close relative first rather than the PwMS (Robinson 1988, 50) now reserved for special cases.

Second, the length of time it can take to secure a formal MS diagnosis, from 12 months to 30 years (Edwards et al. 2008, Maw 2011) with all the anxiety that may engender. Third, the problems of securing the appropriate information in the right quantity at the right time (Robinson et al. 1996, 76; Johnson 2003, 55; Edwards et al. 2008, 462) and, finally the understandable possible emotional responses to being given a diagnosis of an incurable progressive disease such as MS (Johnson 2003, Burgess 2010b), of perhaps anger, sorrow and fear, all sensitively reviewed by Benz and Reynolds (2005).

Once the MS diagnosis has been confirmed a further issue needs to be confronted, who to tell? Some such as the novelist MJ Hyland (2012) initially tried to keep their MS a secret from as many people as possible because in her case it made her feel a failure, too close to how she viewed her inadequate family, hiding her symptoms by saying she had an ingrowing toenail or a climbing accident. Similarly, Gill Green (2009, viii–ix), a professor of sociology at Essex University, decided not to wear her diagnosis in public and initially only tell her immediate family and friends because she may need their support. She did not want to be labelled sick, or as 'the one with MS', or a tragic case and, because her MS had so far taken a benign trajectory she did not want to be viewed as a fraud. And, finally, she did not want to be regarded as a 'poor bet' for the future with the implications that may have for her career; an issue many PwMS in work may agonise over for some time.

MS Nurses. Since their initial introduction in Canada in the 1970s MS specialist nurses have played an increasingly important role in the care of PwMS in many parts of the world. Their main reason for existence initially was to help their patients self-inject with the new DMDs but since then research has demonstrated how their role has become increasingly complex in three distinct ways. First, the range of care needs for which they may be responsible has increased (Porter and Keenan 2003, Gutteridge 2006, Corry et al. 2011) with While et al. (2009) identifying 39 ranging from relapse management to emotional support. Second, the settings in which they carry out their activities can vary from a clinic in an acute hospital neurology unit to undertaking house calls in a community setting or any combination of the two. And, third the case load may be extremely high (Johnson et al. 2001a, Ward-Abel et al. 2010) varying according to the UK National Audit Office (2011, 36) from 220 in the East of England Strategic Health Authority (SHA) to 650 in the North West SHA. But, at the same time these posts have become under threat from financial restraint and attempts at amalgamating them into general neurological nurses.

Research effort has therefore become increasingly focussed on demonstrating that MS nurses make a positive contribution to the care of PwMS in three different ways. First, it has been shown that MS nurses are held in high regard by their client group and receive a very positive appraisal from them (Ward-Abel et al. 2010, Heinonen and Dorning 2011). Second, it has been shown that MS nurses have been successful at specific aspects of patient care such as for example, cutting expected GP and hospital referrals, preventing complications such as pressure ulcers and helping PwMS become more responsible for their own care; in other words demonstrating MS nurses are cost effective (Gutteridge 2006, Warner et al. 2005, Johnson et al. 2001b, Mynors et al. 2012). However, third, attempts at a major evaluation of MS nursing practice by comparing places that had recently appointed MS nurse with those that did not have been far from convincing (Forbes et al. 2006a). Nevertheless, according to Mynors and colleagues (2012, 23) empirical evidence on how MS nurses improve patient care is weak and that in order to promote their case for support they need to be more proactive in collecting evidence of what they do, the standards to which they adhere and the experience of their patients.

Self-help courses. Given the necessity of PwMS in the recent past to look after themselves with the help of relatives and friends because formal medicine had little to offer them it would be reasonable to expect them to be ideal candidates for self-help programmes such as the Expert Patients Programme in the England (Expert Patients Programme/Community Interest Company, undated) and 'Getting to Grips with MS' type courses as offered by many MS Society chapters and branches. Indeed, they have often been enthusiastic attendees. This has led directly to problems with demonstrating a positive impact of such courses for two related reasons. First, because many of the attendees had already taken part in similar courses and second because as a result they were already effective self- managers. These courses therefore were preaching to the converted. Thus, any measurable increase in the abilities of attendees as a result of a course would be small. In fact many PwMS saw such courses simply as a way of topping up their existing skills (Barlow et al. 2009a). Nevertheless, research in this field did demonstrate a gender difference in the reasons for attending a self-help course: men primarily for information gathering; women for reassurance through interaction with other people in a similar situation (Barlow et al. 2009b, Chaplin et al. 2012). But, a note of caution was also added regarding the self-advocacy objective of these courses because of the presence of cognitive impairment, of memory, concentration and lack of insight in a large minority of PwMS that could make them unsuitable to be their own advocates. Thus, a policy of self-advocacy, especially in terms of symptom management may not be applied to the majority of PwMS (Wade and Green 2001, 65; Zajicek et al. 2007, 176).

Rehabilitation. Rehabilitation is concerned with interventions that help people maintain physical, emotional and social health (Thompson 2005, Walton 2009) and regarded as a necessary component of quality health care for PwMS (Kraft et al. 2008). As such for any particular person with MS it is an evolving process that may cover a large range of different therapies and procedures over their life time. Delivering a rehabilitation service therefore will involve a range of different specialists, including physiotherapists, continence advisers, occupational therapists and neuro-psychologists (Rossiter and Thompson 1995) that may exist as a multidisciplinary team in an acute hospital in a large urban area. But, elsewhere it may be extremely challenging to assemble and may require the patient to visit a number of different sites for effective treatment. Research in this area of medicine has proved extremely challenging for many reasons (Kraft et al. 2008, Khan et al. 2008). These must include heterogeneous MS populations, difficulties of measuring interventions and their outcomes, patient attrition, control group specification and defining an appropriate study or follow-up time period. Nevertheless, there have been a number of attempts to assess the importance of a rehabilitation service with its bundle of interventions compared to 'standard care'. This has shown that when PwMS have been subjected to a consolidated rehabilitation programme then positive outputs have been observed in disability, motor functioning, emotional wellbeing and quality of life compared to controls (Craig et al. 2003) and that this was even true for seriously disabled people too (Freeman et al. 1999). But, it was not so convincing in a randomised wait-list controlled study in Melbourne where although improvements in disability and motor function were better than in the control group, no difference was found in quality of life measures. This may have been because, as Kraft et al. (2008) have suggested, much better outcome measures are required in this area of research. However, the gains from such programmes of rehabilitation were limited in time; lost in less than a year unless associated with a good on-going community care and regular top-up sessions (Freeman et al. 1999); perhaps an unrealistic aspiration in places where funding is limited and rehabilitation capacity in short supply.

Palliative care. Palliative care techniques in their concern for symptom control, psychological wellbeing and end-of-life issues (Plumb

2006) may be of help in relieving the suffering of significantly disabled PwMS of say EDSS 8 and above. Such a view was tested through a set of research projects in South East London during the first decade of the twenty-first century (Higginson and Hart 2006, Edmonds et al. 2007a and 2007b) that culminated in a phase II clinical trial (Higginson et al. 2008 and 2009, Edmonds et al. 2010). This research effort produced three particularly important results. First, it revealed the poor state of formal care for severely disabled PwMS in this area. Care lacked coordination and continuity, with information in short supply on services, benefits and end-of-life issues; the experience of which leading to one of the iconic MS aphorisms of that time, 'fighting for everything' (Edmonds et al. 2007b). This finding was unexpected not only because the individuals concerned were the most disabled and vulnerable PwMS in the area but also because by UK standards this area was supposed to have well-resourced neurological service. There was a large neurology centre with five MS nurses and neurologists interested in MS. The second, and most important finding was that this research demonstrated that a palliative care service could have a positive role in relieving the suffering of PwMS and their carers through the comparison of two groups of eligible patients, a fast track group that was offered an intensive three-month palliative care service immediately and a control that had to wait three months for the service. In this case the fast track group revealed much better outcomes in symptom relief and carer burden than the control group. Furthermore, it was demonstrated that the fast track group was more cost effective than the control group (Higginson et al. 2009). However, the third important finding was that the benefits of the palliative care intervention soon began to wane, to be lost completely within three months. To maintain their benefits therefore an educational top-up regime would be required regularly.

Respite care. Another aspect of care in which the benefits may soon fade is in respite care; the opportunity to have a break from the daily routine of caring for someone, or of receiving care (McNally et al. 1999). The benefits of a respite break for a carer are well known and include relieving carer strain so they can continue with their caring duties, a chance for social contacts, holidays and hobbies and carrying out domestic DIY. There may be benefits of equal importance for the person receiving care too. In the case of visiting an established respite centre these may include socialising, having access to equipment and trained staff that limits the impact of their disabilities and permitting trips out. However, for some carers and for their charges taking part in respite care may also incur a psychological cost of guilt for the former and anger for the latter when they do not approve (Mullen et al. 2011).

7.5 Conclusions

This chapter began by detailing the large range of care services used by PwMS; their needs matching the needs of society generally across a full range of specialist areas. The dominant contacts PwMS made for their care outside their immediate family in the UK were their GP, the consultant neurologist, the physiotherapist and latterly the MS Nurse. However, what could not be made clear from the research evidence were the legitimate demands for care that could not be met either by the available health or social care services, that is the care services PwMS had to do without or try to satisfy through their own and their family's efforts. The analysis then moved on to outline the standards of care for PwMS that had been proposed by both the charitable and the government sectors in the UK, particularly from the MS Society, NICE and the Department of Health, that is the standards of care PwMS ought to be able to receive. Unfortunately, when audits of these standards were undertaken very poor compliance was discovered. Admittedly much of this research suffered from a number of methodological difficulties mainly because of its principal mode of data collection by self-selected questionnaire. Nevertheless, it indicated that during the first decade of the twenty-first century large numbers of PwMS in the UK received a substandard service. Indeed, this point received added emphasis when specific elements of care were investigated. Access to rehabilitation was called a matter of chance, MS nursing posts were being threatened and axed, people needed to resort to CAM because of ineffective standard therapies, and fighting for everything was necessary for the seriously disabled in south east London. What was even more depressing was that when good practice was discovered the authors often regarded it more as a result of effective individual local champions rather than the result of normal health-care staff behaviour.

From their audit of care services for PwMS in Oxfordshire at the end of the last century Wade and Green (2001, 170) commented that 'Patients have a right to better care than has been described in this report'. That would seem to apply to the results presented in this analysis too for the first few years of the twenty-first century and would concur with the conclusions of Forbes and colleagues (2007, 12) in their review of the care research evidence. Audits of care service provision in other developed countries are now needed to discover whether the British experience is the exception or the rule.

The text considered a number of specific issues directly related to the care of PwMS. For example, during the diagnostic phase although there would still appear to be serious issues around the time it may take, the manner in which it is given and information availability, if existing guidelines are followed then these problems should be increasingly minimised. Investigating this issue via the participants of self-help 'Getting to Grips with MS' type courses should perhaps be considered in the future.

It may be that after attending self-help courses some PwMS will be able to become effective expert patients but, because of the symptoms many PwMS may experience as a direct result of their condition such as cognition difficulties, pain and fatigue, it was suggested this might not be appropriate for the majority.

The research on informal care givers indicated that most were middle-aged married men and, although this was n heterogeneous group, evidence on some sectors of it such as the young and the infirmed older carers was particularly sparse. Many suffered from carer strain of both a physical and an emotional nature that permeated all aspects of their lives. But, in their caring tasks it would appear women tended to suffer more than men; the latter more able to reserve time and space in their lives for their own interests. In addition, this material tended to reinforce the view that in terms of coping with their illness most PwMS had to rely most of the time on themselves and their nearest family members.

The research on MS nurses revealed the huge diverse nature of the job and the large caseloads most experienced. In particular, it demonstrated MS Nurses were very good as a contact point for PwMS and their families, at securing appointments with specialists, information provision, promoting independence and managing specific symptoms such as pressure ulcers.

The research on the use of DMDs demonstrated first their increasing variety and second their uneven international geography of use in which the wealthiest nations benefitted most. It also showed that although these drugs could change the course of the disease for the better compared to what would have been expected to happen in terms of relapse rates and revealed brain lesion load, it was unclear whether such measures of disease activity had any relevance in assessing what should be the principal aim of any MS therapy, the prevention of sustained irreversible disability. For example, there was, and still is, a definite need to decide the significance of relapses in disability progression in both the short and long term and to the tipping point into SPMS. That may require the establishment of a long-term DMD clinical trial as well as the production of a meaningful control group. The point at which DMD therapies should begin also needs to be clarified. What this discussion did make clear, however, was why many PwMS do not have access to any DMD therapy in the UK. There were three important reasons. The first and most important reason was that the majority of DMDs have only been demonstrated to have an impact on early stage RRMS and are of no benefit what-so-ever on progressive forms of MS. The second reason was that many people stop taking them because of their side effects and impotence for some PwMS. The third reason was because of their lack of cost effectiveness according to the imperfect model used by NICE that initially led to them not being allowed to be purchased by the NHS. This latter reason was to some extent overcome by the Risk Assessment Scheme for the first four DMDs but still applies to the more recent preparations. Exceptions to this position include people with highly active disease who can access more powerful DMDs such as Tysabri and Fingolimod.

The review of research on CAM pointed out how little was known of the degree to which PwMS make use of these treatments, although given the number and growth of self-help books, magazines and their recommended preparations and interventions it must be assumed to be extensive. The text then focussed on two new developments, stem cell therapy and the relief of CCSVI, the first of which is under intensive research, the second shown to be irrelevant. Nevertheless, both are on offer by unscrupulous doctors in many places around the world more for reasons of financial gain than any real hope of clinical success generating a new form of medical tourism that preys on the fears of vulnerable PwMS.

The work on rehabilitation that mainly focussed on research undertaken at the NHNN in London noted the effectiveness of such a service when delivered by a multidisciplinary team, but pointed out that it may be difficult to set up and coordinate such activity outside a major well-resourced hospital. It also noted that the positive impacts of a rehabilitation programme diminish with time necessitating regular refresher sessions to maximise effectiveness; a condition that makes their resourcing problematic in many places. This section also highlighted vocational rehabilitation, the possible ways of assisting PwMS to return to work if they have had to leave and retain their employment as their MS develops by managing performance and managing expectations.

On the demand and supply of respite care along with its use and benefits there was little available evidence. What did seem to be particularly favoured, however, by both the PwMS using respite care and their carers was the expert MS nursing that could be accessed in these centres in addition to the opportunities for socialising and the trips out they could offer. They were therefore viewed as important social resources by both the PwMS who used them and their carers.

In a very similar manner to rehabilitation, palliative care for PwMS was also shown to have a generally positive impact in the short term and especially in symptom management but that these gains soon began to wane. Thus, in order to maintain effectiveness a top-up programme would be required regularly.

Perhaps the most disturbing feature of this review of the research on the care of PwMS was not the limited amount of work that has been undertaken in this area, but the ease with which it was possible to question many of the results. Some of this emanated from a lack of basic infrastructure for research on PwMS such as sampling frames and data bases. Other still unresolved problems stem from a lack of understanding of the variables that need to be collected and over what time period. But, some preventable issues came from poor decision making that almost doomed the research to produce problematic results. For example, the testing of the effectiveness of an expert patient programme with people who had already attended 'Getting to Grips with MS' type courses and the testing of the impact of MS Nurses or a palliative care programme in areas that already had a relatively good neurology service. In both cases showing a significant positive impact in the short term over what already existed was always going to be difficult. Even so, in the latter seriously disabled PwMS in south east London were shown to experience a poorly coordinated, unresponsive service. PwMS in many places deserve much better care than they appear to be receiving during the early twenty-first century and much better research to guide the development of that care.

8
Conclusion

8.1 General observations

The principal objective of this book was to present a review of the research evidence on people with Multiple Sclerosis (PwMS) and the lives they lead, to include a collection of the available evidence and an evaluation of its veracity. Unfortunately, little original research on this subject had been completed in the recent past in any of the expected cognate academic disciplines of sociology, psychology, economics or human geography. This may not have been a surprise given MS is a relatively uncommon illness, but its potentially profound impact on a person's life may have been expected to have commanded some interest. It has attracted very little. Thus, a great deal of the material presented did not come from traditional social science research but from neurology and related healthcare studies, often as a subsidiary element of the work and not as its main focus. There is therefore an almost empty research territory waiting to be occupied, a colonisation that should be relatively easy to achieve by the increasing availability of MS-related empirical evidence through a number of growing databases and a highly compliant MS clientele with an excellent record of cooperation with research requests.

It had been hoped that a number of generalities about PwMS in the United Kingdom (UK) may have been possible to extract from the available research, but again this was usually not possible for two reasons. The first reason was simply because the appropriate research had not been carried out whereas the second reason was that when it had been attempted methodological errors often interceded to question its usefulness.

The most reliable general characteristics from any cohort of people, short of a total population survey, are obtained through random, and therefore representative, samples. Such surveys have never been undertaken for PwMS in the UK because to do so would necessitate a national sampling frame of all PwMS and such a list has never existed. Instead for such work surrogates have had to be used which has usually relied on the membership list of the largest MS charity in the UK, the MS Society. Unfortunately, when such a list of PwMS had been used the randomness of the sample, and therefore its representativeness, was often corrupted by the adding of self-selected elements, limiting the general statements that could be made with any confidence from them.

One of the major objectives of this review was critically to interrogate the research that had been published on PwMS in the UK to decide on the degree to which its results were trustworthy. In this context one generalisation was possible; in the majority of the research reviewed in this book, the results were not as robust as they had been reported. The problems with much of the research using random sampling techniques has already been noted, but the issues are potentially much worse in the use of self-selecting samples that have often been used to investigate health-care experiences. In these cases the results were by definition biased, but in uncertain ways. As a result their findings should be treated with the utmost scepticism. Similar caution should also be applied to research based on very small cohorts, often termed pilot studies. It may be perfectly reasonable to carry out such work as a preliminary exercise to a potentially much larger study, or when the issue is particularly complex or where resources are scare. But, no matter how plausible their findings may be, their samples are usually much too small for the basis of any general observations and on which to base policy prescription or behavioural change.

8.2 Demographic characteristics

An area in which there was some unanimity across the research effort on PwMS in the UK was in terms of their demographic characteristics. There were two principal sources of demographic data described in this book, regional prevalence studies in which the total ascertainment of all cases of MS was attempted and the surveys of the membership of the MS Society. The former may present accurate portraits of MS communities, but each regional survey related to only one place at one particular point in time. Nevertheless, despite these material displaying minor variations between regions, it was characterised by remarkable unanimity in recorded demographic attributes. For example, relating to the gender balance of PwMS there was agreement across all regional cohort studies that women dominated in a ratio of at least 2:1 and that in the recent past this dominance had been increasing. How long this trend may continue was unknown as were its causes other than to intone the MS research cliché of a complex interaction between genetic, environmental and lifestyle factors. But, what this does mean is that MS was becoming an increasingly female condition; an observation that raises important research questions as to how the experience of MS fits into the changing roles of women and men in society, on their roles as spouses, partners, home-makers, bread-winners, workers and parents. And, more prosaically, how do PwMS cope with the many necessary visits to different health-care professionals needed to manage their condition with their familial and economic responsibilities? It is a question that from a consumer perspective might be phrased as how can the delivery of the health-care needed by PwMS best be organised to allow them to carry out as normal a life as possible?

On the ages of PwMS in the UK, a number of clear generalities emerged too. The disease began, or when the first clinical signs appeared, on average when a person was in their early 30s. Thus, MS in general was not a disease of childhood or early adulthood although paediatric and teenage cases have been found. For the majority of sufferers MS symptoms began after the school and further/higher education years and most likely during the early years of a chosen career and the forming of an expected long-term relationship with another person. It is on these nascent and inchoate personal and economic relationships that MS will begin to impose unanticipated strains.

For most regional cohorts the mean age of PwMS was 50 or 51 years, the decade in their lives when many begin to enter a secondary progressive phase of the illness, when acquired disabilities become permanent. This is a time in the life a person with MS, especially if mobility and cognitive disability is involved, when employment opportunities may be seriously compromised and when difficult and perhaps emotionally painful decisions have to be made about how they will try to live the rest of their lives in the knowledge they will probably have no disease modifying drug (DMD) to help slow the progression of their condition and limited support at ameliorating their symptoms. Successful adjustment at this time therefore will depend to a large degree on the strength of the relationships they have already developed with partners, family members, employers, friends and medical staff and their response to becoming increasingly dependent on the use of medical aids and pharmacological support. Thus, the middle years of someone's life with MS may provide a number of new challenging physical and psychological strains. This is a seriously under-researched area of the lives of PwMS.

From the regional age distribution evidence there would appear to have been fewer individuals in the older age bands, and especially in the 80 years and above category, than would have been expected from national trends. This may have been indicative of PwMS dying younger than would have been expected. What is more in the older age bands the female to male balance tended to increase suggesting that in MS as in the UK society more generally women tend to live longer than men.

The regional surveys also supported the view that in the UK MS was essentially a disease of white Caucasians with fewer than 5 per cent of cases coming from other ethnic groups. However, such an assertion demands an important note of caution in that some cultures of particularly Asian and Islamic origin may provide powerful cultural forces that could lead to their PwMS being excluded from the UK state's healthcare services and therefore from being recorded on hospital and General Practitioner (GP) databases. Careful and sensitive research is therefore required in known ethnic concentrations in the UK such as in the cities on the Pennine fringe, Birmingham or London to discover the degree to which this may occur. Such an enquiry may also help to discover the rate at which protection against MS provided by non-white ethnicity diminished through the generations as some commentators have predicted.

Finally, the regional studies offered evidence that MS prevalence at both the small area census and individual scales was inversely related to deprivation or standard of living, especially in Scotland. An explanation for such a phenomenon may be provided by the hygiene hypothesis, but no other support for such a view had been found elsewhere either in the UK or in Europe.

The national surveys of members of the MS Society served three important functions demographically. First of all they added support to the regional evidence in terms of there being far more women than men with MS in the UK, on average ages, ethnicity and the relationship of MS with deprivation. Second, where demographic differences were found between the regional studies and the MS Society member surveys, they indicated how the latter may differ from PwMS in the UK generally. This led to the suggestion that MS Society members were on average slightly older than PwMS generally and tended to be over-represented by women. The third important function of the national surveys of MS Society members was that they provided evidence on other demographic characteristics of PwMS in the UK, most notably on family constitution, divorce, employment and education. However, much of this material cannot be said to be representative of MS Society members or of PwMS in the UK generally. Nevertheless, what it did indicate was that large numbers of PwMS, and probably the vast majority of them, lived with a spouse or partner and as a result did not live alone and was not divorced. In addition, large numbers of PwMS in the UK were well educated, although probably not conclusively to a higher standard than the UK population generally, and of those of working age many more than would have been expected were either unemployed or had retired early because of their MS even when level of disability was held constant statistically. Given employment is usually regarded as a crucial component of personal material and psychological wellbeing, this above average propensity for PwMS to be unemployed and be retired early needs to be understood in much more detail. This could allow strategies to be developed to help PwMS stay in work longer and return to work more successfully if they had been initially forced to retire early.

8.3 Frequency and geography

This book presented a review of research evidence on the number of PwMS in the UK and concluded that the estimate of Thomas et al. (2009) of 100,000 adopted by the MS Society was too frugal and should be at least 10 per cent higher at 110,000. The General Practice Research Database (GPRD) work by Mackenzie and colleagues (2014) suggested an even higher figure of 127,000 with prevalences for the 4 separate countries of the UK all higher than for any of the earlier regional studies within their borders except for Orkney and Shetland, that in turn might support the view that there had been more PwMS in the UK than the regional evidence had so far suggested.

The range of regional prevalences revealed by epidemiological research in the UK over the last 30 years or so was from a maximum of 410/100,000 in Orkney in 2009 to a minimum of 74/100,000 in Guernsey in 1991. Attempting to account for this geographical variation was never going to be achieved satisfactorily because of the inconsistent nature of the regions involved; for example, different types, functionalities, sizes and dates. However, an understanding of the geography of MS became possible separately for the countries of England and Scotland when hospital admissions evidence became available for health authority areas for the first few years of the twenty-first century. In both countries there was a tendency for the highest rates of MS hospital admissions to be in the more northerly areas that may suggest an explanation based on UV exposure and vitamin D deficiency. However, this could not be the whole explanation because there were clear exceptions to a longitudinal gradient of MS cases and correlation coefficients were far from unity. One other possibility this evidence suggested was that large urban areas tended to record relatively low rates of MS compared to their adjacent regions. There were a number of possible reasons that could account for such a trend that would include the geographical distributions of ethnic minorities and relatively impoverished neighbourhoods that both tended to record relatively low rates of MS. In addition, it may also be the case that the people in such large relatively crowded places developed a natural immunity more easily than their rural counterparts to the sorts of infections that may trigger an MS response. These possible relationships need much more careful examination.

When repeat surveys of regions were undertaken increases in prevalence invariably took place and sometimes substantially so. For example, in South Glamorgan between 1988 and 2005 MS prevalence increased from 100/100,000 to 146/100,000, in SE Cambridgeshire between 1990 and 1993 from 112/100,000 to 131/ 100,000 and in north Northern Ireland between 1996 and 2004 from 168/100,000 to 231/100,000 that all led to absolute increases in the number of PwMS in their respective regions. Thus, there was support for the view that in the recent past both the prevalence rate and the frequency of PwMS in the UK had been increasing.

Such increases came about as the net result of new cases of the disease (incidence), deaths of PwMS, the net-migration of PwMS and the longevity of those who remained in situ. The limited evidence available on each of these 'components of change' was reviewed in turn that suggested that the principal component of change in each regional case was a rise in incident cases of MS. However, in some places it was not at all clear the degree to which people moving into an area with MS, that is in-migrants, were part of these incident totals. Nevertheless, annual incidence rates varied widely between the regions investigated and over time from 4.4/100,000 in Leeds between 1995 and 1996 to 12.00/100,000 for Lothian/Borders between 1992 and 1995, but generally were thought to have increased. What is more these increases were shown to be accounted for by a much higher rate of increase in the incidence of MS among women often at more than twice the rate among men. Many authors commentated on the reasons for the increasing rate of MS among women that included both genetic and life-style factors. But, increases in the rate of MS have also been taking place for men too, yet there has been no consideration of the possible genetic, environmental or life-style factors that could account for this phenomenon.

Evidence on the causes of the death of PwMS is particularly sparse and usually dependent on death certificates that need not record a person had MS, only if it was the primary cause of a person's death or made a significant contribution to their death. Indeed, up to half of all deaths of PwMS may not have MS noted on their death certificates at all. But, no matter how inadequate the limited evidence in this area may have been it tended to support the view that PwMS died at an earlier age than people generally, and that death rates from MS were higher in Scotland and Northern Ireland than in Wales and England. However, the evidence on gender differences between MS death rates was too imperfect to call. As the proximate cause of death MS would appear to play a relatively modest role, but in increasing the difficulties of trying to beat other potentially life-threatening medical challenges such as respiratory infections MS may play a very significant role indeed. The ways in which MS may affect life chances needs to be explained much more clearly to PwMS so they can take appropriate steps if they so wish. The potentially highly toxic nature of smoking on the lives of PwMS was noted in Chapter 2. Are there any other such elements of daily living that PwMS could be advised to either avoid or embrace? Finally, on suicide as a cause of death of PwMS in the UK, while some have taken their own lives the numbers have been very small and there was no evidence to suggest suicides among PwMS were any higher than among the UK population generally. This may not be the case in other countries, however.

International migration studies have made assertions about the likelihood of a migrant developing MS being dependent on the prevalences of their destination and departure areas and on the age at which migration took place. Some have suggested that a critical age exists of between 15 and 20 years below which a migrant would adopt the chances of getting MS of their destination area, after which they would keep the chances of getting MS of their region of departure.

Regional epidemiological research in MS in the UK that attempted to enumerate all possible cases of the illness almost ceased in the twenty-first century, with the notable exception of Aberdeen city and the northern isles of Scotland. There was also work published on South Glamorgan and north Northern Ireland, and it is to be hoped that their established regional data bases of PwMS and ones like them will be maintained in the future. Their potential elimination would be unfortunate for two main reasons. The first reason is that they provide one of the ways in which the components of change of MS numbers can be established. For example, is the number of PwMS still increasing and is it female incidence rates that are still the primary driving factor? The second reason is that they offer a mechanism for calculating the magnitude of any MS phenomenon, demographic, health-care or behavioural, either through its direct recording during their primary data collection phase or through the use of a regional list of PwMS as a sampling frame. The self-selecting surveys of the proto UK MS Register or the South West Impact of MS Project (SWIMS) database cannot offer such an option because they are by definition partial, in that not everyone with MS need take part, and biased because certain groups of people may either choose not to take part or not be able to do so. The nature of such biases needs to be carefully defined and may be particularly worrying if these databases were found systematically to under-represent certain groups of PwMS such as the significantly disabled, the cognitively impaired, the old or the poor. Such potential findings would limit the data sets usefulness in two additional and fundamental ways. The first way would be because they would not cover the full range of possible types of PwMS and therefore limit the use for research that related demographic, clinical, behavioural and health-care attributes to one another. The second limitation would be in being able to offer limited evidence on the sorts of PwMS who may be having most difficulty coping with their illness and need the greatest degree of support. To help overcome these problems it is to be hoped that the evolving UK MS Register will attempt to collect either the GP records and/or the hospital records of all PwMS in a number of individual regions. As explained in Chapter 3 these two sources will include the vast majority of PwMS in any locality and may be regarded as an 'expected' number against which the 'observed' number from the existing self-selected evidence already in the Register could be compared.

8.4 The impact of MS

PwMS may experience a wide range of symptoms during their lives that can impact sometimes very seriously on their ability to carry out normal activities of daily living and secure gainful employment. These may include symptoms that can be difficult to hide such as physical disablement and incontinence to symptoms that can be practically 'invisible' such as pain, fatigue and depression. Unfortunately, a lack of available evidence made it impossible to quantify with any precision either the number of PwMS who may be experiencing a particular symptom at any point in time or the overall person years of suffering it may cause over any given period of time. All that could be said was that for some symptoms the number of people involved was likely to be large with, for example, mobility difficulties of various degrees likely to as high as 50 per cent of all those with the affliction, or approximately 50,000 people in the UK, at the start of the twenty-first century.

In the early phases of MS symptoms such as blurred vision or foot dragging will most likely be single events that last a few days or weeks, a relapse, and then virtually disappear or remit. However, as PwMS get older and move into a more progressive form of the disease, symptoms regularly fail to remit so that they begin to be experienced in bundles. Thus, the longer a person has been diagnosed as having MS the greater the number of symptoms they are likely to face. However, this need not be exclusively so. Some people with very aggressive disease may soon become very disabled indeed. For example, in the palliative care study in South East London, the mean age of the 51 significantly disabled people involved was only 53 years.

It follows directly from these observations that many middle-aged PwMS will require not one form of symptom relief but many simultaneously. It is also worth remembering that this is the time in many people's MS careers when they receive a firm diagnosis of secondary progressive MS (SPMS), when they begin to realise that any functional losses caused by their MS are likely to be permanent. It is a time when their life course becomes seriously challenged, their expected biographies disrupted, when relationships and employment prospects may become seriously jeopardised. Yet there is very little research that focusses on this potentially MS-induced mid-life crisis. There has been some interest shown in the impact of an MS diagnosis on a person's life and the immediate post-diagnosis period, but almost nothing on this equally important time in the life of a PwMS when important strategic decisions about the future may have to be made. What sorts of changes take place in peoples' lives at this time and what strategies are employed to help them cope? Furthermore, to what extent does the severity of such changes vary by gender, age, disability or by any other characteristic of their lives? Such a project could be seen in a wider context of what PwMS do with their lives after diagnosis? There are two particularly important reasons why such research could be important. First of all it might help to demonstrate that life with MS for probably most people with the illness for most of the time may not be as difficult, unrewarding and tragic as many both with or without the disease may have first thought. The second reason is to demonstrate that PwMS, even when seriously disabled and unemployed, can still lead meaningful and rewarding lives not only in their own terms but in terms of benefitting their wider society too.

One of the more optimistic findings of the research on the quality of life of PwMS was that it was not necessarily directly related to disability; some highly disabled PwMS were able to regard themselves as having a relatively high quality of life. The opposite was, however, also possible; people with low disability regarding their lives as thoroughly miserable. Research is required to discover why these extreme positions are possible and if any lessons can be learned from them to help people generally lead more satisfying and meaningful lives. One of the difficult issues to tackle in this context is how wellbeing should be measured in ways that have meaning and relevance to people with MS and their carers and perhaps also to their health-care professionals and researchers too (Noble et al. 2012). And, because it is an issue that is fraught with so many methodological problems, it might be that there is not one solution, with a range of different constructs required for different purposes.

8.5 The care of PwMS

The general view that must be adopted from the research on the care of PwMS in the UK is that although standards of care have been established by both official and charitable organisations, they were rarely achieved by health and care services. Furthermore, surveys of PwMS regularly reported an inadequate provision and experience of care. This may simply be a reflection of the generally poor provision of care services for neurological and long-term conditions in the UK that may well persist for some time given future economic policy prescriptions for the nation. Nevertheless, given this context it is important that examples of good practice are discovered and promoted and places that are having problems in delivering a proper service are supported. For example, geographically are the best chances of receiving an adequate service for PwMS essentially dependent on living within easy commuting distance of a major neurology centre in a large urban area? And, as a corollary, does provision get increasingly poor with increased rurality and physical isolation?

Research into a number of specific therapeutic interventions such as a palliative care service, a rehabilitation programme and respite care were all shown to have positive impacts in the short term, but for these gains to be maintained they would all have required regular top-ups. However, the research into MS nurse provision could not show unambiguously a positive impact due mainly to either inadequate or over-ambitious research designs. This situation now needs urgent ameliorative action. Research therefore needs to be undertaken that describes how MS specialist nurses spend their time, but more importantly this research also needs to show how MS specialist nurses reduce actual and potential physical and psychological harm and thereby save time for doctors and money for health-care providers.

Research output from investigations of DMD usage presented some potentially confusing messages especially for lay PwMS. There appeared to be agreement among neurologists that taking DMDs reduced the rate of relapses and MRI-revealed brain lesion loads compared to what would have been expected to happen in people with early phase relapsing remitting MS (RRMS) even though the early results from the British Risk Sharing Scheme did not support this view. However, there was no unanimity on whether DMD therapy reduced disability in the longer term or delayed entry into SPMS. Nor was there agreement on when DMD therapy should commence. These matters need to be unequivocally resolved as soon as possible so that doctors and especially patients can make properly informed decisions about their future treatment. One further issue with DMD therapy was that while it appeared to be positive and well-tolerated by some PwMS, it appeared not to work at all with intolerable side-effects for others. An important research question for the future therefore is to be able to decide the types of PwMS who will benefit from a certain DMD treatment and those who will not without the need for a wasteful and often uncomfortable trial and error regime.

8.6 The view of MS in the UK press

In the introduction to this book a number of dire predictions about life with MS were presented that had been printed recently in the UK press. In this material it was stated that compared to a member of the general public a person with MS had a greater chance of

1. Dying younger
2. Taking their own life
3. Being unemployed
4. Living in poverty
5. Being dependent on state benefits
6. Being divorced
7. Living alone/being isolated
8. Not starting a family.

The research evidence presented in this book allowed these assertions to be tested. Although in most cases the research was of questionable worth and the evidence of limited general applicability, it did support two of these contentions, and probably the most serious ones that PwMS in the UK tended to die younger and have a higher rate of unemployment than their general public counterparts. However, it was also explained that the reasons for shorter lives were not properly understood and could be the result of factors that can be altered by either medical intervention or life-style changes. It therefore need not necessarily follow that such a difference should persist in the future. The reasons for the second potentially serious consequence of having MS, higher unemployment, related to disability are well understood, but there were other elements to this relationship that were not, where appropriate vocational rehabilitation may help to reduce the disparity. As a result, this difference need not necessarily be so stark in the future; it is up to British society to make the appropriate changes. In three other realms, living alone, divorce and suicide, the evidence suggested that PwMS were at least no worse off than the general population and may well be better off. However, in relation to poverty, dependency on state benefits and family deferral the evidence simply did not exist to come to even the most tentative conclusions. It was wrong therefore to claim that PwMS stood a greater chance than members of the British public of being disadvantaged in these areas.

8.7 The average person with MS and beyond

If it is reasonable to try to define an average person with MS in the UK, then according to the evidence reviewed in this book they would be female, white Caucasian, middle-aged, living in their own home with a spouse or partner, whose disability was at the point of needing an aid to walk, not in work and if employed at the point of retirement because of their disability relative to the demands of their employment. Such a stereotype serves at least two useful purposes. First of all it helps to define a group of PwMS about which most is probably known or can be inferred, yet about which much more is required because they are a group of people going through one of the most fundamental changes of their lives; they are going through the MS-induced mid-life crisis of entering secondary progression. The second use of this stereotypical description of a person with MS is that it helps to define the PwMS about whom least is known, namely those at the extremes of the attributes used in this definition, especially the aged, the poor, the socially and physically isolated, the severely disabled, characteristics that individually and especially in combination can make life exceedingly challenging. It is people with these characteristics who are least likely to join an MS society or the UK MS Register and who are most difficult to access. Yet, it is these sorts of PwMS along with those who care for them for whom dedicated research is required better to understand their particular problems and experiences so that ameliorative action can be developed to try to help them lead less difficult and more rewarding lives.

Notes

1 Introduction

1. This lecture achieved temporary notoriety when it was improperly published in the May/June *New Pathways* magazine (Issue 49) as 'what are the myths and what are the facts about MS?' The impropriety came from the fact that the article had not been written by Alistair Coles but in fact by Judy Graham, the editor of *New Pathways*, from notes taken from Coles' lecture. She quite properly printed an apology for this error on page four of the next *New Pathways* (Issue 50). The notoriety came from the reaction to the lecture. Certainly judging from the letters to the *New Pathways* Magazine, many PwMS appeared to be either genuinely unaware, or unwilling to countenance, some of the disease's more serious implications.
2. For example, in the analysis of the costs of early DMDs by Chilcott et al. (2003) the withholding of evidence for commercial reasons was noted, while the lengthy withholding of evidence may be inferred in the time it took for the first results from the Risk Sharing Scheme to become available. This scheme began recruiting MS patients in 2002 yet it took seven years for the first preliminary and disappointing results to be published in Boggild et al. (2009).

2 Multiple Sclerosis: A Brief Overview of the Illness

1. See Robertson et al. (1996a) for a review of earlier British research on MS familial inheritance.
2. For a thorough critical review of a bio-medical approach to MS, see the review article by Compston and Coles (2008), the scholarly tome by Compston et al. (2005) *McAlpine's Multiple Sclerosis* and the briefing volume by Scolding and Wilkins (2012). For the briefest of competent descriptions of the natural history of the disease see Burgess (2010a) and for an excellent treatment of the biology of MS suitable for the lay reader see Amor and van Noort (2012). Unfortunately, the latter's attempted discussion of the social impacts of MS is poor.

3 Research on People with MS: Definitions, Data Sources and Methodologies

1. See Murray (2005, 320–1) for the Schumacher diagnostic criteria that classified patients with MS as either those with relapses and remission or those with progression, either from the beginning or after a number of relapses.
2. Statistical evidence derived from the Cornwall and Devon county websites, accessed 17/03/2011.

4 What Type of Person Suffers from MS?

1. Social Classes based on occupations:
    I. Professional (including doctors, solicitors, chemists, university professors and clergymen).
    II. Managerial and technical occupations (including school teachers, computer programmers, personnel managers, nurses, actors and laboratory technicians).
    III. skilled occupations
        (N) Non-manual including typists, clerical workers, photographers, sales representatives and shop assistants.
        (M) Manual including cooks, bus drivers, railway guards, plasterers, bricklayers, hairdressers and carpenters.
    IV. Partly skilled (including bar staff, waitresses, gardeners and caretakers).
    V. Unskilled (including refuse collectors, messengers, lift attendants and labourers).

5 How Many People Have MS? A Case Study of the UK

1. I applied to the MS Society to read the original research report by Thomas and colleagues so I could comment on their work in this book but was refused on confidentiality grounds because they did not want to jeopardise the possibility of its publication.
2. The age range 30–44 years is included because it was the nearest available census category to the peak prevalence age range, 35–44, in the McDonnell and Hawkins (1998, 425) study.
3. By the beginning of the eighteenth century, many of the descendants of these early settlers in Ulster were themselves on the move westwards across the Atlantic to America. Between 1718 and 1775, more than 100,000 men and women made the perilous journey, making them the most populous ethnic group to make this sea crossing barring slaves from Africa. Although these Presbyterians of Scottish descent had fought to oppose the forces of James II in Ireland and helped in the long reconstruction of the north after the devastation of the war, they failed to gain the political respect and power they had expected and believed they deserved, never legally the equals of members of the established Church of Ireland (Griffin 2001). Added to this a number of failed harvests at the beginning of the eighteenth century meant that many people in Ulster were willing to take the risk of trying to make a new life for themselves in an entirely new country. In so doing they may well have been one of the important vectors for the importation of the MS susceptibility genes into North America.
4. It is also worth observing that an average annual incidence rate of 4.0/100,000 between 1960 and 1972 was calculated by Dean et al. (1976) for Greater London after a trawl of all hospital records. Such a result should be regarded as relatively high for a time 20 years before most of the material considered for this analysis, especially so given the likely biases in the mode of ascertainment.

6 The Impact of MS

1. A useful source of recently developed measures in this area can be found on the Neuro-QOL website (http://www.neuroqol.org/default.aspx), an American initiative to develop a clinically relevant and psychometrically robust health-related quality of life assessment tool for adults and children.
2. It may well be possible to consider PwMS as having certain positive traits, or develop them because of their illness, such as self-reliance, resourcefulness, creativity and independence because the medical profession until very recently could offer them very little to relieve their suffering. Similarly, the qualities of altruism, social responsibility and care especially for their fellow sufferers may be included. If indeed this is true, then why dwell on loss when one could count such positive gains?
3. For a formal discussion of the problems of rating scales in neurological research, see Hobart et al. (2007).
4. The earlier and very clear analysis by Blumhardt and Wood (1996) also shows the heavy economic burden borne by the person with MS and their family.

7 The Care of People with MS

1. The full range of the sources of care and support PwMS may need can be usefully found in a report by the UK's National Audit Office (2011, 15) for neurological conditions generally.
2. This is now a well-developed argument for both the UK and US health-care services that drugs are over- and wrongly prescribed by doctors (see Welch et al. 2011). The reasons for this are many but they include the eagerness of doctors to give their patients something to keep them happy with the added bonus of the placebo effect and the eagerness of the drug companies to sell their wares through persuasive research and advertising.
3. See the update on Cannon White's stem cell treatment in *New Pathways* Issue 60, March/April, 22–3.
4. A further death was reported of a Canadian woman following CCSVI treatment in California in *New Pathways* July/August 2010, Issue 68, 46.

References

Ackroyd J (2003) *Where do you think you're going. Report of the John Grooms inquiry into the needs of young disabled people.* John Grooms, London.

Al-Hashel J, Besterman Ad and Wolfson C (2008) The prevalence of MS in the Middle East. *Neuroepidemiology* 31(2), 129–37.

Albert PJ, Proal AD and Marshall TG (2009) Vitamin D: the alternative hypothesis. *Autoimmunity Reviews* 8(8), 639–44.

Allison RS (1931) Disseminated sclerosis in North Wales: an inquiry into its incidence, frequency, distribution and other etiological factors. *Brain* 53(4), 391–430.

Allison RS and Millar JHD (1954) Prevalence and familial incidence of disseminated sclerosis in Northern Ireland. *Ulster Med J* 23, 5–27.

Alonso A and Hernan MA (2008) Temporal trends in the incidence of MS: a systematic review. *Neurology* 71(2), 129–35.

Alonso A, Jick SS, Olek MJ and Hernan MA (2007) Incidence of MS in the UK: findings from a population based cohort. *J Neurol* 254, 1736–41.

Amor S and van Noort H (2012) *Multiple Sclerosis*. OUP, Oxford.

Archibald K, Coleman R and Foster C (2011) Open letter to UK Prime Minister David Cameron and Health Secretary Andrew Lansley on safety of medicines. *Lancet* 377(9781), 1915.

Ascherio A and Munger KL (2007) Environmental risk factors for MS. Part II: non-infectious factors. *Ann Neurol* 61(6), 504–13.

Ashfield T (2005) Cannabis use in multiple sclerosis. *Primary Health Care* 15(6), 25–9.

Baird W, Jackson R, Ford H, Evangelou N, Busby M, Bull P and Zajicek J (2009) Holding personal information in a disease specific register: the perspectives of people with MS and professionals on consent and access. *J Med Ethics* 35, 92–6.

Bakshi R, Thompson AJ, Rocca MA, Pelletier D, Dousset V, Barkhof F, Inglese M, Guttmann CRG, Horsfield MA and Filippi M (2008) MRI in MS: current status and future prospects. *Lancet Neurol* 7(7), 615–25.

Ballas D and Dorling D (2007) Measuring the impact of major life events on happiness. *Int J Epidemiol* 36, 1244–52.

Banwell B, Ghezzi A, Bar-Or A, et al. (2007) MS in children: clinical diagnosis, therapeutic strategies and future directions. *Lancet Neurol* 6(10), 887–902.

Barclay E (2009) Stem-cell experts raise concerns about medical tourism. *Lancet* 373, 883–4.

Bardon J (1992) *A history of Ulster.* Blackstaff Press, Belfast.

Barlow J, Edwards R and Turner A (2009a) The experience of attending a lay-led, chronic disease self-management programme from the perspective of participants with multiple sclerosis. *Psychol Health* 24, 1167–80.

Barlow J, Turner A, Edwards B and Gilchrist M (2009b) A randomised controlled trial of lay-led self-management for people with multiple sclerosis. *Patient Educ Counsel* 77, 81–9.

Bartley M, Sacker A and Clarke P (2004) Employment status, employment conditions and limiting illness: prospective evidence from the British household panel survey 1991–2001. *J Epidemiol Community Health* 58, 501–6.

Bates D (2011) Summary: registry data. *Neurology* 76 (Suppl. 1), S39–S41.

Bazelier MT, van Staa T, Uitdehaag BMJ, Cooper C, Leufkens HGM, Vestergaad P, Bentzen J and de Vries F (2011) The risk of fracture in patients with multiple sclerosis: the UK general practice database. *J Bone Miner Res* 26, 2271–9.

Beaumont JG (2004) The MS symptom impact diary (MSSID): psychometric evaluation of a new instrument to measure the day to day impact of multiple sclerosis. *J Neurol Neurosurg Psychiatry* 75, 526–7.

Bennetto L, Burrow J, Sakai H, Cobby J, Robertson NP and Scolding N (2011) The relationship between relapse, impairment and disability in multiple sclerosis. *Mult Scler J* 17(10), 1216–24.

Benz C and Reynolds R (2005) *Coping with MS*. Vermillion, London.

Berer K and Krishnamoorthy G (2012) Commensal gut flora and brain autoimmunity: a love or hate affair? *Acta Neuropathol* 123(5), 639–51.

Bhopal R (2002) *Concepts of epidemiology*. OUP, Oxford.

Blackford KA (1999) A child's growing up with a parent who has multiple sclerosis: theories and experiences. *Disability and Society* 14(5), 673–85.

Blumhardt LD and Wood C (1996) The economics of multiple sclerosis: a cost of illness study. *Br J Med Econ* 10(2), 99–118.

Boal FW (1969) Territoriality and the Shankill/Falls divide, Belfast. *Irish Geography* 6(1), 30–50.

Boeije RH and van Doorne-Huiskes A (2003) Fulfilling a sense of duty: how men and women giving care to a spouse with MS interpret this role. *Community, Work and Family* 6(3), 223–44.

Boggild M, Palace J, Barton P, Ben-Schlomo Y, Bregenzer T, Dobson C et al. (2009) Multiple sclerosis risk sharing scheme: two year results of clinical cohort study with historical comparator. *BMJ* 339:b4677.

Bogosian A, Moss-Morris R, Yardley L and Dennison L (2009) Experiences of partners in the early stages of multiple sclerosis. *Mult Scler J* 15, 876–84.

Bogosian A, Moss-Morris R and Hadwin J (2010) Psychological adjustment in children and adolescents with a parent with multiple sclerosis: a systematic review. *Clin Rehabil* 24(9), 789–801.

Bogosian A, Moss-Morris R, Bishop FL and Hadwin J (2011) How do adolescents adjust to their parent's multiple sclerosis?: an interview study. *Br J Health Psychol* 16(2), 430–44.

Bowen C and MacLehose A (2009) Living with progressive MS in the family. *Open Door*, Aug, 10–1.

Bowen C, MacLehose A and Beaumont JG (2010) Advanced multiple sclerosis and the psychosocial impact on families. *Psychology and Health* 26(1), 113–27.

Bowling AC (2007) *Complementary and alternative medicine and multiple sclerosis*. Second Edition. Demos, New York.

Brazier J, Roberts J, Tsuchya A and Busschbach J (2004) A comparison of the EQ-5D and SF-6D across seven patient groups. *Health Economics* 13(4), 873–84.

Bronnum-Hansen H, Koch-Henriksen N and Stenager E (2004) Trends in survival and cause of death in Danish patients with MS. *Brain* 127(4), 844–50.

Bronnum-Hansen H, Stenager E, Stenager EN and Koch-Henriksen N (2005) Suicide among Danes with multiple sclerosis. *J Neurol Neurosurg Psychiatry* 76(10), 1457–9.

Brustad M, Sandanger T, Aksnes L, et al. (2004) Vitamin D status in a rural population of northern Norway with high fish liver consumption. *Public Health Nutr* 7(6), 783–9.

Burgess M (2002) *MS, theory and practice for nurses*. Whurr, London.

—— (2010a) Shedding greater light on the natural history and prevalence of multiple sclerosis. *Br J Neurosci Nurs* 6(1), 7–11.

—— (2010b) The process of adjustment: providing support after a diagnosis of multiple sclerosis. *Br J Neurosci Nurs* 6(4), 156–60.

Burnfield A (1985) *Multiple sclerosis: a personal exploration*. Souvenir Press, London.

Bury M (1982) Chronic illness as biographical disruption. *Sociology of Health and Illness* 4, 167–82.

Carstairs V and Morris R (1991) *Deprivation and health in Scotland*. Aberdeen University Press, Aberdeen.

Chalmers I (2007) The lethal consequences if failing to make use of all relevant evidence about the effects of medical treatments: the need for systematic reviews. In Rothwell P (Ed.) *Treating individuals: from randomised trials to personalised medicine*. The Lancet, London, 395–404.

Chalmers I and Glasziou P (2009) Avoidable waste in the production and reporting of research evidence. *Lancet* 374, 86–9.

Chao MJ, Ramagopalan SV, Herrera BM, Orton SM, Handunnetthi L, Lincoln MR, Dyment DA, Sadovnick AD and Ebers GC (2011) MHC transmission: insights into gender bias in MS susceptibility. *Neurology* 76, 242–6.

Chaplin H, Hazan J and Wilson P (2012) Self-management for people with long-term neurological conditions. *Br J Community Nursing* 17(6), 250–7.

Chataway J, Schuerer J, Alsanousi A, et al. (2014) Effect of high dose simvastatin on brain atrophy and disability in secondary progressive multiple sclerosis (MS-STAT): a randomised, placebo-controlled, phase 2 trial. *Lancet* 383, 2213–21.

Chesson R (2003) *Who's there for the carers?* Report from the MS Society Scotland, Edinburgh.

Chilcott J, McCabe C, Tappenden P, O'Hagan A, Cooper NJ, Abrams K and Claxton K (2003) Modelling the cost-effectiveness of interferon beta and glatiramer acetate in the management of multiple sclerosis. *BMJ* 326, 522–9.

Chipchase SY and Lincoln NB (2001) Factors associated with carer strain in carers of people with multiple sclerosis. *Disabil Rehabil* 23(17), 768–76.

Coles A (2008) What are the myths and what are the facts about MS. *New Pathways* 49, 19–20.

Coles AJ and Compston A (2014) Product licences for alemtuzumab and multiple sclerosis. *Lancet* 383(9920), 867–8.

Coles AJ, Fox E, Vladic A, Gazada SK, Brinar V, Selmaj KW, Bass AD, Wynn DR, Margolin DH, Lake SL, Moran S, Palmer J, Smith MS and Compston DAS (2011) Alemtuzumab versus interferon beta-1a in early relapsing-remitting multiple sclerosis: a post-hoc subset analysis of clinical efficiency outcomes. *Lancet Neurol* 10, 338–48.

Compston DAS (1990a) The dissemination of multiple sclerosis: the Langdon-Brown lecture 1989. *J Royal College of Physicians* 24, 207–18.

―――― (1990b) Risk factors for multiple sclerosis: race or place. *J Neurol Neurosurg Psychiatry* 53, 821–3.
―――― (1997) Genetic epidemiology of multiple sclerosis. *J Neurol Neurosurg Psychiatry* 62, 553–61.
―――― (2009) Multiple sclerosis. In Donaghy M (Ed.) *Brain's diseases of the nervous system*. OUP, Oxford.
―――― (2011) The family way. *MS Matters* 97, 18–19.
Compston A and Coles A (2008) Multiple Sclerosis. *Lancet* 372, 1502–17.
Compston A, Lassmann H, Wekerle H et al. (2005) *McAlpine's multiple sclerosis*, 4th edition. Elsevier, Philadelphia.
Confavreux C and Vukusic S (2008) The clinical epidemiology of MS. *Neuroimaging Clinics of North America* 18(4), 589–622.
Confavreux C, Vukusic S, Moreau T and Adeleine P (2000) Relapses and progression of disability in multiple sclerosis. *New Engl J Med* 343, 1430–8.
Confavreux C, Vukusic S and Adeleine P (2003) Early clinical predictors and progression of irreversible disability in multiple sclerosis: an amnesic process. *Brain* 126, 770–82.
Cook I (2008) Is there an MS personality? *New Pathways* 49, 40–1.
―――― (2010) CCSVI: where to be tested and treated in the UK and overseas. *New Pathways* 62, Jul–Aug, 44–6.
Cook SD, Cromarty JI, Tapp W, Poskanzer D, Walker JD and Dowling PC (1985) Declining incidence of MS in the Orkney Islands. *Neurology* 35, 545–51.
Cooke A (2001) *A guide to finding quality information on the Internet: selection and evaluation strategies*. Library Association, London.
Cornwall Council (2009) *Cornwall 2009: demographic evidence base*. Community Intelligence Department, Cornwall Council.
Cornwell J (1984) *Hard-earned lives: accounts of health and illness from East London*. Tavistock, London.
Corry M, McKenna M and Duggan M (2011) The role of the clinical nurse specialist in MS: a literature review. *Br J Nurs* 20(2), 86–93.
Corthals AP (2011) Multiple sclerosis is not a disease of the immune system. *Quarterly Review of Biology* 86(4), 287–321.
Courts NF, Newton AN and McNeal LJ (2005) Husbands and wives living with multiple sclerosis. *J Neurosci Nurs* 37(1), 20–7.
Coyle PK (2005) Gender issues. *Neurol Clin* 23(1), 39–60.
Craig J, Young CA, Ennis M, Baker G and Boggild MA (2003) A randomised controlled trial comparing rehabilitation against standard therapy in multiple sclerosis patients receiving intravenous steroid treatment. *J Neurol Neurosurg Psychiatry* 74, 1225–30.
Cross T and Rintell D (1999) Children's perceptions of parental MS. *Psychology, Health and Medicine* 4, 355–60.
Cuthbert K (2010) *Keeping balance: a psychologist's experience of chronic illness and disability*. Matador, London.
Cutter G, Yadavalli R, Marrie RA et al. (2007) Changes in the sex ratio over time in multiple sclerosis. *Neurology* 68, A162.
Dalton CM, Brex PA, Miszkiel KA, Hickman SJ, MacMannus DG, Plant GT, Thompson AJ and Miller DH (2002) Application of the new McDonald criteria to patients with clinically isolated syndromes suggestive of MS. *Ann Neurol* Jul 52(1), 47–53.

Dean G and Elian M (1997) Age at immigration to England of Asian and Caribbean immigrants and the risk of developing MS. *J Neurol Neurosurg Psychiatry* 63, 565–8.

Dean G, McLoughlin H, Brady R, Adelsyein AM and Tallett-Williams J (1976) Multiple sclerosis among immigrants in Greater London. *BMJ* 1, 861–4.

Degenhardt A, Ramagopalan SV, Scalfari A and Ebers GC (2009) Clinical prognostic factors in multiple sclerosis: a natural history review. *Nat Rev Neurol* 5, 672–82.

del Pilar Cortes Nino M, Tampieri D and Melancon D (2010) Endovascular venous procedures for multiple sclerosis. *Mult Scler J* 16(7), 771–2.

DeLuca GC, Ramagopalan SV, Herrera BM, Dyment DA, Lincoln MR, Montpetit A, Pugliatti M, Barnardo MC, Risch NJ, Sadovnick AD, Chao M, Sotgiu S, Hudson TJ and Ebers GC (2007) New association discovered between genes and MS. *Proceedings of the National Association of Sciences* USA Dec 26, 104(52), 20896–901.

Dennison L and Moss-Morris R (2010) Cognitive behavioural therapy: what benefits can it offer people with multiple sclerosis? *Expert Rev Neurotherapeutics* 10(9), 1383–90.

Dennison L, Moss-Morris R and Chalder T (2009) A review of psychological correlates of adjustment in patients with multiple sclerosis. *Clinical Psychology Rev* 29(2), 141–53.

Dennison L, Yardley L, Devereux A and Moss-Morris R (2010) Experiences of adjustment to early stage multiple sclerosis. *J of Health Psychology* 16(3), 478–88.

Department of Health (2005) *The national service framework for long-term conditions*. Department of Health, London.

—— (2010) *Equity and excellence: liberating the NHS*. DoH, London.

Dilorenzo TA, Becker-Feigeles J, Halper J and Picone MA (2008) A qualitative investigation of adaptation in older individuals with multiple sclerosis. *Disabil Rehabil* 30(15), 1088–97.

Dobson R, Ramagopalan S and Giovannoni G (2012) Bone health and multiple sclerosis. *Mult Scler J* 18(11), 1522–8.

Doidge D (2008) *The brain that changes itself: stories of personal triumph from the frontiers of brain science*. Penguin, London.

Dolan P, Gudex C, Kind P and Williams A (1995) A social tariff for Euro Qol: results from a UK general population survey. *Dept. Economics, University of York Discussion Paper 138*.

Donaghy M (2009, Ed.) *Brain's diseases of the nervous system*, 12th Edition. OUP, Oxford.

Donnan PT, Parrat JDE, Wilson SV, Forbes RB, O'Riordan JI and Swingler RJ (2005) Multiple sclerosis in Tayside: detection of clusters using a spatial scan statistic. *Mult Scler J* 11, 403–8.

Dorling D (2010) All connected?: geographies of race, death, wealth, votes and births. *Geographical Journal* 176(3), 186–98.

Dyck I (1995) Hidden geographies: the changing lifeworlds of women with MS. *Soc Sci Med* 40(3), 307–20.

Ebers GC (2008) Environmental factors and MS. *Lancet Neurol* 7(3), 268–77.

Ebers GC, Heigenhauser L, Daumer M, Lederer C and Noseworthy JH (2008) Disability as an outcome in MS clinical trials. *Neurology* 71, 624–31.

Ebers GC, Traboulsee A, Li D, Langdon D, Reder AT, Goodin DS et al. (2010) Analysis of clinical outcomes according to original treatment groups 16 years after the pivotal IFNB-1b trial. *J Neurol Neurosurg Psychiatry* 81, 907–12.

Edmonds P, Vivat B, Burman R, Silber E and Higginson IJ (2007a) Loss and change: experiences of people severely affected by multiple sclerosis. *Palliative Medicine* 21, 101–7.

Edmonds P, Vivat B, Silber E, Burman R and Higginson IJ (2007b) 'Fighting for everything': service experiences of people severely affected by MS. *MS* 13, 660–7.

Edmonds, Hart S, Gao W, Vivat B, Burman R, Silber E and Higginson IJ (2010) Palliative care for people severely affected by multiple sclerosis: evaluation of a novel palliative care service. *Mult Scler J* 16(5), 627–36.

Edwards RG, Barlow JH and Turner AP (2008) Experiences of diagnosis and treatment among people with MS. *J Eval Clin Pract* 14, 460–4.

Elian M and Dean G (1983) Need for and use of social and health services by multiple sclerosis patients living at home in England. *Lancet* 1, 1091–3.

—— (1987) Multiple sclerosis among the United Kingdom-born children of immigrants from the West Indies. *J Neurol Neurosurg Psychiatry* 50, 327–32.

—— (1993) Motor neuron disease and multiple sclerosis among immigrants to England from the Indian subcontinent, and east and west Africa. *J Neurol Neurosurg Psychiatry* 56, 454–7.

Elian M, Nightingale S and Dean G (1990) MS among UK-born children of immigrants from the Indian subcontinent, Africa and the West Indies. *J Neurol Neurosurg Psychiatry* 53, 906–11.

Esmonde L and Long AF (2008) Complementary therapy use by persons with multiple sclerosis: benefits and research priorities. *Complementary Therapies in Clinical Practice* 14, 176–84.

Evans C et al. (2013) Incidence and prevalence of multiple sclerosis in the Americas: a systematic review. *Neuroepidemiology* 40(3), 195–210.

Expert Patients Programme /Community Interest Company (undated) Self-care reduces costs and improves health. Expert Patients Programme, London. See website www.expertpatients.co.uk.

Feinstein A (1997) MS: depression and suicide. *BMJ* 315, 691–2.

Filippi M and Rocca MA (2011) The multiple sclerosis mystery: is there a vascular component. *Lancet Neurol* 10, 597–8.

Fischer S, Huber CA, Imhof L, Maher Imhof R, Furter M, Ziegler SJ and Bosshard G (2008) Suicide assisted by two Swiss right-to-die organisations. *J Med Ethics* 34(11), 810–4.

Fleming JD and Cook TD (2006) MS and the hygiene hypothesis. *Neurology* 67, 2085–6.

Fog M and Hyllested K (1966) Presence of disseminated sclerosis in the Faroes, the Orkneys and Shetland. *Acta Neurol Scand* 42, 9–11.

Forbes A, While A, Mathes L and Griffiths P (2006a) Evaluation of a MS specialist nurse programme. *Nursing Studies* 43, 985–1000.

—— (2006b) Health problems and health-related quality of life in people with multiple sclerosis. *Clin Rehabil* 20(1), 67–78.

Forbes A, While A and Mathes L (2007) Informal carer activities, carer burden and health status in multiple sclerosis. *Clin Rehabil* 21, 563–75.

Forbes RB, Wilson SV and Swingler RJ (1999) The prevalence of MS in Tayside, Scotland: do latitudinal gradients really exist? *J Neurol* Nov 246(11), 1033–40.

Ford CD, Jones KH, Middleton RM, Lockhart-Jones H, Maramba IDC, Noble GJ, Osborne LA and Lyons RA (2012) The feasibility of collecting information from people with Multiple Sclerosis for the UK MS Register via a web portal: characterising a cohort of people with MS. *BMC Medical Informatics and Decision Making* 12:73 doi:10.1186/1472-6947-12-73.

Ford HL (2006) The effect of consent guidelines on a multiple sclerosis register. *MS* 12, 104–7.

Ford HL, Gerry E, Airey CM, Vail A, Johnson MH and Williams DRR (1998) The prevalence of MS in the Leeds Health Authority. *J Neurol Neurosurg Psychiatry* 64, 605–10.

Ford H, Gerry E, Johnson M and Williams DRR (2000) *Health needs assessment in a population-based cohort of people with MS*. Nuffield Institute for Health, Leeds.

Ford HI, Gerry E, Johnson MH and Tennant A (2001a) Health status and quality of life of people with multiple sclerosis. *Disabil Rehabil* 23, 516–21.

Ford HL, Gerry E, Tennant A, Whalley D, Haigh R and Johnson MH (2001b) Developing a disease-specific quality of life measure for people with MS. *Clin Rehabil* 15, 247–58.

Ford HL, Gerry E, Johnson MH and Williams DR (2002) A prospective study of the incidence, prevalence and mortality of MS in Leeds. *J Neurol* 249, 260–5.

Ford HL, Johnson MH and Rigby AS (1996) Variations between observers in classifying MS. *J Neurol Neurosurg Psychiatry* 61, 418.

Ford HL, Tennant A and Johnson MH (1997) The Leeds MSQoL scale: a disease specific measure of quality of life in MS. *J Neurol Neurosurg Psychiatry* 62, 210.

Forsyth E (1988) *Multiple sclerosis: exploring sickness and health*. Faber and Faber, London.

Fox CM, Bensa S, Bray I and Zajicek JP (2004) The epidemiology of MS in Devon: a comparison of the new and old classification criteria. *J Neurol Neurosurg Psychiatry* 75, 56–60.

Freeman J and Thompson A (2000) Community services in multiple sclerosis: still a matter of chance. *J Neurol Neurosurg Psychiatry* 69(6), 728–32.

Freeman J, Langton DW, Hobart JC and Thompson AJ (1999) Inpatient rehabilitation in MS: do the benefits carry over into the community? *Neurology* 52, 50–6.

Freeman DM, Dosemeci M and Alavanja MC (2000) Mortality from MS and exposure to residential and occupational solar radiation: a case controlled study based on death certificates. *Occup Environ Med* 57, 418–21.

Freeman J, Ford H, Mattison P, Thompson A, Ridley J and Haffenden S (2002) *Developing MS healthcare standards: evidence based recommendations for service providers*. MS Society and the MS Professional Network, London.

Friedmann P and Wattjes MP (2013) Chronic venous insufficiency in multiple sclerosis: the final curtain. *Lancet* 383(9912), 106–8.

Gale CR and Martyn CN (1995) Migrant studies in MS. *Prog Neurobiol* 47, 425–48.

Gatrell AC and Elliott SJ (2009) *Geographies of health: an introduction*. 2nd Edition. Wiley, Chichester.

Gesler WM (1992) Therapeutic landscapes: medical issues in light of the new cultural geography. *Soc Sci Med* 34, 735–46.

Gershuny J (1978) *After industrial society? The emerging self-service economy*. Palgrave Macmillan, London.

Gilmore CP, Cottrell DA, Scolding NJ, Wingerchuk Dm, Weinshenker BG and Boggild M (2010) A window of opportunity for no treatment in early multiple sclerosis. *Mult Scler J* 16(6), 756–9.

Giovannoni G and Ebers G (2007) MS: the environment and causation. *Curr Opinion Neurol* 20(3), 261–8.

Giovannoni G, Cook S, Rammohab K, Rieckmann P, Sorensen PS, Vermersch P, Hamlett A, Viglietta V, Greenberg S, on behalf of the CLARITY study group (2011) Sustained disease-activity free status in patients with relapsing-remitting multiple sclerosis treated with cladribine tablets in the CLARITY study: a post-hoc and subgroup analysis. *Lancet Neurol* 10, 329–37.

Glantz MJ, Chamberlain MC, Liu Q, Hsieh C, Edwards KR, Van Horn A and Recht L (2009) Gender disparity in the rate of partner abandonment in patients with serious medical illness. *Cancer* 115, 5237–42.

Goldacre MJ, Seagroatt V, Yeates D and Acheson ED (2004) Skin cancer in people with MS: a record linkage study. *J Epidemiol Community Health* 58, 142–4.

Goodin DS (2009) The causal cascade to MS: a model for MS pathogenesis. *PLoS ONE* 4(2), e4565. doi:10.1371/journal.pone.0004565.

Goodkin DE, Cookfair D, Wende K, Bourdette D, Pulicino P, Scherokman B, et al. (1992) Inter- and intrarater scoring agreement using grades 1.0 to 3.5 of the Kurtzke expanded disability status scale (EDSS). Multiple Sclerosis Collaborative Research Group. *Neurology* 42, 859–63.

Graham J (2010) *Managing multiple sclerosis naturally: a self-help guide to living with MS*. Healing Arts Press, Rochester.

Grant RM, Carver AD and Sloan RL (1998) MS in Fife. *Scott Med J* 43, 44–7.

Gray M (2011) Is that supposed to be me? *MS Matters* 100, Nov/Dec, 22–3.

Gray OM, McDonnell GV and Hawkins SA (2008) Factors in the rising prevalence of MS in the North-East of Ireland. *Mult Scler J* 14, 880–6.

Green G (2009) *The end of stigma: changes in the social experience of long-term illness*. Routledge, Abingdon.

Green G and Todd J (2008) 'Restricting choices and limiting independence': social and economic impact of MS upon households by level of disability. *Chronic Illn* 4(3), 160–72.

Green G, Todd J and Pevalin D (2007) Biographical disruption associated with MS: using propensity scoring to assess the impact. *Soc Sci Med* 65(3), 524–35.

Greenhaigh J, Ford H, Long AF and Hurst K (2004) The MS symptom impact diary (MSSID): psychometric evaluation of a new instrument to measure the day to day impact of multiple sclerosis. *J Neurol Neurosurg Psychiatry* 75, 577–82.

Griffin P (2001) *The people with no name*. Princeton University Press, Princeton.

Gruenewald DA, Higginson IJ, Vivat B, Edmonds P and Burman RE (2004) Quality of life measures for palliative care of people severely affected by MS: a systematic review. *Mult Scler* 10, 690–725.

Gutteridge V (2006) Addressing economic realities: how to maintain the benefits of MS specialist nursing. *Br J Neurosci Nurs* 2(10), 499–504.

Hakim EA, Bakheit AM, Bryant TN, Roberts MW, McIntosh-Michaelis SA, Spackman AJ, Martin JP and McLellan DL (2000) The social impact of MS: a study of 305 patients and their relatives. *Disabil Rehabil* 22(6), 288–93.

Hammond SR, McLeod JG, Millingen KS, Stewart-Wynne EG, English D, Holland JT and McCall MG (1988) The epidemiology of multiple sclerosis in three Australian cities: Perth, Newcastle and Hobart. *Brain* 111, 1–25.

Hammond SR, McLeod JG, Macaskill P and English DR (1996) MS in Australia: socio-economic factors. *J Neurol Neurosurg Psychiatry* 61, 311–3.

Hammond SR, English DR and McLeod JG (2000) The age-range of risk of developing multiple sclerosis: evidence from a migrant population in Australia. *Brain* 123, 968–74.

Handel AE, Handunnetthi L, Ebers G and Ramagopalan SV (2009a) Type 1 diabetes mellitus and multiple sclerosis: common etiological features. *Nat Rev Endocrinol* 5(12), 655–64.

Handel AE, Jarvis L, McLaughlin R, Fries A, Ebers G and Ramagopalan SV (2009b) The epidemiology of multiple sclerosis in Scotland: inferences from hospital admissions. *PLoS ONE* 6(1), e14606. doi:10.1371/journal.pone.0014606.

Handel AE, Williamson AJ, Disanto G, Handunnetthi L, Giovannoni G and Ramagopalan SV (2010) An up-dated meta-analysis of multiple sclerosis following infectious mononucleosis. *PLoS ONE* 5(9), e12496. doi:10.1371/journal.pone.0012496.

Handel AE, Williamson AJ, Disanto G, Dobson R, Giovannoni G and Ramagopalan SV (2011) Smoking and multiple sclerosis: an updated meta-analysis. *PLoS ONE* 6(1), e16149. doi:10.1371/journal.pone.0016149.

Havrdova E, Galetta S, Hutchinson M, Steafaski D, Bates D, Polman CH, O'Connor PW, Giovannoni G, Phillips JT, Lublin FD, Pace A, Kim R and Hyde R (2009) Effect of natalizumab in clinical and radiological disease activity in multiple sclerosis: a retrospective analysis of the Natalizumab safety and efficiency in relapsing-remitting multiple sclerosis (AFFIRM) study. *Lancet Neurol* 8, 254–60.

Hawkes CH and Giovannoni G (2010) The McDonald criteria for multiple sclerosis: time for clarification. *Mult Scler J* 16(5), 566–75.

Hawkins S and Kee F (1988) Updated epidemiological studies of MS in N. Ireland. *J Neurol* 235: S86, note 176.

Hawton K and van Heeringen K (2009) Suicide. *Lancet* 373, 1372–81.

Heinonen R and Dorning H (2011) *Experiences of people using MS specialist nurse services*. MS Society, London.

Hemmett L, Holmes J, Barnes M and Russell N (2004) What drives quality of life in multiple sclerosis? *QJM* 97, 671–6.

Hennessy A, Swingler RJ and Compston DA (1989) The incidence and mortality of MS in south east Wales. *J Neurol Neurosurg Psychiatry* 52, 1085–9.

Hepworth M and Harrison J (2004) A survey of the information needs of people with multiple sclerosis. *Health Informatics J* 10, 49–69.

Hermann BP, Vickrey B, Hays RD, Cramer J, Devinsky O, Meador K, Perrine K, Myers LW and Ellison GW (1996) A comparison of health related quality of life in patients with epilepsy, diabetes and multiple sclerosis. *Epilepsy Research* 25, 113–8.

Hernan MA, Jick SS, Logroscino G, Olek MJ, Asherio A and Jick H (2005) Cigarette smoking and the progression of MS. *Brain* 128, 1461–5.

Higginson IJ and Hart S (2006) Symptom prevalence and severity in people severely affected by multiple sclerosis. *J Palliative Care* 22(3), 158–65.

Higginson IJ, Hart S, Burman R, Silber E, Saleem T and Edmonds P (2008) Randomised controlled trial of a new palliative care service: compliance, recruitment and completeness of follow-up. *BMC Palliat Care* 7:7.

Higginson IJ, McCrone P, Hart SR, Burman R, Silber E and Edmonds PM (2009) Is short-term palliative care cost-effective in multiple sclerosis? A randomised phase II trial. *J Pain Symptom Manage* 38(6), 816–26.

Hignell A (2011) *Higgy: matches, microphones and MS*. Bloomsbury, London.
Hirst CL, Ingram G, Swingler R, Compston A, Pickersgill TP and Robertson NP (2008a) Change in disability in patients with MS: a 20 year prospective population based analysis. *J Neurol Neurosurg Psychiatry* 79, 1137–43.
Hirst CL, Swingler R, Compston A, Ben-Shlomo Y and Robertson NP (2008b) Survival and cause of death in MS: a prospective population based study. *J Neurol Neurosurg Psychiatry* 79, 1016–21.
Hirst CL, Ingram G, Pearson O Pickersgill T, Scolding N and Robertson N (2008c) Contribution of relapses to disability in MS. *J Neurol* 255(2), 280–7.
Hirst C, Ingram G, Pickersgill T, Swingler R and Compston DAS (2009) Increasing prevalence and incidence of MS in South East Wales. *J Neurol Neurosurg Psychiatry* 80, 386–91.
Hobart JC and Cano S (2009) Improving the evaluation of therapeutic interventions in MS: the role of new psychometric methods. *Health Technol Assess* 13(12), 1–200.
Hobart J, Lamping D, Fitzpatrick R, Riazi A and Thompson A (2001) The Multiple Sclerosis Impact Scale (MSIS-29): a new patient-based outcome measure. *Brain* 124, 962–73.
Hobart JC, Riazi A, Lamping DI, Fitzpatrick R, and Thompson AJ (2003) Measuring the impact of MS on walking ability. The 12-item MS Walking Scale (MSWS-12). *Neurology* 60(1), 31–6.
Hobart JC, Cano SJ, Zajicek JP and Thompson AJ (2007) Rating scales as outcome measures for clinical trials in neurology: problems, solutions, and recommendations. *Lancet Neurol* 6, 1094–105.
Hollowell J (1997) The general practice research database: quality of morbidity data. *Population Trends* 87, 36–40.
Holmes J, Madgwick T and Bates D (1995) The cost of MS. *Br J Med Econ* 8, 181–93.
Honigsbaum M (2009) The patient's view: John Donne and Katharine Anne Porter. *Lancet* 374, 194–5.
Hughes N, Locock L and Ziebland S (2013) Personal identity and the role of 'carer' among relatives and friends of people with multiple sclerosis. *Soc Sci Med* 96, 78–85.
Hurwitz BJ (2011a) Registry studies of long-term multiple sclerosis outcomes: description of key registries. *Neurology* 76 (Suppl. 1), S3–S6.
—— (2011b) Analysis of current multiple sclerosis registers. *Neurology* 76 (Suppl. 1), S7–S13.
Hutchinson M (2011) Relapses do not matter in relation to long-term disability: commentary. *Mult Scler J* 17, 1417.
Hyland MJ (2012) Hardy animal. *Granta* 120, 29–46.
Ingram G, Colley E, Ben-Shlomo Y, Crossburn M, Hirst CL, Pickersgill TP and Robertson NP (2010) Validity of patient-derived disability and clinical data in multiple sclerosis. *Mult Scler J* 16(4), 472–9.
ISSCR (International Society for Stem Cell Research) (2008) *Patient handbook on Stem Cell Therapies*. ISSCR, www.isscr.org.
Jennum P, Wanscher B, Frederiksen J and Kielberg J (2012) The socioeconomic consequences of multiple sclerosis: a controlled national study. *European Neuropsychopharmacology* 22(1), 36–43.

Jick H, Jick SS and Derby LE (1991) Validation of information recorded on general practitioner based computerised data resource in the United Kingdom. *BMJ* 302, 766–8.

Jobin C, Larochette C, Parpal H, Coyle PK and Duquette P (2010) Gender issues in multiple sclerosis: an update. *Women's Health* 6(6), 797–820.

Johnson J (2003) On receiving the diagnosis of multiple sclerosis: managing the transition. *Mult Scler J* 9, 82–8.

Johnson J, Goldstone L and Smith P (2001a) *Evaluation of MS Specialist Nurses. A review and development of the role. Part I Report on the national survey of MS Specialist Nurses in the UK.* South Bank University of London and MS Research Trust.

Johnson J, Goldstone L and Smith P (2001b) *Evaluation of MS Specialist Nurses. A review and development of the role. Part II Case study of a new MS Specialist Nurse service in West Berkshire.* South Bank University of London and MS Research Trust.

Jones KH, Ford DV, Jones PA, John A, Middleton RM, Lockhart-Jones H, Osborne LA and Noble GJ (2012) A large scale study of anxiety and depression in people with multiple sclerosis: a survey via the web portal of the UK MS Register. *PLoS ONE* 7(7), e41910. doi:10.1371/journal.pone.0041910.

Julian LJ, Vella L, Vollmer T, Hadjimichael O and Mohr DC (2008) Employment in multiple sclerosis. Exiting and re-entering the work force. *J Neurol* 255, 1354–60.

Karampampa K, Gustavsson A, Miltenburger C and Eckert B (2012) Treatment experience, burden and unmet needs (TRIBUNE) in MS: results from five European countries. *Mult Scler J* 18(6) (Suppl. 2), 7–15.

Kapoor R, Furby J, Hayton T, Smith KJ, Daniel R, Altmann DR, Brenner R, Chataway J, Hughes RAC and Miller DH (2010) Lamotrigine for neuroprotection in secondary progressive multiple sclerosis: a randomised, double-blind, placebo-controlled, parallel-group trial. *Lancet Neurol* 9, 681–8.

Karenberg A (2008) MS on screen: from disaster to coping. *Mult Scler J* 14(4), 530–40.

Khan F, Ng L and Turner-Stokes L (2008) Effectiveness of rehabilitation intervention in persons with multiple sclerosis: a randomised controlled trial. *J Neurol Neurosurg Psychiatry* 79, 1230–5.

Kingston M (2010) *The MonSter and the Rainbow: memoir of a disability.* Jay walker Writing, Newport.

Kobelt G, Lindgren P, Parkin D, Francis D, Johnson M, Bates D and Jonsson B (2000) Costs and quality of life in MS: a cross-sectional observational study in the UK. *Stockholm School of Economics Working Paper Series in Economics and Finance*, Stockholm.

Kobelt G, Berg J, Lindgren P, Kerrigan J, Russell N and Nixon R (2006a) Costs and quality of life of multiple sclerosis in the United Kingdom. *Eur J Health Econ* 7, S96–S104.

Kobelt G, Berg J, Lindgren P, Fredrickson S and Jonsson B (2006b) Costs and quality of life of patients with multiple sclerosis in Europe. *J Neurol Neurosurg Psychiatry* 77, 918–26.

Koch M, Uyttenboogaart M, van Harten AM and Keyser J (2008a) Factors associated with the risk of secondary progression in MS. *Mult Scler J* 14, 799–803.

Koch M, De Keyser J and Tremlett H (2008b) Timing of birth and disease progression in MS. *Mult Scler J* 14(6), 793–8.

Koch M, Kingwell E, Rieckmann P, Tremlet H and UBC MS Clinic Neurologists (2011) The natural history of secondary progressive multiple sclerosis. *J Neurol Neurosurg Psychiatry* 81, 1039–43.

Koch-Henriksen N and Sorensen PS (2010) The changing demographic pattern of multiple sclerosis epidemiology. *Lancet Neurol* 9, 520–32.

―――― (2011) Why does the north-south gradient of incidence of multiple sclerosis seem to have disappeared on the Northern hemisphere? *J Neurol Sci* 311, 58–63.

Koch-Henriksen N, Ramussen S, Stenager E and Madsen M (2001) The Danish MS registry: history, data collection and validity. *Dan Med Bull*, 48, 91–4.

Koffman J, Gao W, Goddard C, Burman R, Jackson D, Shaw P, Barnes F, Silber E and Higginson I (2013) Progression, symptoms and psychosocial concerns among those severely affected by multiple sclerosis: a mixed-methods cross-sectional study of black Caribbean and white British people. *PLoS ONE*. doi: 10.1371/journal.pone.0075431.

Kraft GH, Johnson KL, Yorkston K, Amtmann D, Bamer A, Bombardier C, Ehde D, Fraser R and Starks H (2008) Setting the agenda for multiple sclerosis rehabilitation research. *Mult Scler J* 14, 1292–7.

Kurtzke JF (1967) On the fine structure of the distribution of MS. *Acta Neurol Scand* 43, 257–82.

―――― (1983) Rating neurological impairment in multiple sclerosis: an expanded disability status scale (EDSS). *Neurology* 33, 1444–52.

Lake J and Evans R (2007 Eds) *MS talent*, Volume 1. Jasmine Cottage, England.

―――― (2009 Eds) *MS talent*, Volume 2. Jasmine Cottage, England.

Lalmohamed A, Bazelier MT, van Staa TP, Uitdehaag BMJ, Leufkens HGM, De Boer A and De Vries F (2012) Causes of death in patients with multiple sclerosis and matched reference subjects: a population-based cohort study. *Eur J Neurol* 18(7), 1007–14.

Lancet Neurology, Leading Edge Comment (2010) A new voice for global neurology. *Lancet Neurology* 9(1), 1.

Lancet Neurology Editorial (2011a) UK neurological care: time to confront the crisis. *Lancet Neurol* 10(8), 671.

―――― (2011b) Balancing the benefits and risks of new drugs for MS. *Lancet Neurol* 10(6), 491.

Langer-Gould A et al. (2013) Incidence of MS in multi-racial and ethnic groups. *Neurology* 80(19), 1734–9.

Lawlor DA and Stone T (2001) Public health and data protection: an inevitable collision or potential for a meeting of minds? *Int J Epidemiol* 30(6), 1221–5.

Lawson DH, Sherman V and Hollowell J (1998) The GPRD. *QJM* 445–52.

Le Blond S (2008) *Down to a sunless sea*. YouWriteOn.com.

Lebrun C, Bensa C, Debouviere M, De Seze J, Wiertlievski S, Brochet B, Clavelou P, Brassat D, Labouge P and Roullet E (2008) Unexpected multiple sclerosis: follow-up of 30 patients with magnetic resonance imaging and clinical conversion profile. *J Neurol Neurosurg Psychiatry* 79, 195–8.

Lee D, Newell R, Ziegler L and Topping A (2008) Treatment of fatigue in MS: a systematic review of the literature. *Int J Nurs Pract* 14(2), 81–93.

Lily O, McFadden E, Hensor E, Johnson M and Ford H (2006) Disease-specific quality of life in multiple sclerosis: the effect of disease modifying treatment. *Mult Scler J* 12, 808–13.

Lockyer MJ (1991) Prevalence of MS in five rural Suffolk practices. *BMJ*, 303, 347–8.

Loder C (1996) *Standing in the sunshine.* Random House, London.

Lonergan R, Kinsella K, Fitzpatrick P, Brady J, Murray B, Dunne C, Hagan R, Duggan M, Jordan S, McKenna M, Hutchinson M and Tubridy N (2011) Multiple sclerosis prevalence in Ireland: relationship to vitamin D status and HLA genotype. *J Neurol Neurosurg Psychiatry* 82, 317–22.

Lublin FD, Baier M and Cutter G (2003) Effect of relapses on development of residual deficit in multiple sclerosis. *Neurology* 61, 1528–32.

MacDonald BK, Cockerell OC, Sander JWAS and Shorvon SD (2000) The incidence and life-time prevalence of neurological disorders in a prospective community-based study in the UK. *Brain* 123, 665–76.

Mackenzie, IS, Morant SV, Bloomfield GA, MacDonald TM and O'Riordan J (2014) Incidence and prevalence of multiple sclerosis in the UK 1990–2010: a descriptive study in the General Practice Research Database. *J Neurol Neurosurg Psychiatry* 85, 76–84.

MacLurg K, Reilly P, Hawkins S, Gray O, Evason E and Whittington D (2005) A primary care-based needs assessment of people with multiple sclerosis. *Br J Gen Pract* 55(514), 378–83.

Manouchehrinia A and Constantinescu CS (2012) Cost-effectiveness of disease-modifying therapies in multiple sclerosis. *Curr Neurol Neurosci Rep* 12(5), 592–600.

Markby DP (1987) The distribution of multiple sclerosis in the United Kingdom. *J Neurol Neurosurg Psychiatry* 50(4), 505–6.

Martyn CN and Osmond C (1989) The prevalence of multiple sclerosis in south east Wales (letter). *J Neurol Neurosurg Psychiatry* 52, 1017.

Matthews P (2008) Meeting the challenge of new drug development for MS. *Research Matters,* Issue 1, 22–3, MS Society.

Maw S (2011) The impact of the NICE guidelines on people's experience of being diagnosed with multiple sclerosis. *Way Ahead* 15(4) Oct, 8–9.

Mayer JD (1981) Geographical clues about multiple sclerosis. *Ann Assoc Am Geogrs* 71(1), 28–39.

Mayor S (2009) Alan Thompson: opening doors for patients with MS. *Lancet Neurol* 8(3), 230.

McCabe C, Claxton K and Culyer AJ (2008) The NICE cost-effectiveness threshold and what that means. *Pharmacoeconomics* 26(9), 733–44.

McCabe C, Chilcott J, Claxton K, Tappenden P, Cooper C, Roberts J, Cooper N and Abrams K (2010) Continuing the multiple sclerosis risk sharing scheme is unjustified. *BMJ* 340:c1786.

McCrone P, Heslin M, Knapp M, Bull P and Thompson A (2008) MS in the UK: service use, costs, quality of life and disability. *Pharmacoeconomics* 26(10), 847–60.

McDonald WI, Compston A, Edan G, Goodkin D, Hartung HP, Lublin FD, McFarland HF, Paty DW, Holman CH, Reingold SC, Sandberg-Wollheim M, Sibley W, Thompson A, van den Noort S, Weinshenker BY and Wolinsky JS (2001) Recommended diagnostic criteria for MS: guidelines from the international panel on the diagnosis of MS. *Ann Neurol* 50, 121–7.

McDonnell GV and Hawkins SA (1998) An epidemiologic study of MS in Northern Ireland. *Neurol* 50, 423–8.

——— (1999) High incidence and prevalence of MS in south east Scotland: evidence of a genetic predisposition. *J Neurol Neurosurg Psychiatry* 66, 411.
——— (2001) An assessment of the spectrum of disability and handicap in MS: a population-based study. *Mult Scler J* 7(2), 111–7.
McDowell L (2009) *Working bodies: interactive service employment and workplace identities*. Wiley-Blackwell, Chichester.
McGuigan C, McCarthy A, Quigley C, Bannan L, Hawkins SA and Hutchinson M (2004) Latitudinal variation in the prevalence of MS in Ireland, an effect of genetic diversity. *J Neurol Neurosurg Psychiatry* 75, 572–6.
McHugh JC, Galvin PL and Murphy RP (2008) Retrospective comparison of the revised McDonald criteria in a general neurology practice in Ireland. *Mult Scler J* 14(1), 81–5.
McLeod JG, Hammond SR and Kurtzke JF (2011) Migration and multiple sclerosis in immigrants to Australia from United Kingdom and Ireland: a reassessment. 1. Risk of MS by age at immigration. *J Neurol* 258, 1140–9.
McNally S, Ben-Shlomo Y and Newman S (1999) The effects of respite care on informal carers' well-being: a systematic review. *Disabil Rehabil* 21, 1–14.
Millar JHD (1980) MS in N. Ireland. In Rose FC (Ed) *Clinical neuroepidemiology*. Pitman Medical, Tunbridge Wells, England.
Miller A (2008) Everybody needs good neighbours. *Open Door*, May, 10–1.
Miller D, Weinshenker B, Filippi M, Banwell B, Cohen J, Freedman M, Galetta S, Hutchinson M, Johnson r, Kappos l, Kira J, Lublin F, McFarland H, Montalban X, Panitch H, Richert J, Rheingold S and Polman C (2008) Differential diagnosis of suspected MS: a consensus approach. *Mult Scler J* 14(9), 1157–74.
Miller DH and Leary SM (2007) Primary progressive MS. *Lancet Neurol* 6(10), 903–12.
Monks J and Robinson I (1989) The characteristics of a national register of people with MS: a comparison between the ARMS register and 10 British MS populations. *J Epidemiol Community Health* 43, 179–86.
Montgomery SM, Bahmanyar S, Hillert J, Ekbom A and Olsson T (2008) Maternal smoking during pregnancy and MS among offspring. *Eur J Neurol* 15(12), 1395–9.
Moore P, Hirst C, Harding KE et al. (2012) Multiple sclerosis and depression. *J Psychosom Res* 73(4), 272–6.
Moore P, Harding K, Clarkson H, Pickersgill TP, Wardle M and Robertson NP (2013) Demographic and clinical factors associated with changes in employment in multiple sclerosis. *Mult Scler* 19(12), 1647–54.
MORI (2003) *Measuring up: experiences of people with MS of health services*. MS Society, London.
Morgan O and Baker A (2006) Measuring deprivation in England and Wales using 2001 Carstairs scores. *Health Statistics Quarterly* 31, 28–33.
Mowry EM, Deen S, Malikova I, Pelletier J, Bacchetti P and Waubant E (2009a) The onset location of MS predicts the location of subsequent relapses. *J Neurol Neurosurg Psychiatry* 80(4), 400–3.
Mowry EM, Pesic M, Grimes B, Deen S, Bacchetti P and Waubant E (2009b) Demyelinating events in early MS have inherent severity and recovery. *Neurology* 72(7), 602–8.
Mullen F, Acheson K and Coates V (2011) Assessing multiple sclerosis patients' and carers' views of respite care. *Br J Neurosci Nurs* 7(3), 547–52.

MSIF (undated) *Principles to promote the quality of life of people with MS.* MSIF, London.
—— (2010) *MSIF survey on employment and MS.* MSIF, London.
—— (2013) *Atlas of MS 2013.* MSIF, London.
Multiple Sclerosis Society of Great Britain and Northern Ireland (undated) Symptom Management Survey. MS Society, London.
MS Society (2002) *Are we being served? Health care experiences of people with MS.* MS Society, London.
—— (2003) *Cannabinoid-based medicines for symptom relief: consultation with people with MS.* MS Society, London.
—— (2008) *What is Primary Progressive MS?* MS Society, London.
—— (2010a) *What is MS?* MS Society, London.
—— (2010b) *Stem cell therapies in MS.* MS Society, London.
—— (2013) Top 10 research priorities. At mssociety.org.uk/ms-news/2013/09/top-10-ms-research-priorities-identified.
—— (2014a) Fatigue. *MS Essentials 14.* MS Society, London.
—— (2014b) The new guideline for MS – what does it mean? MS Society website accessed 17/10/14, http://www.mssociety.org.uk/get-involved/campaigns/campaigns-blog/2014/10/new-guidelins-ms-E2%80%93-what-does-it-mean.
MS Society and the National Hospital for Neurology and Neurosurgery (1997) *Standards of healthcare for people with MS.* MS Society, London.
MS Trust (2004) *MS explained.* MS Trust, Letchworth.
—— (2008) *Falls.* MS Trust, Letchworth.
—— (2015) Management of MS in primary and secondary care – NICE Clinical Guideline 186: an analysis of how it measures up. *Way Ahead* 19(1), 11–5.
Mumford CA, Fraser MB, Wood NW and Compston DA (1992) MS in the Cambridge health district of East Anglia. *J Neurol Neurosurg Psychiatry* 55, 877–82.
Murphy N, Confravreux C, Haas J, Konig N, Roullet E, Saller M, Swash M, Young C, Merlot J-L and the Cost of Multiple Sclerosis Study Group (1998) Economic evaluation of multiple sclerosis in the UK, Germany and France. *Pharmacoeconomics* 13, 607–22.
Murray S, Bashir K, Penrice G and Wormersley J (2004) Epidemiology of MS in Glasgow. *Scott Med J* 49, 100–4.
Murray TJ (2005) *Multiple sclerosis: the history of a disease.* Demos, New York.
Mutch K (2010) In sickness and in health: experience of caring for a spouse with MS. *Br J Nurs* 19(4), 214–9.
Mynors G, Perman S and Morse M (2012) *Defining the value of MS specialist nurses.* MS Trust, Letchworth.
Naci H, Fleurence R, Birt J and Duhig A (2010) The impact of increasing neurological disability of multiple sclerosis on health utilities: a systematic review of the literature. *J Med Econ* 13(1), 78–89.
National Audit Office (2011) *Department of health: services for people with neurological conditions.* The Stationary Office, London.
NHS National Workforce Projects (2008) *Long-term neurological conditions: a good practice guide to the development of the multidisciplinary team and the value of the specialist nurse.* National Workforce Projects, Manchester.
National end of life care Intelligence Network NEoLCIN (2010) Deaths from neurodegenerative diseases in England, 2002 to 2008. *NEoLCIN Bulletin* 1. NHS.

Neurological Alliance (2003) Neuro numbers: a brief overview of the numbers of people in the UK with a neurological condition. Neurological Alliance, London. Website – www.neural.org.uk.

Neurological Commissioning Support (2010) *Halfway through – are we halfway there?* Neurological Commissioning Support, London.

NICE (2002) *Beta interferon and galtiramer acetate for the treatment of multiple sclerosis.* Technical Appraisal Guidance No 32, NICE, London.

——— (2003) *Management of MS in primary and secondary care.* NICE, London.

——— (2014) *Multiple sclerosis: management of multiple sclerosis in primary and secondary care.* NICE clinical guideline 186. NICE, London.

Nicholas R and Wilkie D (2011) Oral disease modifying treatments in the management of MS. *Open Door*, Aug, 6–7.

Nicholl L, Hobart JC, Cramp AFL and Lowe-Strong AS (2005) Measuring quality of life in multiple sclerosis: not as simple as it sounds. *Mult Scler J* 11, 708–12.

Nielson NM, Frisch M, Rostgaard K, Wohlfahrt J, Hjalgrim H, Koch-Henriksen N, Melbye M and Westergaard T (2008) Autoimmune diseases in patients with MS and their first-degree relatives: a nationwide cohort study in Denmark. *Mult Scler J* 14(6), 823–9.

Noble JG, Osbourne LA, Jones KH, Middleton RM and Ford DV (2012) Commentary on Disability outcome measures in multiple sclerosis clinical trials. *Mult Scler J* 18(12), 1718–20.

Nortvedt MW and Riise T (2003) The use of quality of life measures in multiple sclerosis research. *Mult Scler J* 9, 63–72.

O'Brien MT (1993) MS: stressors and coping strategies in spousal caregivers. *J Community Health Nursing* 10, 123–35.

O'Connor RJ et al. (2005) Factors influencing work retention for people with multiple sclerosis: cross-sectional studied using qualitative and quantitative methods. *J Neurol* 252(8), 892–6.

O'Hara L, de Souza L and Ide L (2004) The nature of care giving in a community sample of people with multiple sclerosis. *Disabil Rehabil* 26, 1401–10.

Oliver M (1996) *Understanding disability: from theory to practice.* Palgrave Macmillan, Basingstoke.

Orme M, Kerrigan J, Tyas D, Russel N and Nixon R (2007) The effect of disease, functional status, and relapses on the utility of people with MS in the UK. *Value in Health* 10(1), 54–60.

Orton SM, Herrera BM, Yee IM, Valdar W, Ramagopalan SV and Eber GC for the Canadian Collaborative Study Group (2006) Sex ratio of MS in Canada: a longitudinal study. *Lancet Neurol* 5, 932–6.

Osborne LA et al. (2012) Sources of discovery, reasons for registration and expectations of an Internet-based register for MS. *International Journal of Healthcare Information Systems and Informatics* 7(3), 27–43.

Osoegawa M, Kira J, Fukazawa T, Fujihara K, Kikuchi S, Matsui M, Kohriyama T, Sobue G, Yamamura T, Itoyama Y, Saida T, Sakata K, Ochi H, Matsuoka T: the Research Committee of Neuroimmunological Diseases (2009) Temporal changes and geographical differences in MS phenotypes in Japanese: nationwide survey results over 30 years. *Mult Scler J* 15(2), 159–73.

Page SA and Mitchell I (2006) Patients' opinions on privacy, consent and the disclosure of health information for medical research. *Chronic Dis Can* 27(2), 60–7.

Parcker G (2008) *Disability poverty in the UK*. Leonard Cheshire Disability, London.
Parkin D, McNamee P and Jacoby A (1998) A cost-utility analysis of Interferon β for multiple sclerosis. *Health Technol Assess* 2, 1–58.
Parkin D, Jacoby A, McNamee P, Miller P, Thomas S and Bates D (2000) Treatment of multiple sclerosis with interferon β: an appraisal of cost-effectiveness and quality of life. *J Neurol Neurosurg Psychiatry 68*, 144–9.
Parmelee MD (2009) *Awkward bitch: my life with MS*. AuthorHouse, Milton Keynes.
Parr H (2002) New body geographies: the embodied spaces of health and medical information on the Internet. *Environment and Planning D: Society and Space* 20, 73–95.
Paty DW and Ebers GC (1998, Eds.) *Multiple sclerosis*. FA Davis, Philadelphia.
Payne A (2012) Your food, your diet. Should we take a fresh approach? *Open Door*, Feb, 6–7.
Persad G, Wertheimer A and Emanuel EJ (2009) Principles for the allocation of scarce medical resources. *Lancet* 373(9661), 423–31.
Peterson EW, Cho CC and Findlayson ML (2007) Fear of falling and associated activity curtailment among middle-aged and older adults with multiple sclerosis. *Mult Scler J* 13, 1168–75.
Peterson EW, von Koch L, Cho CC and Findlayson ML (2008) Injurious falls among middle-aged and older adults with MS. *Archives of Physical Medicine and Rehabilitation* 89(6), 1031–7.
Petit-Zeman (2010) Giving people what they want. Want to know which treatments work best? Try asking patients. *Prospect*. Jul, 58.
Peuckmann-Post V, Elsner F, Krumm N, Trottenberg, P and Radbruch L (2010) Efficacy of pharmacological treatments for fatigue associated with advanced disease. *Cochrane Database of Systematic Reviews*, Issue 11.
Pfleger C, Koch-Henriksen N, Stenager E, Flachs E and Johansen C (2009) Head injury is not a risk factor for MS: a prospective cohort study. *Mult Scler J* 15(3), 294–8.
Pfleger CCH, Flachs EM and Koch-Henriksen N (2010a) Social consequences of multiple sclerosis: clinical and demographic predictors – a historical prospective cohort study. *Eur J Neurol* 17, 1346–51.
―――― (2010b) Social consequences of multiple sclerosis. Part 2. Divorce and separation: a historical prospective cohort study. *Mult Scler J* 16(7), 878–82.
Phadke JK (1987) Survival pattern and cause of death in patients with multiple sclerosis: results from an epidemiological survey in north east Scotland. *J Neurol Neurosurg Psychiatry* 50, 523–31.
Phadke JK and Downie AW (1987) Epidemiology of MS in the north east (Grampian region) of Scotland – an update. *J Epidemiol Community Health* 4, 5–13.
Plumb S (2006) *MS and Palliative Care: a guide for health and social care professionals*. MS Society, London.
Polman CH, Rheingold SC, Banwell B, Clanet M, Cohen JA, Filippi M, Fujihara K, Havrdova E, Hutchinson M, Kappos L, Lublin FD, Montalban X, O'Connor P, Sandberg-Wollheim M, Thompson AJ, Waubant E, Weinshenker B and Wolinsky JS (2005) Diagnostic criteria for MS: 2005 revisions to the MacDonald criteria. *Ann Neurol* 58(6), 840–6.
Pompili M, Forte A, Palermo M et al. (2012) Suicide risk in multiple sclerosis: a systematic review of current literature. *J Psychosom Res* 73(6), 411–7.

Porter B and Keenan E (2003) Nursing at a specialist diagnostic clinic for multiple sclerosis. *Br J Nurs* 12(11), 650–6.
Poskanzer DC, Schapira K and Miller H (1963) Epidemiology of MS in the counties of Northumberland and Durham. *J Neurol Neurosurg Psychiatry* 26, 368–76.
Poskanzer DC, Walker AM, Yonkondy J and Sheridan JL (1976) Studies of epidemiology in Orkney and Shetland Islands. *Neurology* 26, 14–7.
Poskanzer DC, Prenney LB, Sheriden JL and Kondy JY (1980) MS in the Orkney and Shetland Islands. 1: Epidemiology, clinical factors and methodology. *J Epidemiol Community Health* 34, 229–39.
Poser CM (1995) Viking voyages: the origin of multiple sclerosis? An essay in medical history. *Acta Neurol Scand* Suppl. 16(1), 11–22.
Poser CM, Paty DW and Scheinberg L (1983) New diagnostic criteria for MS: guidelines for research protocols. *Ann Neurol* 13, 227–31.
Prasad A and Bell L (2008) *'I've got nothing to lose by trying it': weighing up claims about cures and therapies for long-term conditions.* Sense about Science, London.
Prunty M, Sharpe L, Butow P and Fulcher G (2008) The motherhood choice: themes arising in the decision-making process for women with multiple sclerosis. *Mult Scler J* 14, 701–4.
Pugliatti M, Sotgiu S and Rosati G (2002) The worldwide prevalence of MS. *Clinical Neurology and Neurosurgery* 104, 182–91.
Qiu J (2010) Venous abnormalities and multiple sclerosis: another breakthrough claim. *Lancet Neurol* 9(5), 464–5.
Ragonese P, Aridon P, Salemi G, D'Amelio M and Savettieri G (2008) Mortality in MS: a review. *Eur J Neurol* 15(2), 123–7.
Ramagopalan SV, Dyment DA, Valdar W, Herrera BM, Criscuoli M, Yee IML, Sadovnick AD and Ebers GC (2007) Autoimmune disease in families with MS: a population-based study. *Lancet Neurol* 6, 694–710.
Ramagopalan SV, Dobson R, Meier U and Giovannoni G (2010) Multiple sclerosis: risk factors, prodromes and potential causal pathways. *Lancet Neurol* 9, 727–39.
Ramagopalan SV, Handel AE, Giovannnoni G, Rutherford Siegel S, Ebers GC and Chaplin G (2011a) Relationship of UV exposure to prevalence of multiple sclerosis in England. *Neurology* 76, 1410–4.
Ramagopalan SV, Hoang U, Seagroatt V, Handel A, Ebers GC, Giovannoni G and Goldacre MJ (2011b) Geography of hospital admissions for multiple sclerosis in England and comparison with the geography of hospital admissions for infectious mononucleosis: a descriptive study. *J Neurol Neurosurg Psychiatry* 82, 682–7.
Ramagopalan SV, Seinog O, Goldacre R and Goldacre M (2012) Risk of fractures in patients with multiple sclerosis: record-linkage study. *BMC Neurology* 12, 135.
Rhodes M (2011) *CCSVI as the Cause of Multiple Sclerosis. The science behind the controversial therapy.* McFarland, London.
Riazi A, Hobart JC, Fitzpatrick R, Freeman JA and Thompson AJ (2003) Sociodemographic variables are limited predictors of health status in multiple sclerosis. *J Neurol* 250, 1088–93.
Riazi A, Thompson AJ and Hobart JC (2004) Self-efficacy predicts self-reported health status in multiple sclerosis. *Mult Scler J* 10, 61–6.
Richards RG, Sampson FC, Beard SM and Tappenden P (2002) *A review of the natural history and epidemiology of MS: implications for resource allocation and health economic models.* Health Technol Assess, 6(10).

Rice CM, Kemp K, Wilkins A and Scolding NJ (2013) Cell therapy for multiple sclerosis: an evolving concept with implications for other neurodegenerative diseases. *Lancet* 382(9899), 1204–13.

Rice-Oxley M, Williams ES and Rees JE (1995) A prevalence survey of MS in Sussex. *J Neurol Neurosurg Psychiatry* 58, 27–30.

Roberts E (2007) *Stumbling along: a journey with the master of surprises*. Writersworld, Enstone Oxfordshire.

Roberts MHW, Martin JP, McLellan DL, McIntosh-Michaelis SA and Spackman AJ (1991) The prevalence of MS in Southampton and South West Hampshire Health Authority. *J Neurol Neurosurg Psychiatry* 54, 55–9.

Robertson N (2000) Enumerating neurology. Editorial. *Brain* 123, 663–4.

Robertson N and Compston A (1995) Surveying MS in the UK. *J Neurol Neurosurg Psychiatry* 58, 2–6.

Robertson N, Deans J, Fraser M and Compston DA (1995) MS in the North Cambridgeshire districts of East Anglia. *J Neurol Neurosurg Psychiatry* 59, 71–6.

Robertson NP, Fraser M, Deans J, Clayton D, Walker N and Compston DAS (1996a) Age-adjusted recurrent risk of relatives of parents with multiple sclerosis. *Brain* 119(2), 449–55.

Robertson N, Deans J, Fraser M and Compston DA (1996b) MS in South Cambridgeshire: incidence and prevalence based on a district register. *J Epidemiol Community Health* 50, 274–9.

Robinson I (1988) Reconstructing lives: negotiating the meaning of multiple sclerosis. In Anderson R and Bury M (Eds) *Living with chronic illness: the experiences of patients and their families*. Unwin Hyman, London.

—— (1991) The context and consequences of communicating the diagnosis of MS: some brief findings from a survey of 900 people. In Wietholter H (Ed.) *Current concepts in multiple sclerosis*. Elsevier Science, Amsterdam.

Robinson I and Hunter M (1998) *Views from the other side: everyday perspectives on living and working with people with MS by those concerned with their informal and formal (health) care*. MS Research Unit, Brunel University, Uxbridge England.

Robinson I, Hunter M and Neilson S (1996) *A dispatch from the frontline: the views of people with MS about their needs*. MS Research Unit, Brunel University, Uxbridge England.

Rose FC, Neilson S and Robinson I (2000) *MS at your fingertips*. Class publishing, London.

Rossiter D and Thompson AJ (1995) Introduction of integrated care pathways for patients with MS in an inpatient neurorehabilitation setting. *Disabil Rehabil* 17(8), 443–8.

Rothwell PM (1998) Quality of life in multiple sclerosis. *J Neurol Neurosurg Psychiatry* 65(4), 433.

Rothwell PM and Charlton D (1998) High incidence and prevalence of MS in south east Scotland: evidence of a genetic predisposition. *J Neurol Neurosurg Psychiatry* 64, 730–5.

Rovaris M, Riccitelli G, Judica E, Possa F, Caputo D, Ghezzi A, Bertolotto A, Capra R, Falautano M, Mattioli F, Martineli V, Comi G and Filippi M (2008) Cognitive impairment and structural brain damage in benign MS. *Neurology* 71, 1521–6.

Royal College of Physicians and the MS Trust (2008) *National audit of services for people with MS 2008: Summary report*. RCP, London.

Royal College of Physicians, National Council for Palliative Care and Society for Rehabilitative Medicine (2008) *Long-term neurological conditions: management of the interface between neurology, rehabilitation and palliative care.* Concise Guidance to Good Practice Series No. 10. Royal College of Physicians, London.

Rudick RA, Miller D, Clough JD, Gragg LA and Farmer RG (1992) Quality of life in MS: comparison with inflammatory bowel disease and rheumatoid arthritis. *Archives of Neurology* 49, 1229–37.

Sadovnick AD, Eisen K, Ebers GC et al. (1991) Cause of death in patients attending multiple sclerosis clinics. *Neurology* 41, 1193–6.

Sapey B, Stewart J and Donaldson G (2005) Increases in wheelchair use and perceptions of disablement. *Disability and Society* 20(5), 489–505.

Sawcer S (2008) The complex genetics of multiple sclerosis: pitfalls and prospects. *Brain* 131(12), 3118–31.

Scalfari A, Neuhaus A, Degenhardt A, Rice GP, Muraro PA, Daumer M and Ebers GC (2010) The natural history of multiple sclerosis, a geographically based study 10: relapses and long-term disability. *Brain* 133, 1914–29.

Schwid SR, Covington M, Segal BM and Goodman AD (2002) Fatigue in MS: current understanding and future directions. *J Rehab Res and Development* 39, 211–24.

Scolding N (2009) Stem cells: the hype and the hope. *Open Door*, Aug, 8–9.

Scolding N and Wilkins A (2012) *Multiple sclerosis.* OUP, Oxford.

Scottish Needs Assessment Project (2000) *Multiple sclerosis.* Office for Public Health in Scotland, Glasgow.

Segal Quince and Partners (1985) *The Cambridge phenomenon: the growth of high technology industry in a university town.* Segal Quince and Partners, Cambridge.

Shakespeare T and Watson N (2001) Disability, politics and recognition. In Albrecht GL, Seelman K and Bury M (Eds) *Handbook of Disability Studies.* Sage, Thousand Oaks, California.

Sharac J, McCrone P and Sabes-Figuera R (2010) Pharmacoeconomic considerations in the treatment of multiple sclerosis. *Drugs* 70(13), 1677–91.

Sharpe G, Price SE, Last A and Thompson RJ (1995) Multiple sclerosis in island populations: prevalence in the Bailiwicks of Guernsey and Jersey. *J Neurol Neurosurg Psychiatry* 58, 22–6.

Shaw M, Dorling D, Gordon D and Davey-Smith G (2000) *The widening gap: health inequalities and policy in Britain.* Policy Press, Bristol.

Shaw M, Bentham T, Davey-Smith G and Dorling D (2008) *The Grim Reaper's Road Map: an atlas of mortality in Britain.* Policy Press, Bristol.

Shepherd DI (1999) Macs with multiple sclerosis. *J Neurol Neurosurg Psychiatry* 66, 410–1.

Shepherd DI and Downie AW (1978) Prevalence of MS in north-east Scotland. *BMJ* 2, 314–6.

Shepherd DI and Summers A (1996) Prevalence of MS in Rochdale. *J Neurol Neurosurg Psychiatry* 61, 415–7.

Shirani A, Zhao Y, Karim ME, Evans C, Kingswell E, van der Kop ML, Oger J, Gustafson P, Petkau J and Tremlett H (2012) Association between use of interferon beta and progression of disability in patients with relapsing-remitting multiple sclerosis. *JAMA* 308(3), 247–56.

Simmons RD (2010) Life issues in multiple sclerosis. *Nat Rev Neurol* 6, 603–10.

Simpson Jr S, Blizzard L, Otahal P, Van der Mei I and Taylor B (2011) Latitude is significantly associated with the prevalence of multiple sclerosis: a meta-analysis. *J Neurol Neurosurg Psychiatry* 82, 1132–41.

Skegg DC, Corwin PA, Craven RS, Malloch JA and Pollock M (1987) Occurrence of multiple sclerosis in the north and south of New Zealand. *J Neurol Neurosurg Psychiatry* 50, 134–9.

Skelton L (2009) *Measuring social wellbeing in the UK*. Working Paper, ONS, London.

Skranbanek P and McCormick J (1992) *Follies and fallacies in medicine*. Tarragon Press, Chippenham.

Sloka JS, Pryse-Phillips WE and Stefanelli M (2008) The relation of ultraviolet radiation and MS in Newfoundland. *Can J Neurol Sci* 35(1), 69–74.

Smeltzer SC (2002) Reproductive decision making in women with multiple sclerosis. *J Neurosci Nurs* 34(3), 145–57.

Smith DM (1977) *Human Geography: a welfare approach*. Edward Arnold, London.

Smith EJ (2009) MS presenting with erotomanic delusions in the context of 'Don't ask, don't tell'. *Mil Med* 174(3), 297–8.

Somers EC, Thomas SL, Smeeth L and Hall AJ (2006) Autoimmune diseases co-occurring within individuals and within families: a systematic review. *Epidemiology* 17, 202–17.

——— (2009) Are individuals with an autoimmune disease at higher risk of a second autoimmune disorder? *Am J Epidemiol* 169, 749–55.

Somerset M, Campbell R, Sharp DJ and Peters TJ (2001) What do people with MS want and expect from health care services? *Health Expectations* 4(1), 29–37.

Somerset M, Sharp D and Campbell R (2002) Multiple sclerosis and quality of life: a qualitative investigation. *J Health Services Research and Policy* 7(3), 151–9.

Sprangers MAG, de Regt EB, Andries F, van Agt HME, Bijl RV, de Boer JB, Foets M, Hoeymans N, Jacobs AE, Kempen GIJM, Miedema HS, Tijhuis MAR and de Haes HCJM (2000) Which chronic conditions are associated with better or poorer quality of life? *J Clinical Epidemiology* 53, 895–907.

Strategy Unit (2005) *Improving the life chance of disabled people*. Cabinet Office, London.

Sundstrom P, Nystrom L and Hallmans G (2008) Smoke exposure increases the risk of MS. *Eur J Neurol* 15(6), 579–83.

Sutherland JM (1956) Observations on the prevalence of MS in Northern Scotland. *Brain* 79, 635–54.

Sweetland J, Riazi A, Cano SJ and Playford ED (2007) Vocational rehabilitation services for people with MS: what patients want from clinicians and employers. *Mult Scler J* 13(9), 183–9.

Sweetland J, Howse E and Playford ED (2012) Systematic review of research undertaken in vocational rehabilitation for people with multiple sclerosis. *Disabil Rehabil* 34(24), 2031–8.

Swingler RJ and Compston D (1986) The distribution of multiple sclerosis in the United Kingdom. *J Neurol Neurosurg Psychiatry* 49, 1115–24.

——— (1988) The prevalence of MS in south east Wales. *J Neurol Neurosurg Psychiatry* 51, 1520–4.

——— (1990) Demographic characteristics of multiple sclerosis in South East Wales. *Neuroepidemiology* 9, 68–77.

Tardieu M and Mikaeloff Y (2008) MS in children: environmental risk factors. *Bull Acad Natl Med* 192(3), 507–9.

The International Genetics Consortium and the Wellcome Trust Case Control Consortium (2011) Genetic risk and a primary role for cell-mediated immune mechanisms I multiple sclerosis. *Nature* 476, 214–9.

Thomas S, Williams R, Williams W and Hall A (2009) Estimates of the prevalence of multiple sclerosis in the United Kingdom. Report to the MS Society Public Briefing http://www.mssociety.org.uk/sites/default/files/MS_prevalence_study_briefing.pdf.

Thomas S, Davies A and Peel C (2010) A mid-term review of the NSF for long-term neurological conditions. *Br J Neurosci Nurs* 6(8), 366–70.

Thompson AJ (2005) Neurorehabilitation in multiple sclerosis: foundations, facts and fiction. *Curr Opinion Neurol* 18, 267–71.

Thompson AJ and Hobart JC (1998) Multiple sclerosis: assessment of disability and disability scales. *J Neurol* 245, 189–96.

Thompson AJ, Toosy AT and Ciccarelli O (2010) Pharmacological management of symptoms in multiple sclerosis: current approaches and future directions. *Lancet Neurol* 9, 1182–99.

Timpson D (2010) *MS: The gloves are off*. Sandars Print People, Northampton, England.

Tomassini V (2008) Imaging brain plasticity in MS. *Way Ahead* 12(4), 8–9.

Townsend G (2008) Supporting people with MS in employment: a United Kingdom survey of current practice and experience. *Br J Occ Ther* 71(3), 103–11.

Tremlett H, Zhao Y and Devonshire V (2008a) Natural history of secondary progressive MS. *Mult Scler J* 14(3), 314–24.

Tremlett H, van der Mei IA, PittasF, Blizzard L, Paley G, Mesaros D, Woodbaker R, Nunez M, Dwyer T, Taylor BV and Ponsonby AL (2008b) Monthly ambient sunlight and relapse rates in MS. *Neuroepidemiology* 31(4), 271–9.

Tripoliti C, Campbell C, Pring T and Taypor-Goh S (2007) Quality of life in MS: should clinicians trust proxy ratings. *Mult Scler J* 13(9), 1190–4.

Trisolini M, Honeycutt A, Wiener T and Lesesne S (2010) *Global economic impact of MS*. MSIF, London.

Tyas D Kerrigan J, Russell N and Nixon R (2007) The distribution of the cost of multiple sclerosis in the UK. How do costs vary by illness severity? *Value in Health* 10(5), 386–9.

van der Linden FAH, D'hooghe MB, Nagels G, Van Nunen A, Polman CH and Uitdehaag BMJ (2008) Proxy ratings from multiple of sources: disagreement on the impact of MS on daily life. *Eur J Neurol* 15(9), 933–9.

van Kessel K and Moss-Morris R (2006) Understanding multiple sclerosis fatigue: a synthesis of biological and psychological factors. *J Psychosom Res* 61, 583–5.

Van Staa T-P and Abenhaim L (1994) The quality of information recorded on a UK database of Primary Care Records: a study of hospitalisations due to hypoglycaemia and other conditions. *Pharmacoepidemiol Drug Safety* 3, 15–31.

Visser EM, Wilde K, Wilson JF, Yong KK and Counsell CE (2012) A new prevalence study of multiple sclerosis in Orkney, Shetland and Aberdeen city. *J Neurol Neurosurg Psychiatry* 83, 719–24.

Vukusic S, Van BV et al. (2007) Regional variations in MS prevalence in French farmers. *J Neurol Neurosurg Psychiatry* 78(7), 707–9.

Wade DT and Green Q (2001) *A study of services for MS. Lessons for managing chronic disability*. Royal College of Physicians, London.

Wall P (2000) *Pain: the science of suffering*. Columbia UP, New York.

Walley T and Mantgani A (1997) The UK General Practice Research Database. *Lancet* 350, 1097–9.

Walton K (2009) Take your place in the system. *MS Matters* 86, Aug/Jul, 22–4.
Ward-Abel N, Mutch K and Huseyin H (2010) Demonstrating multiple sclerosis specialist nurses make a difference. *Br J Neurosci Nurs* 6(7), 319–24.
Ward-Abel N, Vernon K and Warner R (2014) An exciting era of treatments for relapsing-remitting multiple sclerosis. *Br J Neurosci Nurs* 10(1), 21–8.
Warner R, Thomas D and Martin R (2005) Improving service delivery for relapse management in multiple sclerosis. *Br J Nurs* 14(14), 746–53.
Wark P (2009) Stem cells: will hope triumph over hype? *The London Times*, 9 Apr.
Welch HG, Schwartz LM and Woloshin S (2011) *Overdiagnosed: making people sick in the pursuit of health*, Beacon Press, Boston Massachusetts.
Weinshenker BG, Bass B, Rice GPA, Noseworthy J, Carriere W, Baskerville J and Ebers GC (1989) The natural history of MS: a geographical based study 1. Clinical course and disability. *Brain* 112(1), 133–46.
Weinstock–Guttman B, Jacobs LB, Brownscheidle CM, et al. (2003) Multiple sclerosis characteristics in African-American patients in the New York State multiple sclerosis consortium. *Mult Scler J* 9, 293–8.
While A, Forbes A, Ullman R and Mathes L (2009) The role of specialist and general nurses working with people with multiple sclerosis. *J Clin Nurs* 18(18), 2635–48.
Wilkins A and Scolding N (2008) Protecting axons in MS. *Mult Scler J* 14(6), 1013–25.
Williams ES and McKernan RO (1986) Prevalence of MS in a south London borough. *BMJ*, 293, 237–9.
Williams ES, Jones DR and McKernan RO (1991) Mortality rates from multiple sclerosis: geographical and temporal trends revisited. *J Neurol Neurosurg Psychiatry* 54, 104–9.
Woodroffe K, Stevens E, Garside D and Holloway E (undated) *MS Society Respite Care Review. A survey of people with MS and their carers. Addressing the needs and aspirations of people with MS, their families and carers, now and in the future.* MS Society, London.
World Health Organisation and the MS International Federation (2008) *Atlas: MS resources in the world*. WHO, Geneva.
Young C (2008) What's going to happen to me. *MS Matters* 77 Jan/Feb, 14–5.
Zamboni P, Galeotti R, Menegatti E et al. (2009) The chronic cerebrospinal venous insufficiency in patients with multiple sclerosis. *J Neurol Neurosurg Psychiatry* 80, 392–9.
Zajicek J (2007) The epidemiology of MS: letter to the editor. *J Neurol* 254, 1742.
Zajicek JP, Ingram WM, Vickery J, Creanor S, Wright DE and Hobart JC (2010) Patient-orientated longitudinal study of multiple sclerosis in south west England (The South West Impact of Multiple Sclerosis Project, SWIMS) 1: protocol and baseline characteristics of cohort. *BMC Neurology* 10:88.
Zajicek JP, Hobart JC, Slade A, Barnes D, Mattison PG et al. (2012) Multiple Sclerosis and Extract of Cannabis: results of the MUSEC trial. *J Neurol Neurosurg Psychiatry* 83(11), 1125–32.
Zajicek J, Fox P, Sanders H, Wright D, Vickery J, Nunn A, et al., UK MS Research Group (2003) Cannabinoids for the treatment of spasticity and other symptoms related to multiple sclerosis (CAMS study): multi-centre randomised placebo-controlled trial. *Lancet* 362, 1517–26.

Zajicek J, Freeman J and Porter B (2007) *MS Care: a practical manual*. OUP, Oxford.
Zivadinov R, Iona L, Monti-Bragadin L, Bosco A, Jurjevic A, Taus C Cazzato G and Zorzon M (2003) The use of standardised incidence and prevalence rates in epidemiological studies of MS. *Neuroepidemiology* 22, 65–74.
Zivadinov R, Weinstock-Guttman K, Hashmi N, Aldelrahman M, Stosic M, Dwyer S, Hussien J, Durfee J and Ramanathan M (2009) Smoking is associated with increased lesion volumes and brain atrophy in multiple sclerosis. *Neurology* 73, 504–10.

Websites accessed

Action on Smoking and Health (ASH), accessed 10 February 2012.
Census of population for Northern Ireland, accessed on various dates.
Clinical Practice Research Datalink, accessed 12 September 2012.
Cornwall County website, accessed 17 March 2011.
Devon County website, accessed 17 March 2011.
Diabetes UK, accessed 06 May 2012.
Expert Patients Programme, London (www.expertpatients.co.uk), accessed 04 March 2012.
GPRD accessed 25 June 2009.
MS Society, accessed 17 March 2011, 13 May 2011, 30 March 2012, 24 April 2012, 12 June 2012.
MS National Therapy Centres, accessed 04 July 2012.
MS Scotland, accessed 20 October 2009.
MS Trust on news items, accessed 18 May 2009, 01 August 2009, 24 October 2009, 19 June 2010.
National Ankylosing Spondylitis Society, accessed 06 May 2012.
NHS Scotland, Data Quality Assurance, Department of Information Services, accessed 20 March 2011.
National Rheumatoid Arthritis Society, accessed 06 May 2012.
National Statistics Online for the census of population, accessed numerous times.
Neuro-QOL website (http://www.neuroqol.org/default.aspx), accessed 06 September 2012.
NICE, accessed 04 December 2010.
Office for National Statistics, Health Statistics, accessed 16 November 2009, 19 February 2010.
Office for Health Economics, accessed 20 February 2010.
Population Trends, accessed numerous times.
Regional Trends, accessed numerous times.
Social Trends, accessed numerous times.
The Information Standard, accessed 23 April 2012.

Index

Numbers in **bold** refer to maps and diagrams.

activities of daily living, 189–91, 193–5
age (of people with MS), 62, 84, 93–9, 262–3, 274
Americas (The), 41
ascertainment (of people with MS)
  charity sector, 56, 72–9
  disability units, 56
  GPs, 56–9, 70–1, 118, 125, 141, 215, 217, *see also* GPRD
  hospitals, 56–8
  sources (of), 56–9
Atlas of MS, 41, 50, 111
Audits of Services, 164, 216–17, *see also* standards of care
Australia, 93, 104, 107, 113, 115, 154, 156, 207, 240, 244, 249, 254
  Tasmania, 34, 93, 113
Austria, 225
auto-immune disease, 13–14, 30, 32
axonopathy, 26

Baghdad, 244
biographical disruption, 162, 193–6
biographies of patients, 16–18, 174–6, 252
brain plasticity, 20
British Household Panel Survey, 200–1

Canada, 34, 38–9, 66, 77, 88, 90 111, 231, 240, 248, 252, 275
  British Columbia, 25, 60, 171, 175
  Labrador, 34
  Newfoundland, 34
  Ontario, 60, 93, 169, 171, 236
cannabis, 8, 36, 242–3
care services (used by PwMS), 215–18, 269–70, 275
carer strain (or burden), 226–7
Cari Loder, 8, 16, 243
caring (for someone with MS), 78, 224–8

Chronic Cerebrospinal Venous Insufficiency (CCSVI), 39, 247–9, 275
clinical trials, 7–8, 229, 233–6, 255
Clinically Isolated Syndrome (CIS), 21, 42, 230
Cognitive Behavioural Therapy (CBT), 180
Complementary and Alternative Medicine (CAM), 141–9
components of change, 110–11, 127, 134, 136, 138–9, 142–57, 265–6
  deaths, 145–52, 266
  incidence (new cases), 142–5, 265
  migrants, 130, 132, 152–7, 266
  stayers, 157
confidentiality (of personal data), 65–6
coping strategies, 177–8
Costa Rica, 249
costs (of MS), 201–5
  direct costs, 202–4
  indirect costs, 202–3, 225
  intangible costs, 204–5
  out-of-pocket (private) costs, 206
  Per Quality Adjusted Life Year (QALY), 202, 236–9
  relapse costs, 205
  service costs, 202–4

Danish Register of People with MS, 61, 90, 103, 107
data bases, *see* research approaches, registers
death, *see also* mortality
  causes of death, 147–50
Death Certificates, 145–50
Denmark, 2, 34, 38–9, 61, 90, 93, 103, 107
depression, 170
deprivation and social class, 102–3, 141, 263, 274

diagnosis (of MS), 21, 59, 251–2, *see also* MS diagnostic criteria
  delivery of, 49, 251
  disclosure of, 252
  impact of, 54
diet, 35–6
disability, 25, 167–76
  milestones, 25, 42, 167
  progression of, 25–30, 170, 232–3
Disease Modifying Drugs, 10, 20–1, 25, 30, 51, 187, 228–41, 270, 273
  availability (access), 229
  clinical trials, 232–5
  cost effectiveness, 231, 235–9
  international comparisons of use (geography), 229, 231
  side effects of, 229–30, 235
  types, 23, 229, 234
  when to start taking?, 230–2
divorce, *see* marital status
drug testing, 7–9

economic impacts of MS, 201–5, *see also* costs
education, 105–6
Eiona Roberts (poet), 16–17
employment (of people with MS), 92–3, 103–5, 167, 175, 195
England, 67, 71, 81, 96, 113–15, 136–42
  Brighton and Mid-Downs, 46–7, 55, 57, 86, 94, 96–8, **117**, 120, 142–3
  Cambridgeshire, 22, 27, 31, 47–8, 55, 57–60, 86, 93–4, 96, 99–100, 116–17, 120, 123–5, 137, 143, 147, 152, 157
  Cornwall and Devon, 62, 65, 84, 164, 217, 273
  Guernsey, 31, 37, 55, 57, 86–7, 94, **117**, 120, 122–4, 137, 264
  Hampshire, 47, 56–8, 84, 86, 94, 106, 113, **117**, 120, 123–4, 143
  Jersey, 31, 37, 55, 57, 85–7, 94, **117**, 120, 122–4, 137
  Leeds, 28, 31, 47, 52, 55, 57, 59–60, 66, 71, 84–6, 94, 99–100, 116–18, 120, 123–4, 142, 147, 150, 157, 164, 247
  London, 37, 72, 78, 82, 84, 108, 139–41, 155, 188, 225, 246, 250, 258, 274
  New Forest, 118–19
  Nottingham, 39
  Oxfordshire, 164, 216–17
  Plymouth, 28, 47, 51, 55–9, 85–6, 94, **117**, 118, 120–1, 123–4
  Rochdale, 22, 27, 47, 55, 57–8, 86, 99–100, **117**, 118, 120, 143, 152
  Suffolk, 55, 57, 86, 94, 118, 120, 123
  Sutton (London), 47, 55, 57, 86, 94, 96–8, **117**, 118–20, 123–4, 143
epigenetic effects, 32
Epstein Barr Virus, 37, 92, *see* Glandular Fever
ethnicity (of people with MS), 99–102, 141, 155–6, 263
  Black, 100–1
  Caucasian (White), 38, 88, 99, 152
European Quality of Life Scale (EuroQol, EQ-5D), 182–9, 237
Expanded Disability Status Scale (EDSS), 108, 166–71, 206, 233–4, 254–5
Expert Patient Programme, 78, 253–4, *see* self-help

falling, 172–3
fatigue, 165, 179–80
focus groups, 164, 251
France, 20, 60, 113, 192
  Lyon, 60, 171

gender issues, 78, 210–11
General Household Survey (GHS) in Britain, 100, 103, 106–7, 191–6
General Practice Research Database, 66, 68–72, 87, 114–15, 145, 150, 173, 264
Germany, 61, 167, 192, 241
Glandular Fever, 37

happiness (components of), 197–9
Hospital Admission Statistics, 67, 128–9, 139–41, 150
hygiene hypothesis, 39, 102–3, 141
Hyperbaric Oxygen Therapy, 241, 243

impacts (of MS), 159–212
impairments, *see* symptoms
incidence (of MS)
  incidence rates, 68–70, 86–7, 113, 274
infections, 37–8, 91, 141
Internet, 3, 176
Ireland, 249
  Donegal, 132
  Dublin, 132
  Wexford, 132
Italy, 192, 225

Japan, 35, 37

latitude, 73–4, 91, 113, 116
Leeds MS Quality of Life Scale
  (LMSQoLS), 182–6
Lhermitte's Sign, 45
Liberation treatment, 10, 247–9, *see*
  CCSVI
life course approach, 98
life expectancy, 95
life style, 102–3
Lifeworlds, 175
lumbar puncture, 52

marital status (of people with MS),
  106–8, 195–6, 206–8
medical mistakes, 10–11
Mexico, 240
mid-life crisis (of PwMS), 268
Middle East, 34
migration, 121
  critical age of, 155–6
  international, 126, 154–6
  local, 121
mobility, *see* walking
mortality rates, 145–50
MS in art, 15–16
MS causal model, 30, 39
MS charities (in UK)
  Action MS (in Northern Ireland), 8
  Action into Research for Multiple
    Sclerosis (ARMS), 60
  Federation of MS Therapy Centres, 6
  MS International Federation (MSIF),
    198–9, 250–1
  MS Society (and its members), 6,
    28–9, 62, 64, 69, 72–7, 79, 84,
    89, 104–6, 113–14, 161, 164,
    172, 179, 182–3, 187–96, 203–4,
    218–20, 222, 225–6, 245, 248,
    261, 263–4, 272, 274
  MS Trust (and its members), 6, 28–9,
    60, 76, 81, 84, 89, 95, 105, 169,
    172, 190–2, 202–3, 220–1, 237–8,
    242
  MS-UK (formerly the MS Resource
    Centre), 6–7
MS diagnosis, 43–69
MS diagnostic criteria, 43–55, 273
  Allison and Millar, 43–5, 47, 116,
    127, 130
  McDonald, 43, 49–53, 61, 69, 128
  Polman (2005 revision), 43, 51
  Poser, 43, 459, 61, 87, 116, 120,
    130, 137–8
  Schumacher, 43
MS genes, 30–2, 88, 126, 132
  major histocompatibility complex,
    32
  MS inheritance, 30, 90, 273
  MS susceptibility, 90
MS Impact Diary, 186
MS Impact Scale (MSIS-29), 80, 182–3,
  187–8
MS indicative tests
  cerebro-spinal fluid, 43, *see* lumbar
    puncture
  Magnetic resonance imagery (MRI),
    28, 43, 51, 228
  visual evoked potential, 43, 45
MS in the media
  film, 14–15
  newspapers, 1–3, 270–1
  TV, 14–15
MS nurses, 84, 252–3
  case load, 252
  evaluation (impact), 252–3
  role of, 252
MS prodromes, 20
MS publications
  books, 5
  charity magazines and pamphlets,
    5–7
  journal articles, 3–5
MS Register (UK), 61–3, 84, 95, 100,
  104–5, 267, 272

304 *Index*

MS risk factors
  behavioural (life-style), 35–9
  environmental, 33–6
MS sources of evidence, 3–8
MS (in) twins, 31
MS types, 22–9
  benign, 23, 28–9
  paediatric, 25, 36, 95
  primary progressive, 25, 28–9, 46
  progressive (in general), 25, 45, 164
  relapsing-remitting, 22–4, 28–9, 53–4
  secondary progressive, 25, 28–9

National Audit Office, 216, 223, 252, 275
National end of life care Intelligence Network, 146
National Health Service (UK), 81, 215–18, 238–40
National Hospital for Neurology and Neurosurgery (NHNN), 75, 84, 189, 217–18, 231, 250
National Hospital Registry, 173
National Institute for Health and Care Excellence (formerly National Institute for Health and Clinical Excellence), NICE, 8, 114–15, 162–3, 165, 202, 229, 236–9
National Service Framework for Long-term Conditions, 222–3
Netherlands, 191
neurological disease, 11–13
New Pathways (magazine of MS-UK), 6–7, 214, 244–6, 249, 273, 275
New Zealand, 61
North America, 2, 56, 90, 113, 274
North American Research Committee on MS (NARCOMS), 61, 90, 103–4, 173
Northern Ireland, 46, 48, 88, 96, 113–15, 130–4, 185–6, 193–3, 217, 274
  North Northern Ireland (Ballymena, Ballymoney, Coleraine, Moyle), 28, 31, 47, 51, 53, 55, 57–8, 60, 86, 94–9, 116, **117**, 120–1, 123–4, 130, 143–4, 169
Norway, 35, 90

palliative (end of life) care, 165, 254–5
  delivering a service, 78
physical disablement, *see* falling; walking
population standardisation, 133–4
Poshanker method, 142–3
prevalence (of MS)
  prevalence rates, **112**, 113, 115–25
Progressive Multifocal Leukoencepholopathy (PML), 230
psychological adjustment (to MS), 78, 176–8
psychological distress, 176, *see also* depression
psychological impacts (of MS), 176–9

quality of life, 181–96, 269
  disease specific measures, 77, 182, 187–91, 197–8, 198–9, 275
  generic measures, 182–9
  questionnaire surveys, 72–82, 84, 182, 187–91, 193–6, 224–7

rehabilitation, 254
  vocational rehabilitation service, 78, 249–51
relapses, 22–4
relationships of people with MS, 167, 205–11
  (with) adolescents (teenagers), 209–10
  (with) children, 209
  (with) partners and spouses, 206–7
repeat surveys, 116, 124–5, 137, 265
research approaches, 260–1
  cross-sectional, 42
  longitudinal, 59–72
  mass surveying, 28–9, 72–7, 84, 95, 100, 103–6, 225–7, 263–4
  qualitative methods, 16–17, 77–8, 224, 226–7, 250–1
  regional counts, 28–9, 56–9, 115–25, 201–3
  registers, 42, 59–72, 95
research methodology, 42
residential care, 207–9
respite care, 255
Risk Sharing Scheme, 236–40
Rivermead Mobility Index, 172

Rotterdam, 246
Russia, 240

sample size calculation, 121
sampling techniques
  random (representative), 17, 124, 217, 225
  self-selecting, 74–5, 226
Sativex, 8, 36, 214
Scotland, 35, 48, 67, 72, 96, 111, 113–15, 125–9
  Aberdeen, 50, 55, 57–8, 78, 86, 88, 94, 102, **117**, 120, 127, 169–76
  Borders, **117**, 118, 121, 126, 128
  Fife, 55, 57–8, 86, 94, 96–7, **117**, 118–19, 120, 123
  Glasgow, 55, 57–8, 85–6, 94–5, 100, 102, **117**, 120, 123, 128, 143–4, 249
  Grampian (North East Scotland), 102, 126, 128, 146–8
  Highland, 128
  Lothian, 47, 55, 57, 86, 94, 96–7, **117**, 118, 120–1, 123–4, 127–8, 143
  Orkney, 50, 55, 57–8, 86, 88, 94, 102, **117**, 118, 120, 122–8, 169–76
  Shetland, 50, 55, 57–8, 86, 88, 94, 102, 113, **117**, 118–20, 123–4, 126–8, 169–76
  Tayside, 46–7, 55, 57, 60, 85–6, 94, 96–7, 115, **117**, 119–20, 123–4, 126–7, 142–4
Scots, 130
Scottish MS Register, 61, 126
Scottish surnames, 126
self-efficacy, 215
self-help programmes, 215, 253–4, *see* Expert Patient Programme
severe MS, 107, 164–5, 207–8
sex or gender (of people with MS), 62, 84–93, 98–9, 261–2
simvastatin, 229
smoking, 36–7, 90–1
social class (of people with MS), *see* deprivation

social model of disability, 2
South West Impact of MS (SWIMS) Register, 61–5, 164, 217, 267
standards of care, 218–23
starting a family, 207
stem cell therapy, 10, 244–7
suicide, 150–2, 170
Sweden, 36, 225
Switzerland, 33, 240
symptom burden, 162–5, **166**
symptom relief, 214
  evidence base, 162–5
Symptom Relief Initiative, 161
symptoms (of MS), 1, 21, 23–4, 42, 159–80, 267–8
symptoms in groups, 164–5, 267

United Kingdom, 3, 84, 88–9, 91, 95, 101, 103–4, 111–58, 169, 182–91, 193–6, 203, 226, 241–3, *see also its four constituent countries*
United States of America, 34, 103, 111–13, 173, 240–1, 248–9
  California, 101
  Chicago, 244–5
  Cleveland Ohio, 191
  Olmsted County, 90, 171
UV radiation, 113, 264, *see also* latitude

Veterans MS Database (USA), 60
Vikings, 153
virtual communities, 176
Vitamin D, 33–5, 113, 264

Wales, 48, 113–15, 120, 135–6
  North Wales, 58, 136
  South Glamorgan (Unitary Authority of Cardiff and the Vale of Glamorgan), 25, 28, 47, 51, 53, 55, 57–60, 79, 86–8, 94–100, 116–19, 123–5, 155–6, 142–5, 147–50, 152, 170
walking, 170–3
wheelchair, 174